Rickettsiology and Rickettsial Diseases

Fifth International Conference

ANNALS OF THE NEW YORK ACADEMY OF SCIENCES
Volume 1166

Rickettsiology and Rickettsial Diseases

Fifth International Conference

Edited by
KARIM E. HECHEMY, PHILIPPE BROUQUI, JAMES E. SAMUEL,
AND DIDIER A. RAOULT

Published by Blackwell Publishing on behalf of the New York Academy of Sciences
Boston, Massachusetts
2009

The *Annals of the New York Academy of Sciences* (ISSN: 0077-8923 [print]; ISSN: 1749-6632 [online]) is published 32 times a year on behalf of the New York Academy of Sciences by Wiley Subscription Services, Inc., a Wiley Company, 111 River Street, Hoboken, NJ 07030-5774.

MAILING: The *Annals* is mailed standard rate. POSTMASTER: Send all address changes to *ANNALS OF THE NEW YORK ACADEMY OF SCIENCES*, Journal Customer Services, John Wiley & Sons Inc., 350 Main Street, Malden, MA 02148-5020.

Journal Customer Services: For ordering information, claims, and any inquiry concerning your subscription, please go to interscience.wiley.com/support or contact your nearest office:

Americas: Email: cs-journals@wiley.com; Tel: +1 781 388 8598 or 1 800 835 6770 (Toll free in the USA & Canada).
Europe, Middle East and Asia: Email: cs-journals@wiley.com; Tel: +44 (0) 1865 778315
Asia Pacific: Email: cs-journals@wiley.com; Tel: +65 6511 8000
Information for Subscribers: The *Annals* is published in 32 issues per year. Subscription prices for 2009 are:
Print & Online: US$4862 (US), US$5296 (Rest of World), €3432 (Europe), £2702 (UK). Prices are exclusive of tax. Australian GST, Canadian GST and European VAT will be applied at the appropriate rates. For more information on current tax rates, please go to www3.interscience.wiley.com/aboutus/journal_ordering_and_payment.html#Tax. The price includes online access to the current and all online back files to January 1, 1997, where available. For other pricing options, including access information and terms and conditions, please visit www.interscience.wiley.com/journal-info.

Delivery Terms and Legal Title: Prices include delivery of print publications to the recipient's address. Delivery terms are Delivered Duty Unpaid (DDU); the recipient is responsible for paying any import duty or taxes. Legal title passes to the customer on despatch by our distributors.

Membership information: Members may order copies of *Annals* volumes directly from the Academy by visiting www.nyas.org/annals, emailing membership@nyas.org, faxing +1 212 298 3650, or calling 1 800 843 6927 (toll free in the USA), or +1 212 298 8640. For more information on becoming a member of the New York Academy of Sciences, please visit www.nyas.org/membership. Claims and inquiries on member orders should be directed to the Academy at email: membership@nyas.org or Tel: 1 800 843 6927 (toll free in the USA) or +1 212 298 8640.

Printed in the USA.

The *Annals* is available to subscribers online at Wiley InterScience and the New York Academy of Sciences' Web site. Visit www.interscience.wiley.com to search the articles and register for table of contents e-mail alerts.

ISSN: 0077-8923 (print); 1749-6632 (online)
ISBN-10: 1-57331-750-0; ISBN-13: 978-1-57331-750-4

A catalogue record for this title is available from the British Library.

ANNALS OF THE NEW YORK ACADEMY OF SCIENCES

Volume 1166

Rickettsiology and Rickettsial Diseases

Fifth International Conference

Editors

KARIM E. HECHEMY, PHILIPPE BROUQUI, JAMES E. SAMUEL,
AND DIDIER A. RAOULT

This volume is the result of the **Fifth International Conference on Rickettsiae and Rickettsial Diseases**, held on May 18–20, 2008 in Marseilles, France.

CONTENTS

Foreword

In the past two decades the *Annals of the New York Academy of Sciences* has published a number of the conferences on rickettsia and rickettsial diseases organized by the European Study Group for Coxiella, Anaplasma, Rickettsia and Bartonella (ESCAR) and by the American Society for Rickettsiology. The fifth International Conference for Rickettsiae and Rickettsial Diseases was held in Marseilles, France on May 18–20, 2008. The meeting year coincides with two milestones in the field of rickettsiology, namely the centennial discoveries of *Rickettsia prowazekii*, the causative agent of epidemic typhus by Stanislaus von Prowazek, and Charles Nicolle's discovery that epidemic typhus is transmitted by body lice. The rickettsias and the bacteria formerly associated with the order Rickettsiales, namely, the genus *Coxiella*, are of major importance for the study of obligate intracellular microorganisms and their potential use as biological weapons. In addition, studies on some members of the genus *Bartonella*, which were formerly placed in the order Rickettsiales were also presented. Particularly noteworthy is the increased appreciation in the general biological science world of the obligate intracellular rickettsia's interaction with the eukaryote host cells.

In this volume, because of space limitations, are twenty of the meeting lectures selected for publication. The remaining lecture's slide and poster presentations will be published in a special online issue of *Clinical Microbiology and Infection*, the official journal of the European Society for Clinical Microbiology and Infectious Diseases (ESCMID).

Although the clinical and epidemiologic spectra of rickettsioses have been studied for years, new observations and discoveries are still being made in these two areas of rickettsiology. Advances in the discipline show that predicting levels of pathogenicity of the newly recognized rickettsias and the pathogenicity of "old" rickettsias based on their geographic distribution, even within a narrow area, are multifactorial. It is evident that greater emphases on culture- and molecular-based techniques are essential to identify novel rickettsias around the world, to unlock the mysteries of known rickettsias, and to provide guidelines for the phylogeny of the rickettsias. New experimental systems are needed to determine the physiological changes in rickettsial gene expression immediately after infection of the host. There is also a need to explore further the hypothesis that the rickettsias cannot grow in axenic media because their growth depends on some essential proteins that are synthesized by the eukaryotic cell.

Postgenomic and proteomic analyses of members of the order Rickettsiales and former members promise to unlock the underlying mechanisms of their pathogenicity. For example, members of the genera *Ehrlichia* and *Anaplasma*, upon interaction with the host cell, demonstrate an upregulation of the gene encoding a type IV secretion apparatus. Understanding of the complex interplay between host and these pathogens may lead to the control of the diseases caused by the ehrlichias and anaplasmas. Genomic and proteomic analyses of antibiotic sensitive and relatively antibiotic insensitive isolates of *Orientia* bacteria suggest that drug insensitivity may arise from multiple mechanisms. The relationship between the rickettsias and their vectors and the transovarial interference of

Rickettsiology and Rickettsial Diseases-Fifth International Conference: Ann. N.Y. Acad. Sci. 1166: vii–viii (2009).
doi: 10.1111/j.1749-6632.2009.04532.x © 2009 New York Academy of Sciences.

rickettsial species in the vectors remains a promising area of research that has not been elucidated. While the pathogenicity of the genus *Coxiella*, the causative agent of Q fever, is directly related to its ability to persist within the host cells, the mechanism of host cell infection by the coxiella remains to be defined. The bacterium causes reproductive disorders and can induce a chronic infection that may be exacerbated with repeated gestations. It was reported that long-term cotrimazole therapy prevents the infection from becoming chronic. Members of the genus *Bartonella* have increased dramatically in the last 20 years. It appears that the *Bartonella* species described to date are capable of parasitizing only a limited number of animal species. It also was stated that the bartonellas should be suspected and included in the differential diagnosis of human and animal cases of endocarditis.

The expansion of the basic knowledge in rickettsia will help define the host–parasite relationship, including various modulating factors that lead to parasitism of the eukaryote by the rickettsia and general prokaryote biology. This will engender interest by both established scientists and young scientists who are searching for a rich field of study, as research in rickettsiology encompasses a number of disciplines at the interface between host and parasite, including epidemiology, entomology, pathology, and immunology.

The editors thank the *Annals of the New York Academy of Sciences* for agreeing to publish some of the presentations that were given at the International Conference on Rickettsiae and Rickettsial Diseases held in Marseilles, France. We also thank the current and former staff of the *Annals* who have done a superb job, namely Linda Mehta, Steve Bohall, and Ralph Brown.

KARIM E. HECHEMY
New York State Department of Health
Albany, New York

PHILIPPE BROUQUI
Université de la Méditerranée
Marseille, France

JAMES E. SAMUEL
Texas A&M University
College Station, Texas

DIDIER A. RAOULT
Université de la Méditerranée
Marseille, France

Current Knowledge on Phylogeny and Taxonomy of *Rickettsia* spp.

Pierre-Edouard Fournier and Didier Raoult

Unité des Rickettsies, CNRS-IRD UMR 6236, Université de la Méditerranée, Faculté de Médecine, Marseille, France

Due to improved diagnostic methods and increased interest, the number of representatives of the genus *Rickettsia* has increased dramatically over the past 20 years, with 25 currently validated species. These arthropod-associated intracellular bacteria are now recognized in all parts of the world. The comparison of the phylogenic organizations obtained from the study of several genes with different functions, and more recently from genomic sequences, provided basis to establish a reliable taxonomy of the bacteria included in the genus *Rickettsia*. These data were incorporated into polyphasic consensus guidelines that provide clear recommendations for the taxonomic classification and nomenclature of rickettsiae and rickettsial diseases.

Key words: Rickettsia; taxonomy; phylogeny; review

Introduction

The strictly intracellular life of rickettsiae, and thus the few phenotypic characters that they express, made traditional identification methods used in bacteriology unapplicable. As a consequence, the word "rickettsia" has long served as a generic term for most small and uncultivable bacteria that were not otherwise identified. As a matter of fact, it was not until 1974, in the 8th edition of the Bergey's manual, that the family *Chlamydiaceae* was removed from the order *Rickettsiales* to be placed in the order *Chlamydiales*.[1] However, the introduction of new identification techniques in the past 3 decades, especially molecular methods, has revolutionized the taxonomy of "rickettsiae." Consequently, the term "*Rickettsia*" currently only applies to arthropod-borne bacteria belonging to the genus *Rickettsia* within the family *Rickettsiaceae* in the order *Rickettsiales*, α-*Proteobacteria*. Bacteria within the genus *Rickettsia* are obligate intracellular, short rods that retain basic fuschin when stained by the Gimenez method,[2] grow in association with eukaryotic cells within which they live free, divide by binary fission in the cytoplasm, and may cause diseases in invertebrate hosts (which act as vectors and reservoirs) or vertebrate hosts.[3,4]

Currently, the *Rickettsia* genus contains 25 officially validated species (Table 1), and several dozens of as-yet uncharacterized strains or arthropod-amplicons. The main vectors of these bacteria are ticks, which are also their reservoirs, but some are associated with lice, fleas, or mites. Some members of the genus *Rickettsia* are recognized human pathogens, but the others should rather be considered as species or strains of unknown pathogenicity than as nonpathogenic, especially when associated with arthropods able to bite humans. *Rickettsia* sp. causes rickettsioses, which are amongst the oldest known arthropod-borne diseases.[5] To date, 16 of the 25 validated species are recognized human pathogens, and another 2 are suspected to cause rickettsioses (Table 1). The pathogenicity of members of the *Rickettsia* genus as well as another few phenotypic properties have been the basis for their classification into

Address for correspondence: Pierre-Edouard Fournier, Unité des Rickettsies, CNRS-IRD UMR 6236, Université de la Méditerranée, Faculté de Médecine, Marseille, France. Voice: +33-491-32-43-75; fax: +33-491-38-77-72. Pierre-Edouard.Fournier@univmed.fr

Rickettsiology and Rickettsial Diseases-Fifth International Conference: Ann. N.Y. Acad. Sci. 1166: 1–11 (2009).
doi: 10.1111/j.1749-6632.2009.04528.x © 2009 New York Academy of Sciences.

TABLE 1. Characteristics of Validated *Rickettsia* Species

Species	Type strain	Vector	Geographical distribution	Pathogenic role	Reference
R. aeschlimannii	MC16	*Hy. marginatum, R. appendiculatus, Ha. punctata*	France, Morocco	Unnamed spotted fever	48
R. africae	ESF-5	*Am. hebraeum, Am. variegatum, R. appendiculatus*	Sub-Saharan Africa, Reunion Island, West Indies	African tick-bite fever	49
R. akari	MK	*Al. sanguineus*	USA	Rickettsialpox	50
R. asiatica	IO-1	*I. ricinus*	Japan	Unknown	51
R. australis	Phillips	*I. holocyclus, I. tasmani, I. cornuatus*	Australia	Queensland tick typhus	50
R. bellii	369L42–1	*D. variabilis, D. occidentalis, D. albipictus, Ha. lepopalustris, Am. cooperi, Ornithodoros concanensis Argas cooleyi*	USA, Brazil	Unknown	52
R. canadensis	2678	*Ha. leporispalustris*	USA	Unknown	50
R. conorii subsp. *conorii*	Malish 7	*R. sanguineus, Ha. leachii*	Mediterranean area, Africa	Mediterranean spotted fever	50, 44
R. conorii subsp. *indica*	ITTR	*R. sanguineus, B. microplus, Ha. leachii*	India	Indian tick typhus	44
R. conorii subsp. *caspia*	A-167	*R. sanguineus, R. pumilio*	Chad, Kosovo, Russia	Astrakhan fever	44
R. conorii subsp. *israelensis*	ISTTCDC1	*R. sanguineus*	Israel	Israeli spotted fever	44
R. felis	URRWXCal₂	*Ctenocephalides felis, Ar. erinacei*	Worldwide	Flea spotted fever	53
R. heilongjiangensis	054	*D. silvarum*	China, Russia, Thailand	Far Eastern rickettsiosis	26
R. helvetica	C9P9	*I. ricinus, I. ovatus, I. persulcatus, I. monospinosus*	Europe, Japan	Suspected agent of a rickettsiosis	54
R. honei	RB	*Ap. Hydrosauri, Am. cajennense, I. granulatus*	Australia	Flinders Island spotted fever	55
R. japonica	YH	*D. taivanensis, Ha. flava I. ovatus, H. longicornis,*	Japan	Oriental or Japanese spotted fever	56
R. massiliae	Mtu1	*R. sanguineus, R. turanicus, R. mulsamae, R. lunulatus, R. sulcatus*	France	Unnamed rickettsiosis	57
R. montanensis	M/5–6	*D. variabilis, D. andersoni*	USA	Unknown	58
R. parkeri	Maculatum20	*Am. maculatum, Am. triste, Am. americanum,*	USA	Unnamed rickettsiosis	50
R. peacockii	Skalkaho	*D. andersoni*	USA	Unknown	59
R. prowazekii	Breinl	*Pediculus humanus humanus*	Africa, Russia, South America	Epidemic typhus	50

Continued

TABLE 1. *Continued*

Species	Type strain	Vector	Geographical distribution	Pathogenic role	Reference
R. raoultii	Khabarovsk	*R. pumilio, D. nttalli, D. marginatus, D. silvarum, D. reticulatus*	France, Russia	TIBOLA or DEBONEL	60
R. rhipicephali	3-7-6	*D. occidentalis, R. sanguineus*	Africa, Europe, USA	Unknown	61
R. rickettsii	Sheila Smith	*Am. aureolatum, Am. cajennense, D. andersoni, D. variabilis, R. sanguineus*	Brazil, Mexico, Panama, USA	Rocky mountain spotted fever	50
R. sibirica subsp. *sibirica*	246	*D. nuttalli, D. silvarum, D. marginatus, D. auratus, D. sinicus, D. pictus, Ha. concinna, Ha. yeni, Ha. wellingtoni*	China, Russia	Siberian or North Asian tick typhus	50, 45
R. sibirica subsp. *mongolitimonae*	HA-91	*Hy. asiaticum, Hy. truncatum*	Algeria, China, France, Greece, South Africa	Lymphangitis-associated rickettsiosis	45
R. slovaca	13-B	*D. marginatus, D. reticulatus*	Europe, Russia	TIBOLA or DEBONEL	62
R. tamurae	AT-1	*Am. testudinarium*	Japan	Unknown	63
R. typhi	Wilmington	*X. cheopis, C. felis, L. segnis*	Worldwide	Murine typhus	50

Al. = *Allodermanyssus*; Am. = *Amblyomma*; Ap. = *Aponomma*; Ar. = *Archeopsylla*; B = *Boophilus*; D = *Dermacentor*; Ha. = *Haemaphysalis*; Hy. = *Hyalomma*; I = *Ixodes*; L = *Leptopsylla*; R = *Rhipicephalus*; X = *Xenopsylla*

2 groups, that is, the spotted fever (SFG) and typhus (TG) groups: i) spotted fever group rickettsiae are mainly associated with ticks, but also fleas (*R. felis*) and mites (*R. akari*), cause spotted fevers in humans, have an optimal growth temperature of 32°C, a G+C content between 32 and 33, can polymerize actin and thus move into the nuclei of host cells, and cross-react with *Proteus vulgaris* OX-2;[3,6,7] ii) in contrast, typhus group rickettsiae are associated with human body lice (*R. prowazekii*) or fleas (*R. typhi*), cause typhus in humans, have an optimal growth temperature of 35°C, a G+C content of 29%, cannot polymerize actin and thus cannot enter the nuclei of host cells, are only found in their cytoplasm and cross-react with *Proteus* OX-19[6,7] (Table 1). *Rickettsia* sp. possesses major antigens against which infected humans produce antibodies. These include the lipopolysaccharide (LPS) and outer membrane proteins of the surface cell antigen (SCA) family, mostly the 120-kDa S-layer protein (OmpB or Sca5),[8] rOmpA (or Sca0) only present in spotted fever group rickettsiae,[9] and Sca4.[10] Various methods were used to study *Rickettsia* species but failed to provide easily reproducible identification tools, including complement fixation, toxinic neutralisation, SDS-PAGE, mouse serotyping, Western blot, development of monoclonal antibodies, and DNA-DNA hybridization.[11–17] As a consequence, although initially discovered in the early XXth century, *Rickettsia* sp. remained badly known until the 1990s and the introduction of molecular tools, and still are a matter of debate, in particular, in regarding their taxonomy. In this article, we review the most recent findings about *Rickettsia* sp. in the domains of phylogeny and taxonomy.

Phylogeny

Until the 1990s, phylogenetic studies of rickettsiae were based on the comparison of morphological, antigenic, and metabolic characters. However, phylogenetic relationships based on these criteria were highly unreliable. The

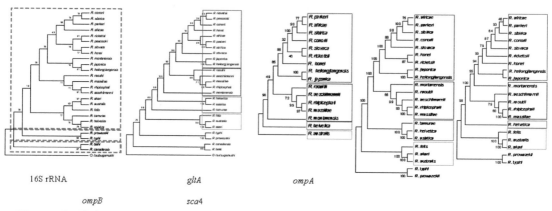

16S rRNA   *gltA*   *ompA*

ompB   *sca4*

Figure 1. Phylogenic organization of *Rickettsia* species based on the comparison of sequences of the 16S rDNA, *gltA*, *ompA*, *ompB*, and *sca4* genes, using the Maximum Parsimony method.

advent of molecular methods allowed phylogenic relationships among intracellular bacteria to be reliably estimated. The use of 16S rRNA gene sequences constituted a major forward in the phylogenetic study of rickettsiae. As a matter of fact, these data showed that several of the bacteria initially classified in the order *Rickettsiales* did not belong to the α-subclass of the *Proteobacteria* phylum. As a consequence, *Coxiella burnetii* and *Rickettsiella grylli* were reclassified within the *Legionellaceae*,[18,19] *Eperythrozoon* sp. and *Haemobartonella* sp. within *Mycoplasmataceae*,[20] *Wolbachia persica* within the γ-subdivision of *Proteobacteria* close to *Francisella* sp.,[18] *Wolbachia melophagi* within the *Bartonellaceae* (Birtles and Molyneux, GenBank accession number X89110), and *Bartonella* sp., *Rochalimaea* sp., and *Grahamella* sp. within the *Bartonellaceae*.[21,22] In addition, *Rickettsia tsutsugamushi*, the agent of scrub-typhus, was found to be distinct enough by 16S rRNA gene sequence comparison to warrant transfer from the genus *Rickettsia* into the genus *Orientia*, which includes a single species, *Orientia tsutsugamushi*.[23]

16S rRNA sequencing enabled the identification of a specific sequence for each rickettsial serotype, but a high degree of sequence similarity (99.9) was observed.[24,25] These studies confirmed the evolutionary unity of the genus (Fig. 1), but since the sequences were almost identical, significant inferences about intragenic phylogeny were not possible. Two

groups were identified: the spotted fever group that contained the largest number of species and the typhus group made of *R. prowazekii* and *R. typhi*. In addition, it was proposed that *R. bellii* and *R. canadensis*, branching outside both groups, diverged prior to the schism between the SFG and the TG.[24] It was also proposed the name "ancestral" group for *R. canadensis* and *R. bellii*. However, because neither *R. canadensis* nor *R. bellii* are ancestors of other *Rickettsia* species, the term "ancestral" group is not justified and should no longer be used. In addition, both species exhibit great genomic divergences, and the consistency of a group that would include them has been discussed.[26,27] Subsequently, phylogenic studies were inferred from sequences from more divergent genes that included *gltA*,[28] the gene encoding the 17-kDa protein,[29] and genes from the autotransporter family *sca*: *ompA*,[9] *ompB*,[30] *sca4*,[10] *sca1*,[31] and *sca2*.[32] Phylogenetic analysis inferred from sequences of the 17-kDa protein-encoding gene provided nonsignificant bootstrap values for most of the nodes.[29] Phylogenic relationships inferred from sequences of the *gltA* gene were supported by significant bootstrap values for all the nodes except those within clusters in the SFG (Fig. 1).[28] Four statistically supported clusters were identified within the SFG. The *R. rickettsii* cluster included: *R. conorii*, *R. peacockii*, *R. honei*, *R. rickettsii*, *R. africae*, *R. parkeri*, *R. sibirica*, *R. slovaca*, *R. heilongjiangensis*, and

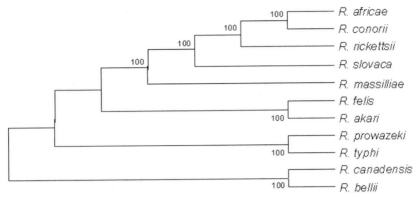

Figure 2. Phylogenic organization of *Rickettsia* species based on the comparison of genome sequences. Six hundred and forty common genes were concatenated prior ro alignment and analysis using the Maximum Parsimony method.

R. japonica. The *R. massiliae* cluster was made of *R. massiliae, R. rhipicephali, R. aeschlimannii, R. raoultii,* and *R. montanensis.* The coherence of the latter cluster was reinforced by the resistance to erythromycin and rifampin of the species it contained.[33] The *R. akari* cluster contained *R. akari, R. felis,* and *R. australis.* The *R. helvetica* cluster, made of *R. helvetica, R. asiatica,* and *R. tamurae,* clustered between the *R. massiliae* and *R. felis* clusters. *R. canadensis* and *R. bellii* clustered neither in the TG nor in the SFG and were shown to be the most outlying rickettsiae. Using *ompA* sequence comparison, the phylogenetic organization in the *R. rickettsii* cluster was well established.[9] The same 3 other clusters were identified (Fig. 1). Significant bootstrap values were found for all nodes except for *R. honei.* However, the *ompA* gene could not be amplified from all *Rickettsia* species.[9] Phylogenetic analysis inferred from sequences of the *ompB* gene confirmed the groups and clusters identified by *gltA* and *ompA* sequencing[30] (Fig. 1). Bootstrap values were significant for most of the nodes with the exception of those inside the cluster including *R. parkeri* and *R. africae.* Sca4 sequence comparison identified 2 well-supported phylogenetic groups (Fig. 1). These included the SFG that consisted of the *R. rickettsii, R. massiliae, R. Helvetica,* and *R. akari* clusters, and the TG. Finally, the phylogenetic organization of *Rickettsia* species inferred from the comparison of sequences of the *sca*1 and *sca*2 genes were similar to those obtained from the analyses of *ompA, ompB,* and *sca4.*[31,32]

The study of intergenic spacer sequences as a genotyping tool also demonstrated to be a potential phylogenetic tool. Using a concatenation of sequences from 3 spacers, (i.e., the *dksA-xerC, mppA-purC* and *rpmE-tRNA*[fMet]), a phylogenetic study obtained an organization similar to those obtained using gene sequences, thus suggesting that intergenic sequences retained some degree of selection pressure.[34]

Over the past 10 years, rickettsial genomics has been an emerging field that rapidly proved its usefulness in a variety of applications. By comparison of 11 rickettsial genome sequences, 640 common genes were identified. By concatenating these 640 genes and using the resulting sequences for phylogenetic analysis, the inferred organization was similar to those previously obtained, but all nodes were supported by elevated bootstrap values (Fig. 2).[35,36] In 2007, the creation of a specific phylogenetic group distinct from the SFG and TG, named transitional group, was proposed for *R. felis* and *R. akari.*[36] However, a cluster including both species and *R. australis* had previously been described within the SFG,[28] and the genome-based phylogeny did not provide any evidence that the creation of a specific group for *R. felis* would be justified. As a consequence, *R. felis, R. akari,* and *R. australis* should be considered as members of the SFG.

Taxonomy

The development of PCR and nucleotide sequencing, particularly the study of 16S rRNA, has considerably modified the taxonomic classification of bacteria, in particular intracellular bacteria that express few phenotypic criteria commonly used for identification and classification. Following the reclassification of several genera, as described above, the order *Rickettsiales* is currently comprised of the genera *Anaplasma, Ehrlichia, Neorickettsia, Orientia, Rickettsia,* and *Wolbachia.*[23,37]

Due to the lack of official rules, defining a species within the *Rickettsia* genus has long been a matter of debate. The guidelines established for extracellular bacteria do not fit well with the strictly intracellular nature of these bacteria. As a matter of fact, the official molecular criteria used for the classification of a bacterial isolates within a vali species, that is, a DNA-DNA hybridization > 70%,[38] a G+C content < 5% and a 16S rRNA divergence < 3%, cannot be applied to *Rickettsia* species. Using these criteria, DNA-DNA hybridization values of > 73% would classify *R. rickettsii, R. conorii, R. sibirica,* and *R. montanensis* within the same species;[17] DNA G+C content values of 32–33% and 29% would classify all SFG and TG rickettsiae, respectively, in only 2 species; a 16S rRNA divergence < 2% would classify all rickettsiae within a single species. In addition, the average nucleotide identity (ANI) method,[39] designed as an alternative of DNA-DNA hybridization for the delineation of bacterial species, is not suitable for rickettsiae as well. Using this criterion, *R. conorii, R. rickettsii,* and *R. sibirica,* with ANI values of > 94%, belong to the same species, as do *R. typhi* and *R. prowazekii.*

Since 1978, mouse serotyping, an immunofluorescent antibody assay with acute phase mouse sera, has been the reference method for the identification of new SFG rickettsiae.[14] This test detects species-specific epitopes of the surface-exposed S-layer proteins (rOmpA and rOmpB), as well as the Sca4 (PS-120) protein, of rickettsiae. Using this method,

a species corresponds to a serotype, with a rickettsial isolate being assumed to belong to a species if both strains exhibit a specificity difference of < 3.[14] Although useful, mouse immunization suffers drawbacks such as a lack of reproducibility and the necessity to compare each new isolate to all previously described species. Other phenotypic methods such as the use of monoclonal antibodies[40,41] and SDS-PAGE did not bring any determinant progress to rickettsial taxonomy. Pulsed-field gel electrophoresis is useful for differentiating rickettsiae, but it suffers from the absence of any database allowing the comparison of PFGE profiles and the lack of reproducibility. Over the last 15 years, a number of genes including those encoding 16S rRNA, citrate synthase (*gltA*), the 17-kDa common antigen, and surface-exposed, high molecular weight antigenic proteins of the *sca* family (*ompA, ompB, sca4, sca1,* and *sca2*), have been used to rapidly and reliably differentiate members of the genus *Rickettsia* either by analysis of restriction fragment length polymorphisms of PCR products (PCR-RFLP) or by direct sequence determination;[9,10,25,28–32] however, it was determined that the identification of bacterial isolates should not rely on the study of a single gene, but rather on the combination of a minimum of 5 genes. The so-called multilocus sequence typing (MLST), initially developed for genotyping purposes, was subsequently proposed as a taxonomic tool.[42] To facilitate the classification of bacterial isolates as rickettsiae at the genus, group, and species levels, genetic criteria based on a MSLT method were developed.[26] The MLST-based criteria used sequences of the 16SrRNA, *gltA, ompA, ompB,* and *sca4* genes (Fig. 3), and were established using a panel of 20 uncontested *Rickettsia* species previously, officially validated using mouse serotyping (*R. prowazekii, R. typhi, R. rickettsii, R. conorii, R. africae, R. sibirica, R. slovaca, R. honei, R. japonica, R. australis, R. akari, R. felis, R. aeschlimannii, R. helvetica, R. massiliae, R. rhipicephali, R. montanensis,* and *R. parkeri*). To incorporate these genetic criteria into the definition of a *Rickettsia* species, an international

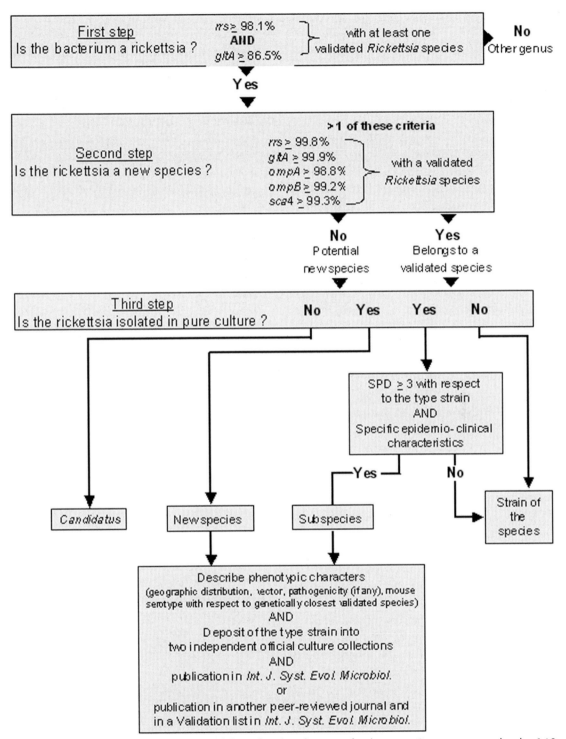

Figure 3. Polyphasic taxonomic guidelines for classification of rickettsiae. Genes: rrs encodes the 16S rDNA; *gltA* encodes the citrate synthase; *ompA* encodes rOmpA; *ompB* encodes rOmpB; *sca4* encodes Sca4. SPD = specificity difference in mouse serotyping.

commitee of expert rickettsiologists proposed rational polyphasic guidelines to classify rickettsial isolates at various taxnonomic levels (Fig. 3) and to clarify the nomenclature within the genus *Rickettsia*.[43] These criteria, incorporating phenotypic, genotypic, and phylogenetic criteria (Fig. 3), were adopted by the International Committee for the Systematics of Prokaryotes through the validation of 4 new *Rickettsia* species: *R. asiatica*, *R. heilongjiangensis*, *R. raoultii*, and *R. tamurae* (Table 1). This polyphasic approach also enabled classification of rickettsial isolates of uncertain taxonomic rank ("*R. mongolotimonae*" within the *R. sibirica* species; *Rickettsia* sp. strain S within the *R. africae* species; *Rickettsia* sp. strain Bar29 within the *R. massiliae* species; *Rickettsia* sp. strain BJ-90 within the *R. sibirica* species; Indian tick typhus rickettsia (ITTR), Astrakhan fever rickettsia (AFR), and Israeli spotted fever rickettsia (ISFR) within the *R. conorii* species). In addition, the taxonomic rank of subspecies was created for members of the *Rickettsia* genus to classify isolates of a species that exhibited specific phenotypic characteristics.[44,45] Four subspecies were created within the *R. conorii* species, that is, *R. conorii* subsp. *conorii*, *R. conorii* subsp. *indica*, *R. conorii* subsp. *caspia*, and *R. conorii* subsp. *israelensis*, and 2 within the *R. sibirica* species, that is, *R. sibirica* subsp. *sibirica* and *R. sibirica* subsp. *mongolitimonae* (Table 1). The subspecies status is currently examined by the International Committee for the Systematics of Prokaryotes.

In an effort to develop a more discriminatory tool able to trace isolates of a single *Rickettsia* species, a sensitive method named multispacer typing (MST) was developed. This method was based on the assumption that intergenic spacers, being noncoding sequences, undergo less evolutionary pressure than coding sequences such as genes, and thus are more variable between strains of a bacterium. MST identified 27 genotypes among 39 *R. conorii* strains,[46] 4 genotypes among 15 *R. prowazekii* strains,[47] 3 genotypes among 10 *R. sibirica* strains,[45] and thus demonstrated to be valuable the discrimination of rickettsiae at the strain level.

Finally, to comply with the requirement from the International Committee for the Systematics of Prokaryotes that isolates of a new bacterial species should be deposited in 2 official culture collections in 2 distinct countries, we created a bacterial strain collection named the Collection de Souches de l'Unité des Rickettsies (CSUR, http://ifr48.timone.univ-mrs.fr/portail2/index.php?option=com_content&task=view&id=96&Itemid=52). This collection was officialized by the World Federation for Culture Collections (WFCC, http://www.wfcc.info/datacenter.html) under number WDCM 874. This collection currently contains 172 rickettsial strains and is able to accept any rickettsial isolates from scientists worldwide.

Conclusions, Perspectives

Molecular biology and modern culture methods have greatly facilitated the study of *Rickettsia* species and the diseases that they cause. However, although 25 *Rickettsia* species are currently validated, several dozens of as-yet unclassified isolates or genotypes are awaiting classification. Access to their genome sequences has provided an essential insight into their evolution and physiology. The discovery of unexpected characteristics such as conjugative properties and the soon-to-be completed collection of rickettsial genomes will allow a better understanding of their phylogenetic and phylogenomic organizations, and thus evolution. These data will also benefit the polyphasic consensus guidelines developed for the taxonomic classification and nomenclature of rickettsiae.

Conflicts of Interest

The authors declare no conflicts of interest.

References

1. Moulder, J.W. 1974. Order I. *Rickettsiales* Gieszczykiewicz 1939, 25. *Bergey's Manual of*

Determinative Bacteriology, 8th edn. R.E. Buchanan & N.E. Gibbons, Eds.: 892–918. The Williams & Wilkins Co. Baltimore, MD.

2. Gimenez, D.F. 1964. Staining rickettsiae in yolk-sac cultures. *Stain Technol.* **39:** 135–140.

3. Teysseire, N., J.A. Boudier & D. Raoult. 1995. *Rickettsia conorii* entry into vero cells. *Infect. Immun.* **63:** 366–374.

4. Burgdorfer, W., R.L. Anacker, R.G. Bird & D.S. Bertram. 1968. Intranuclear growth of *Rickettsia rickettsii*. *J. Bacteriol.* **96:** 1415–1418.

5. Maxey, E.E. 1899. Some observations of the so-called spotted fever of Idaho. *Med. Sentinel.* **10:** 433–438.

6. Heinzen, R.A., S.F. Hayes, M.G. Peacock & T. Hackstad. 1993. Directional actin polymerization associated with spotted fever group *Rickettsia* infection of Vero cells. *Infect. Immun.* **61:** 1926–1935.

7. Teysseire, N., C. Chiche-Portiche & D. Raoult. 1992. Intracellular movements of *Rickettsia conorii* and *R. typhi* based on actin polymerization. *Res. Microbiol.* **143:** 821–829.

8. Ching, W.M., G.A. Dasch, M. Carl & M.E. Dobson. 1990. Structural analyses of the 120-kDa serotype protein antigens of typhus group rickettsiae. Comparison with other S-layer proteins. *Ann. N. Y. Acad. Sci.* **590:** 334–351.

9. Fournier, P.E., V. Roux & D. Raoult. 1998. Phylogenetic analysis of spotted fever group rickettsiae by study of the outer surface protein rOmpA. *Int. J. Syst. Bacteriol.* **48:** 839–849.

10. Sekeyova, Z., V. Roux & D. Raoult. 2001. Phylogeny of *Rickettsia* spp. inferred by comparing sequences of 'gene D', which encodes an intracytoplasmic protein. *Int. J. Syst. Evol. Microbiol.* **51:** 1353–1360.

11. Plotz, H., R.L. Reagan & K. Wertman. 1944. Differentiation between "Fièvre boutonneuse" and Rocky Mountain spotted fever by means of complement fixation. *Proc. Soc. Exp. Biol. Med.* **55:** 173–176.

12. Bell, E.J. & H.G. Stoenner. 1960. Immunologic relationships among the spotted fever group of rickettsias determined by toxin neutralisation tests in mice with convalescent animal serums. *J. Immunol.* **84:** 171–182.

13. Eisemann, C.S. & J.V. Osterman. 1976. Proteins of typhus and spotted fever group rickettsiae. *Infect. Immun.* **14:** 155–162.

14. Philip, R.N. *et al.* 1978. Serologic typing of rickettsiae of the spotted fever group by microimmunofluorescence. *J. Immunol.* **121:** 1961–1968.

15. Gilmore, R.D. Jr. & T. Hackstadt. 1991. DNA polymorphism in the conserved 190 kDa antigen gene repeat region among spotted fever group rickettsiae. *Biochim. Biophys. Acta.* **1097:** 77–80.

16. Anacker, R.L., R.E. Mann & C. Gonzales. 1987. Reactivity of monoclonal antibodies to *Rickettsia rickettsii*

with spotted fever and typhus group rickettsiae. *J. Clin. Microbiol.* **25:** 167–171.

17. Myers, W.F. & C.L. Wisseman, Jr. 1981. The taxonomic relationship of *Rickettsia canada* to the typhus and spotted fever groups of the genus *Rickettsia*. *Rickettsiae and Rickettsial Diseases*. W. Burgdorfer & R.L. Anacker, Eds.: 313–325. Academic Press. New York, NY.

18. Weisburg, W.G. *et al.* 1989. Phylogenetic diversity of the rickettsiae. *J. Bacteriol.* **171:** 4202–4206.

19. Roux, V., M. Bergoin, N. Lamaze & D. Raoult. 1997. Reassessment of the taxonomic position of *Rickettsiella grylli*. *Int. J. Syst. Bacteriol.* **47:** 1255–1257.

20. Neimark, H., K.E. Johansson, Y. Rikihisa & J.G. Tully. 2001. Proposal to transfer some members of the genera *Haemobartonella* and *Eperythrozoon* to the genus *Mycoplasma* with descriptions of 'Candidatus Mycoplasma haemofelis', 'Candidatus Mycoplasma haemomuris', 'Candidatus Mycoplasma haemosuis' and 'Candidatus Mycoplasma wenyonii'. *Int. J. Syst. Evol. Microbiol.* **51:** 891–899.

21. Birtles, R.J., T.G. Harrison, N.A. Saunders & D.H. Molyneux. 1995. Proposals to unify the genera *Grahamella* and *Bartonella*, with descriptions of *Bartonella talpae* comb.nov., *Bartonella peromysci* comb. nov., and three new species, *Bartonella grahamii* sp. nov., *Bartonella taylorii* sp. nov., and *Bartonella doshiae* sp. nov. *Int. J. Syst. Bacteriol.* **45:** 1–8.

22. Brenner, D.J., S.P. O'Connor, H.H. Winkler & A.G. Steigerwalt. 1993. Proposals to unify the genera Bartonella and Rochalimaea, with descriptions of *Bartonella quintana* comb. nov., *Bartonella vinsonii* comb. nov., *Bartonella henselae* comb. nov., and *Bartonella elizabethae* comb. nov., and to remove the family Bartonellaceae from the order *Rickettsiales*. *Int. J. Syst. Bacteriol.* **43:** 777–786.

23. Tamura, A., N. Ohashi, H. Urakami & S. Miyamura. 1995. Classification of *Rickettsia tsutsugamushi* in a new genus, *Orientia* gen nov, as *Orientia tsutsugamushi* comb. nov. *Int. J. Syst. Bacteriol.* **45:** 589–591.

24. Stothard, D.R., J.B. Clark & P.A. Fuerst. 1994. Ancestral divergence of *Rickettsia bellii* from the spotted fever and typhus groups of *Rickettsia* and antiquity of the genus *Rickettsia*. *Int. J. Syst. Bacteriol.* **44:** 798–804.

25. Roux, V. & D. Raoult. 1995. Phylogenetic analysis of the genus *Rickettsia* by 16S rDNA sequencing. *Res. Microbiol.* **146:** 385–396.

26. Fournier, P.E. *et al.* 2003. Gene sequence-based criteria for the identification of new *Rickettsia* isolates and description of *Rickettsia heilongjiangensis* sp. nov. *J. Clin. Microbiol.* **41:** 5456–5465.

27. Ogata, H. *et al.* 2006. Genome sequence of *Rickettsia bellii* illuminates the oole of amoebae in gene exchanges between intracellular pathogens. *PLoS Genet.* **2:** e76.

28. Roux, V., E. Rydkina, M. Eremeeva & D. Raoult. 1997. Citrate synthase gene comparison, a new tool for phylogenetic analysis, and its application for the rickettsiae. *Int. J. Syst. Bacteriol.* **47:** 252–261.

29. Anderson, B.E. & T. Tzianabos. 1989. Comparative sequence analysis of a genus-common rickettsial antigen gene. *J. Bacteriol.* **171:** 5199–5201.

30. Roux, V. & D. Raoult. 2000. Phylogenetic analysis of members of the genus *Rickettsia* using the gene encoding the outer-membrane protein rOmpB (ompB). *Int. J. Syst. Evol. Microbiol.* **50:** 1449–1455.

31. Ngwamidiba, M., G. Blanc, D. Raoult & P.E. Fournier. 2006. Sca1, a previously undescribed paralog from autotransporter protein-encoding genes in *Rickettsia* species. *BMC Microbiol.* **6:** 12.

32. Ngwamidiba, M. *et al.* 2005. Phylogenetic study of *Rickettsia* species using sequences of the autotransporter protein-encoding gene sca2. *Ann. N. Y. Acad. Sci.* **1063:** 94–99.

33. Rolain, J.M., M. Maurin, G. Vestris & D. Raoult. 1998. *In vitro* susceptibilities of 27 rickettsiae to 13 antimicrobials. *Antimicrob. Agents Chemother.* **42:** 1537–1541.

34. Fournier, P.E. & D. Raoult. 2007. Identification of rickettsial isolates at the species level using multispacer typing. *BMC. Microbiol.* **7:** 72.

35. Fournier, P.E. *et al.* 2008. Variations of plasmid content in *Rickettsia felis*. *PLoS ONE* **3:** e2289.

36. Gillespie, J.J. *et al.* 2007. Plasmids and rickettsial evolution: insight from *Rickettsia felis*. *PLoS ONE* **2:** e266.

37. Dumler, J.S. *et al.* 2001. Reorganisation of genera in the families *Rickettsiaceae* and *Anaplasmataceae* in the order *Rickettsiales* : unification of some species of *Ehrlichia* with *Anaplasma*, *Cowdria* with *Ehrlichia* and *Ehrlichia* with *Neorickettsia*, descriptions of six new species combinations and designation of *Ehrlichia equi* and 'HGE agent' as subjective synonyms of *Ehrlichia phagocytophila*. *Int. J. Syst. Evol. Microbiol.* **51:** 2145–2165.

38. Wayne, L.G. *et al.* 1987. Report of the Ad hoc committee on reconciliation of approaches to bacterial systematics. *Int. J. Syst. Bacteriol.* **37:** 463–464.

39. Konstantinidis, K.T. & J.M. Tiedje. 2005. Genomic insights that advance the species definition for prokaryotes. *Proc. Natl. Acad. Sci. USA* **102:** 2567–2572.

40. Walker, D.H. *et al.* 1992. Antigenic diversity of *Rickettsia conorii*. *Am. J. Trop. Med. Hyg.* **47:** 78–86.

41. Xu, W.B. & D. Raoult. 1998. Taxonomic relationships among spotted fever group rickettsiae as revealed by antigenic analysis with monoclonal antibodies. *J. Clin. Microbiol.* **36:** 887–896.

42. Stackebrandt, E. *et al.* 2002. Report of the ad hoc committee for the re-evaluation of the species definition in bacteriology. *Int. J. Syst. Evol. Microbiol.* **52:** 1043–1047.

43. Raoult, D. *et al.* 2005. Naming of rickettsiae and rickettsial diseases. *Ann. N. Y. Acad. Sci.* **1063:** 1–12.

44. Zhu, Y., P.E. Fournier, M. Eremeeva & D. Raoult. 2005. Proposal to create subspecies of *Rickettsia conorii* based on multi-locus sequence typing and an emended description of *Rickettsia conorii*. *BMC. Microbiol.* **5:** 11.

45. Fournier, P.E., Y. Zhu, X. Yu & D. Raoult. 2006. Proposal to create subspecies of *Rickettsia sibirica* and an emended description of *Rickettsia sibirica*. *Ann. N. Y. Acad. Sci.* **1078:** 597–606.

46. Fournier, P.E., Y. Zhu, H. Ogata & D. Raoult. 2004. Use of highly variable intergenic spacer sequences for multispacer typing of *Rickettsia conorii* strains. *J. Clin. Microbiol.* **42:** 5757–5766.

47. Zhu, Y., P.E. Fournier, H. Ogata & D. Raoult. 2005. Multispacer typing of *Rickettsia prowazekii* enabling epidemiological studies of epidemic typhus. *J. Clin. Microbiol.* **43:** 4708–4712.

48. Beati, L., M. Meskini, B. Thiers & D. Raoult. 1997. *Rickettsia aeschlimannii* sp. nov., a new spotted fever group rickettsia associated with *Hyalomma marginatum* ticks. *Int. J. Syst. Bacteriol.* 548–554.

49. Kelly, P.J. *et al.* 1996. *Rickettsia africae* sp. nov., the etiological agent of African tick bite fever. *Int. J. Syst. Bacteriol.* **46:** 611–614.

50. Skerman, V.B.D. & P.H.A. Sneath. 1980. Approved list of bacterial names. *Int. J. Syst. Bacteriol.* **30:** 225–420.

51. Fujita, H. *et al.* 2006. *Rickettsia asiatica* sp. nov., isolated in Japan. *Int. J. Syst. Evol. Microbiol.* **56:** 2365–2368.

52. Philip, R.N. *et al.* 1983. *Rickettsia bellii* sp. nov. : a tick-borne *Rickettsia*, widely distributed in the United States, that is distinct from the spotted fever and typhus biogroups. *Int. J. Syst. Bacteriol.* **33:** 94–106.

53. La Scola, B. *et al.* 2002. Emended description of *Rickettsia felis* (Bouyer et al. 2001) a temperature-dependant cultured bacterium. *Int. J. Syst. Evol. Microbiol.* **52:** 2035–2041.

54. Beati, L. *et al.* 1993. Confirmation that *Rickettsia helvetica* sp. nov. is a distinct species of the spotted fever group of rickettsiae. *Int. J. Syst. Bacteriol.* **43:** 521–526.

55. Stenos, J., V. Roux, D. Walker & D. Raoult. 1998. *Rickettsia honei* sp. nov., the aetiological agent of Flinders Island spotted fever in Australia. *Int. J. Syst. Bacteriol.* **48:** 1399–1404.

56. Uchida, T., T. Uchiyama, K. Kumano & D.H. Walker. 1992. *Rickettsia japonica* sp. nov., the etiological agent of spotted fever group rickettsiosis in Japan. *Int. J. Syst. Bacteriol.* **42:** 303–305.

57. Beati, L. & L. Raoult. 1993. *Rickettsia massiliae* sp.nov., a new spotted fever group rickettsia. *Int. J. Syst. Bacteriol.* **43:** 839–840.

58. Bell, E.J., G.M. Kohls, H.G. Stoenner & D.B. Lackman. 1963. Nonpathogenic rickettsias related to the spotted fever group isolated from ticks, *Dermacentor variabilis* and *Dermacentor andersoni* from Eastern Montana. *J. Immunol.* **90:** 770–781.

59. Niebylski, M.L. *et al.* 1997. *Rickettsia peacockii* sp.nov., a new species infecting wood ticks, *Dermacentor andersoni*, in Western Montana. *Int. J. Syst. Bacteriol.* 446–452.

60. Mediannikov, O. *et al.* 2008. *Rickettsia raoultii* sp. nov., a spotted fever group rickettsia associated with *Dermacentor* ticks in Europe and Russia. *Int. J. Syst. Evol. Microbiol.* **58:** 1635–1639.

61. Burgdorfer, W., L.P. Brinton, W.L. Krinsky & R.N. Philip. 1978. *Rickettsia rhipicephali :* a new spotted fever group rickettsia from the brown dog tick *Rhipicephalus sanguineus. Rickettsiae and Rickettsial Diseases.* J. Kazar, R.A. Ormsbee & I.V. Tarasevich, Eds.: 307–316. House of the Slovak Academy of Sciences. Bratislava.

62. Sekeyova, Z. *et al.* 1998. *Rickettsia slovaca* sp. nov., a member of the spotted fever group rickettsiae. *Int. J. Syst. Bacteriol.* **48:** 1455–1462.

63. Fournier, P.E., N. Takada, H. Fujita & D. Raoult. 2006. *Rickettsia tamurae* sp. nov., isolated from *Amblyomma testudinarium* ticks. *Int. J. Syst. Evol. Microbiol.* **56:** 1673–1675.

Closing the Gaps between Genotype and Phenotype in *Rickettsia rickettsii*

Marina E. Eremeeva and Gregory A. Dasch

Rickettsial Zoonoses Branch, Division of Viral and Rickettsial Diseases, Centers for Disease Control and Prevention, Atlanta 30333, GA

Rocky Mountain spotted fever (RMSF) caused by *Rickettsia rickettsii* is a severe rickettsiosis that occurs in nearly every state of the continental USA. RMSF is endemic in Central and Southern America, with recent well-documented cases in Mexico, Costa Rica, Panama, Colombia, Brazil, and Argentina. RMSF is the most malignant among known rickettsioses causing severe multiorgan dysfunction and high case fatality rates, which can reach 73% in untreated cases. Variations in pathogenic biotypes of *R. rickettsii* isolates have been described, and potential correlations of these differences to various clinical manifestations of RMSF have been suggested. We have recently reported on a method of genetic comparison employing sequence differences in intergenic regions (IGR typing) in isolates of *R. rickettsii* of human, tick, and animal origin. The grouping obtained correlated well with 2 other genotyping systems we have developed, which target the presence and distribution of variable numbers of tandem repeats (TR) and insertion/deletion (INDEL) events. Twenty-five total genotypes of *R. rickettsii* in 4 primary groups could be distinguished: isolates from Montana, isolates associated with *Rhipicephalus sanguineus* ticks and human infections in Arizona, other isolates from the USA where *Dermacentor variabilis* is thought to be the primary vector, and the isolates primarily associated with *Amblyomma* ticks from Central and South America. In addition, isolate Hlp#2, which is often considered to be a nonpathogenic isolate of *R. rickettsii* and closely related serotype 364D, exhibited the most diversity from the other isolates compared, and they differ significantly from each other. Because complex interactions underlie the pathogenesis of *R. rickettsii in vivo*, it is difficult to define the causality of individual events that occur in infected vertebrate hosts and humans. Many microbial factors are likely to contribute to the varied ability of *R. rickettsii* to cause cellular injury; some of them may also contribute importantly to its virulence for vertebrate hosts and may be linked to the variable genetic markers we have identified. Since circulation of *R. rickettsii* in nature includes vertical transstadial and transovarial transmission within tick vectors and horizontal passages through vertebrate hosts, it is plausible that isolates of different virulence arose when they became isolated during adaptation to novel vertebrate and tick hosts. Characterization of the physiologically important changes in rickettsial gene expression that occur immediately after tick-to-human or tick-to-animal transitions may require development of new experimental systems.

Key words: *Rickettsia rickettsii*; genotyping; VNTR; INDEL; intergenic region

Introduction

Address for correspondence: Marina E. Eremeeva, Rickettsial Zoonoses Branch, Mail Stop G-13, National Center for Zoonotic, Vector-borne and Enteric Diseases, Centers for Disease Control and Prevention, 1600 Clifton Road NE, Atlanta GA 30333. Voice: +404-639-4612; fax: +404-639-4436. MEremeeva@cdc.gov

The findings and conclusions described in this manuscript are those of the authors and do not necessarily represent the views of the Centers for Disease Control and Prevention and the Department of Health and Human Services.

Rocky Mountain spotted fever (RMSF) caused by *Rickettsia rickettsii* is a severe rickettsiosis that occurs in nearly every state of the continental USA with average annual incidence of 2.2 cases/million persons.[1] In the USA, *R. rickettsii* is primarily transmitted by *Dermacentor andersoni* and *D. variabilis* in the western and eastern and central parts of the USA, respectively. Although *Rhipicephalus sanguineus* was implicated as a vector of *R. rickettsii* in Mexico in the 1940s, only recently did PCR-based detection and identification, as well as isolation of *R. rickettsii* directly from brown dog ticks and patients in eastern Arizona, confirm and solidify these early observations based on classical methods.[2–5] The presence of *R. rickettsii* in brown dog ticks has been also detected in both California and Georgia,[6,7] suggesting that this association may be more common than had been previously thought. RMSF is endemic in Central and Southern America, with recent well-documented cases in Mexico, Costa Rica, Panama, Colombia, Brazil, and Argentina.[8–15] Transmission of *R. rickettsii* in those regions has been typically associated with *Amblyomma cajennense* and *A. aureolatum*,[16–18] but other tick vectors like *R. sanguineus* cannot be excluded.

RMSF is an acute disease, which manifests after a 3- to 10-day incubation period following a tick bite or an accidental exposure to an aerosol of the rickettsiae.[19] *R. rickettsii* first invade endothelial cells of small and middle-sized vessels, where they multiply and eventually destroy the cells—as do the other rickettsiae.[20] Subsequent invasion of vascular smooth muscle cells by *R. rickettsii* results in more severe tissue necrosis, which is a hallmark of RMSF.[20,21] Primary symptoms of RMSF are very nonspecific and often include high fever, severe headache, and muscle pain, and may be accompanied by nausea, vomiting, abdominal pain, and cough.[1,19] A maculopapular rash appears on the lower extremities after 3 to 5 days of illness. Later during the course of infection, the rash develops into a petechial and even hemorrhagic presentation in severe cases, and it spreads from the palms and soles to the body trunk; however, approximately 10% of RMSF is spotless, particularly in older people.[19,22,23] Neurologic and gastroenteric dysfunctions, retinal injury, cardiopulmonary, and renal deficiency are among the syndromes which can occur during RMSF, further complicating its clinical recognition and, therefore, its diagnosis and treatment.[19,22–25] Gangrene, particularly of the extremities, can develop as the final result of progression of skin lesions from macular rash to hemorrhages and to necrosis.[21] RMSF responds well to doxycycline treatment; however, before antibiotics were introduced the mortality rate could be as high as 73 percent.[26] Based on current passive surveillance data, CDC reported an overall case-fatality rate of 1.4% during 1997–2002;[1] that may increase up to 10% in untreated cases.[19] These reported cases of RMSF based largely on non-species-specific serology, undoubtedly include infections due to exposures to other spotted fever group agents.[27] In Brazil, in active surveillance the reported RMSF case fatality rate in the last decade ranges from 12.5% to 73.3% (median 34.7%) in San Paulo State[28] and 22–24% in 3 other states with fatal cases (Rio de Janeiro, Minas Gerais, and Espirito Santo).[29] At present, delayed diagnosis and inappropriate antimicrobial therapy continue to cause unnecessary fatalities.[4,25,30,31] A high proportion of fatal RMSF cases in North America occurs among patients suffering from spotless forms of the disease and among young children.[10,19,23,30–32]

R. rickettsii is highly infectious by parenteral route, where 1 organism is enough to cause disease. Infections can also occur by aerosol exposure, commonly in laboratory workers.[33,34] RMSF has a rapid onset, and host factors appear to contribute to the likelihood of fulminant disease.[19,22,35] The microorganism is maintained in ticks by transovarial and transstadial transmission and survives well in overwintering ticks and in tick feces,[36,37] although it can decrease tick fecundity and survival.[38] Suburban life styles and recreational activities are important risk factors contributing to the increasing incidence of RMSF in North America.

Phenotypic Variation among Isolates of *Rickettsia rickettsii*

Variations in biotypes of isolates of *R. rickettsii* have been described, and potential correlations of these biological differences to various clinical manifestations of RMSF have been suggested. Anacker and colleagues[39,40] reported differences in the virulence of 6 *R. rickettsii* isolates in the guinea pig model of infection, grouping them into 3 categories: isolates with highest virulence (human isolate Sheila Smith and 2 isolates from *D. andersoni*, Norgaard and Sawtooth from Montana), lesser virulence (patient isolates Morgan and Simpson from North Carolina) and lowest virulence, isolate Hlp. The same authors observed differences in mobilities of proteins from the whole cell lysates of these isolates by 1-dimensional gel SDS-polyacrylamide gel electrophoresis, by Western blotting with sera of guinea pigs infected with isolate Sheila Smith, and precipitation of rickettsial antigens labeled with ^{125}I by pooled guinea pig sera; however, only Hlp was markedly differentiated by this method.[39,40] Strains from North Carolina and Montana also differed in at least 1 epitope of the 120-kDa protein with monoclonal antibodies in an enzyme-linked immunosorbent assay.[41]

Hlp isolate, often referred to in the literature as serotype Hlp—based on its unique characteristics using microimmunofluorescence with mouse immune sera[42]—has a long history of being differentiated from prototypical isolates of *R. rickettsii* including its association with the rabbit tick, *Haemaphysalis leporispalustris*.[43] The original study conducted by Parker and his coworkers recovered 7 Hlp isolates; however, only 2 were referred to by name including group 2 and group 3. It was reported that all 7 Hlp isolates were similar serologically and provided protective immunity to other isolates of *R. rickettsii*; however, there was a marked difference in its lower virulence in the guinea pig infection model. Compared to an unidentified "laboratory strain of Rocky Mountain spotted fever rickettsiae," the Hlp isolates showed increased incubation periods, increased duration and decreased degree of fever, and decreased scrotal reactions.[43] The literature descriptions regarding the experimental usage and passage history of specific Hlp isolates are not very complete;

some authors refer only to using Hlp isolate obtained from Parker, while others refer to isolate Hlp#2. It appears that most published studies used Hlp#2, but this conclusion cannot be confirmed. Phenotypic observations reported by Parker and colleagues[43] about Hlp isolates with low passage histories were subsequently reproduced by other investigators using Hlp isolates passaged for extended period through laboratory animals, embryonated chicken eggs, and cell culture,[39] suggesting the genetic stability of the Hlp#2 avirulent phenotype.

In contrast, another avirulent isolate of *R. rickettsii* Iowa from *D. variabilis* was originally characterized as virulent or mildly virulent for guinea pigs.[44] However, it was subsequently noticed that Iowa isolate displayed various degrees of virulence for guinea pigs following its passage in embryonated chicken eggs.[44] Accordingly, while early passages exhibited mild virulence, which subsequently increased and was comparable with that of prototype virulent isolates of *R. rickettsii*, it eventually displayed an avirulent phenotype for guinea pigs. Detailed analysis of a high-egg passage clone of Iowa isolate showed that the strain was deficient in its ability to lyse Vero cells, and it formed indistinct plaques compared to the clear and well-defined plaques observed for *R. rickettsii* isolate Bitterroot.[45] Iowa isolate was shown to be deficient in processing outer membrane protein B (OmpB) from its 168-kDa precursor into the 120-kDa mature passenger protein and 32-kDa beta barrel of the autotransporter.[45]

Eleven isolates of *R. rickettsii* were different in causing variable and quantifiable amounts of cellular injury *in vitro* as determined by the release of lactate dehydrogenase and alteration of the cellular system of antioxidants of infected cells.[46] The observed clustering of isolates by degree of injury resembles the virulence typing system proposed by Price for isolates recovered from *Dermacentor* ticks collected in Montana and based originally on the guinea pig model of infection (Table 1); these guinea pig phenotypes were reproduced after they were passaged in ticks, embryonated eggs, and susceptible

TABLE 1. Phenotypic Typing of *R. rickettsii* Based upon Variation in Virulence for Guinea Pigs following Intraperitoneal Inoculation as Proposed by W. P. Price (1953)[47]

Strain	Average days of fever	Average height of fever	Scrotal reaction	Percent fatality	Incubation period (days)	Persistence in animals (days)
R	8.1 ± 1.3	40.6 ± 0.12	$++++$	33	2	32
S	4.1 ± 0.65	40.4 ± 0.11	$++$	0	2	26
T	4.0 ± 0.92	40.3 ± 0.15	0	0	2	26
U	0	0	0	0	ND	10

animals such as the guinea pig.[47,48] Type R included a group of isolates expressing the most virulent phenotype with long-lasting fever and scrotal reactions, and mortality in $\sim 30\%$ of infected animals. *D. andersoni* tick isolate Bitterroot and human isolate Sheila Smith from the Bitterroot Valley are typically referred to as the prototype R strains of *R. rickettsii*. Infection with strains of S- or T-type group caused significantly milder symptoms and shorter duration of fever, and several contemporary isolates of *R. rickettsii* may be included in the S category (Morgan and Simpson evaluated by Anacker *et al.*[39]), while extent representative examples for category T are not available except the original Price T isolate from our collection.[46,49] Inoculation of guinea pigs with U strains did not induce any detectable symptoms of rickettsioses, features which led some contemporary investigators to conclude that type U isolates were really *R. montanensis* that had been improperly identified due to the lack of modern genetic tools in the 1950s. Since no Price U isolates are available, this conjecture cannot be confirmed directly.

The varied ability of different eukaryotic cell lines to maintain sustained growth of *R. rickettsii* isolates may alter their phenotypic and biological characteristics upon continued passage.[50,51] Isolates may also express differences in invasiveness as found with the Iowa isolate.[45] Indeed, various cell culture phenotypes may be detected when isolates are inoculated into different human endothelial cell lines (Fig. 1A and B), indicating host specific factor[s] can affect intracellular interactions. Similar observations were made when isolates of *Rickettsia conorii*

were compared in T3, L929, and Vero cell lines.[52,53]

Virulence of *R. rickettsii* may not necessarily be a stable characteristic of the isolate, since it may have an alterable expression under some conditions, changing from low virulence to high virulence for guinea pigs, respectively, in questing and engorged ticks, a transition known as the reactivation phenomenon.[54] Warming can also produce similar reactivation of virulence in *R. rickettsii*,[55] while treatment with para-aminobenzoic acid results in a lowered virulence phenotype for *R. rickettsii*.[56] The latter process is reversible upon supplementation of Coenzyme I (CoI) or Coenzyme A (CoA).[56] Whether reactivation events and transition and adaptations from ticks to animals or passaging between different experimental animals, embryonated eggs, and cell culture may similarly effect changes in phenotype with all genotypes of *R. rickettsii* is not well understood. However, it was clearly demonstrated that reactivation of *R. rickettsii* Bitterroot is accompanied by profound morphological changes in rickettsial cells.[57] The microcapsular protein layer, which is often called a paracrystalline surface protein layer or S-layer, composed of the autotransporter proteins, OmpA, and OmpB, is readily identified by electron microscopy of virulent rickettsiae in engorged ticks as a discrete electron-lucent zone around the rickettsial cell. In starved ticks, the microcapsular layer of avirulent rickettsiae is not detected as a discrete structure, but feeding of ticks or their incubation at $37°C$ results in restoration of a visible S-layer structure and the full pathogenicity and virulence of the rickettsiae for guinea pigs.

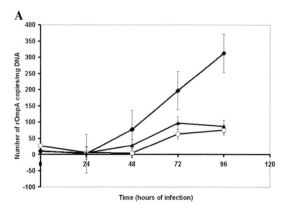

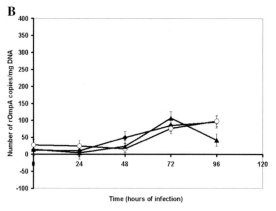

Figure 1. Variable growth kinetics of isolates of *R. rickettsii* in different types of human endothelial cells. (**A**) Human lung endothelial cell line (HULEC), (**B**) Human microvascular endothelia cells (HMEC). Growth of the isolate Bitterroot is indicated by (♦), growth of the isolate Hlp#2 is indicated by (○), growth of the isolate PriceT is indicated by (▲). Endothelial cells were cultivated in 24 well plates to confluence and inoculated in triplicate with each isolate at multiplicity of infection of 1 rickettsial plaque forming unit per cell. Infected monolayers were harvested 1 hr. following inoculation and at 24, 48, 72 and 96 hr. of infection. DNA was extracted and copy numbers of rickettsial DNA was established using SYBR-Green PCR as previously described,[73] total DNA content was measured using PicoGreen assay (Molecular Probes, Eugene, OR, USA).

Once tools became available for comparing the genetic characteristics of isolates of rickettsiae, it became very tempting to try to establish a putative correlation between biological phenotypes and specific genetic markers in *R. rickettsii*. Several types of mutations have been found in several genes of *R. rickettsii* in-

cluding *glt*A,[58,59] the number of repeated 72–75 amino acid sequences in *omp*A,[51,60] and truncation of *omp*B as in the Iowa avirulent clone.[45] Although, numerous differences between the avirulent Iowa clone and virulent Sheila Smith-PP clone genomes were found,[61] which ones might directly contribute to the attenuation of Iowa clone have not been systematically examined and evaluated. Herein, we review the different genetic typing systems we have applied to numerous isolates of *R. rickettsii* and discuss their association with geographic origins and vertebrate host reservoirs and tick vectors. We developed 3 different typing systems targeting variable number of tandem repeat sites (VNTR), polymorphic intergenic regions (IGR), and variable insertion and deletion events (INDEL). Comparisons of the sequenced genomes of different species of *Rickettsia* have demonstrated that a significant level of genetic conservation exists at both the species and genus levels in coding sequences, and many such regions appear too conserved to be very useful for genotyping even at the species level let alone for assessing intraspecies variation.[62] In contrast, intergenic regions appear to be under less stringent selective pressure and hence possess greater sequence diversity than the coding regions.[49,62,63]

We assembled a collection of 38 *R. rickettsii* isolates obtained between 1935 and 2004 from humans, 3 different species of ticks, and 3 animal species in 10 US states, Central and South America, and included 2 other closely related tick isolates, Hlp#2 and 364D serotypes (Table 2). While it is the largest collection of *R. rickettsii* isolates studied to date, it does not necessarily represent an ideal collection of isolates in many ways. The greatest limitation is that some isolates are unique in geographic origin, and many have not been subjected to characterization of phenotype either in guinea pigs or *in vitro*. Some isolates are low passage, but many others underwent extensive but poorly documented passage history under varied conditions in different laboratories and were obtained many decades ago. In contrast, some isolates were obtained in our laboratory in the last several years, so their history and passages are known precisely. Consequently, it is desirable to obtain many more contemporary isolates to ensure that the different genetic groups defined here are fully representative of different populations of *R. rickettsii* as they exist presently in nature. Indeed, it is both entirely possible and likely that additional genetic variants of *R. rickettsii* may exist, and some of these may have novel phenotypes.

Genetic Typing Systems

One primary goal for our comparison of isolates of *R. rickettsii* was to determine if phenotypic variations in isolates of *R. rickettsii* have an underlying genetic or physiological-adaptive basis. We wished to first group representative isolates with similar genetic traits to reduce the number of strains to be investigated by the more laborious phenotypic characterization methods. Since the genetic homogeneity of our isolates was unknown, it would also be necessary to clone stocks of isolates before conducting phenotypic studies, a similarly labor-intensive task. This genetic analysis would provide the first set of markers useful in studying the molecular epidemiology of *R rickettsii*. To ensure that all traits differentiating different groups of *R. rickettsii* were known, this genetic survey would help us to select which isolates would be characterized first by complete genome sequencing. It was hoped that any genetic differences found would reflect early divergence of populations during their geographic separation and association with specific species of tick and animal reservoirs. Further, if these distinct genetic traits could be shown to be associated with specific phenotypic variations in virulence in animals or *in vitro* systems, they might also play roles in the clinical manifestations of disease in humans, adaptations to animal reservoirs and ticks, and even capacity for vertical versus (vs.) horizontal transmission. With the development of improved systems for

genetic manipulation of *Rickettsia*, it might be possible to obtain isogenic mutants to assess the importance of individual differences between isolates differing in phenotype to confirm the importance of those genetic differences.

Different types of genomic loci were evaluated to address these questions including coding regions, tandem repeats, intergenic regions, and sites containing insertions or deletion events (INDEL). Comparison of genomic sequences of several species of *Rickettsia* had revealed that coding regions are more conserved and less useful for genotyping at the isolate level than intergenic regions.[62–65] Only 47 INDEL sites were identified within coding regions of isolates Iowa and Sheila Smith-PP,[61] representing only 33% of a total of 143 deletions identified as a result of comparison of the 2 genomes. The coding sequences (CDS) deletions resulted in gene truncations, in-frame deletions, frameshifts, and total gene deletions, but these apparent differences depend to some degree on the quality of the CDS annotations and accuracy of DNA sequencing of these 2 genomes. Sites containing tandem repeats or INDELs may also be the most useful for isolate typing, since they can be detected without DNA sequencing in many cases as seen in an INDEL in the GltA coding region,[58,59] variations in numbers of tandem repeats of ompA detected in different isolates,[60] and spontaneous loss of repeat elements during *in vitro* passages of isolate Sheila Smith.[51] VNTR and INDEL sites as well as intergenic region divergences may or may not affect virulence depending upon how they alter gene functions or gene regulation.

Typing Based on Variable Numbers of Tandem Repeats

Tandem Repeats (TR) are the sites in the genome where an identical or nearly identical nucleotide sequence is present in 2 or more adjacent copies. If the copy number for such repeats differs in individual isolates they are referred to as variable numbers of TR sites (or VNTR). We previously reported some

TABLE 2. *Rickettsia rickettsii*-like Isolates Used for Genotyping

Isolate, reference	Geographic collection, year of isolation[a]	Source	Origin, collection[b]	Typing system[c]		
				VNTR	IGR	INDEL
AZ-1[5]	Arizona, 2004	*Rhipicephalus sanguineus*	CDC	+	+	ND[a]
AZ-3[5]	Arizona, 2004	Human blood, fatal RMSF	CDC	+	+	+
AZ-4[5]	Arizona, 2004	Human blood, fatal RMSF	CDC	+	+	+
AZ-5[5]	Arizona, 2004	*Rhipicephalus sanguineus*	CDC	+	+	+
AZ-6[5]	Arizona, 2004	Human skin	CDC	+	+	+
AZ-7[5]	Arizona, 2004	*Rhipicephalus sanguineus*	CDC	+	+	ND
AZ-8[5]	Arizona, 2004	*Rhipicephalus sanguineus*	CDC	+	+	+
AZ-9[5]	Arizona, 2004	*Rhipicephalus sanguineus*	CDC	+	+	+
Bitterroot (VR891)[68]	Bitterroot Valley, MT, 1945	*D. andersoni*	ATCC/WRAIR	+	+	+
Brazil[68]	Brazil, before 1943	Human blood	WRAIR	+	+	+
BSF Di6[69]	Hanover County, VA, 1961	*Didelphis marsupialis virginiana*	WRAIR	+	+	+
BSF Mp40[69]	Fairfax County, VA, 1961	*Microtus pennsylvanicus*	WRAIR	+	+	+
BSF Rab1[69]	Prince Edward County, VA, 1960	*Sylvilagus floridans*	WRAIR	+	+	+
Coleman[49]	Charlottesvile, VA, 1969	Fatal RMSF, autopsy materials	McGhee, MCV	+	+	+
Colombia[49]	Colombia, 1935?	Presumably human blood or autopsy specimens from fatal RMSF	Pretzman, ODPH	+	+	+
Costa Rica[11,46]	Costa Rica, 1979?	RMSF patient	L. Fuentes, UCR	+	+	+
Duffey[49]	North Carolina, 1986?	RMSF patient blood	D. Walker (from C. Pretzman, ODPH)	+	+	+
Hauke[49]	Clermont, OH, 1986	Fatal RMSF	C. Pretzman, ODPH	+	+	+
Hino[49]	Oklahoma, 1964	Fatal RMSF	M. Bozeman, WRAIR	+	+	+
Hlp#2[43]	Coyote Gulch, Bitterroot Valley, MT, 27 July 1948	*Haemaphysalis leporispalustris*	G. McDonald, RML/CDC	+	+	+
Iowa[44]	Iowa, 1941	*Dermacentor variabilis*	NA	+	+	+
Lost Horse Canyon (LHC)[37]	Lost Horse Canyon, Bitterroot Valley, MT, 1958	*Dermacentor andersoni*	M. Peacock, RML	+	+	+
Morgan[42]	North Carolina, 1975	RMSF patient blood	G. McDonald, RML	+	+	+
OSU 83–13-4[49]	Clermont County, OH, 1983	*Dermacentor variabilis*	C. Pretzman, ODPH	+	+	+

Continued

TABLE 2. *Continued*

Isolate, reference	Geographic collection, year of isolation[a]	Source	Origin, collection[b]	Typing system[c]		
				VNTR	IGR	INDEL
OSU 84–21C[49]	Franklin County, OH, 1985	*Dermacentor variabilis*	C. Pretzman, ODPH	+	+	+
OSU 85-Lu1[49]	Lucas County, OH, 1985	*Dermacentor variabilis*	C. Pretzman, ODPH	+	+	+
Panama 2004[10]	Panama, 2004	Fatal RMSF	CDC	+	+	+
PriceT[47]	Montana, before 1953	*Dermacentor andersoni*	J. Spielman, HSPH	+	+	+
Sawtooth[70]	Sawtooth Canyon, Bitterroot Valley, MT, 1961	*Dermacentor andersoni*	C. Pretzman (from W. Burgdorfer, RML)	+	+	ND
Sheila Smith[71]	Montana, 1946	RMSF patient	ATCC	+	+	+
Sheila Smith-PP	Montana, 1946	RMSF patient	CWPP	+	+	+
Stewart[49]	Ft. Meade, VA, 1970	RMSF patient blood	M. Bozeman, WRAIR	+	+	+
Sutkiewicz[46]	Frederick, MD, 1973	RMSF patient blood	M. Bozeman, WRAIR	+	+	+
Von Schlemmer[49]	Frederick, MD, 1970	RMSF case	M. Bozeman, WRAIR	+	+	+
364D[72]	Ventura County, CA, 1966	*Dermacentor occidentalis*	RML	+	+	+
76RC[59]	Georgia, 1976	Fatal RMSF, blood	CDC	ND	+	+
78RL[59]	Georgia, 1978	RMSF	CDC	ND	+	+
80JC[59]	Omaha, NE, 1980	RMSF	CDC	ND	+	+
81WA[49]	North Carolina, 1986	RMSF	D. Walker (from C. Pretzman, ODPH)	+	+	+
84JG[46]	North Carolina, 1986	RMSF	D. Walker	+	+	+

[a]?, history uncertain; ND, not determined; analysis of Iowa isolate was *in silico* only.

[b]ATCC, American Type Culture Collection, Manassas, VA; CWPP, plaque purified, from C. Wisseman collection, University of Maryland School of Medicine, Baltimore, MD; CDC, Centers for Disease Control and Prevention, Atlanta, GA; HSPH, Harvard School of Public Health, Cambridge, MA; MCV, Medical College of Virginia, Charlottesville, VA; RML, Rocky Mountain Laboratory, Hamilton, MT; ODPH, Ohio State Department of Public Health, Columbus, OH; WRAIR, Walter Reed Army Institute of Research, Washington, DC; UCR, University of Costa Rica, San Jose, Costa Rica; IAL, Instituto Adolfo Lutz, Sao Paulo, Brazil.

[c]VNTR = variable number of tandem repeats; IGR = intergenic regions; INDEL = insertions or deletion events.

characteristics of TR found in *R. rickettsii* Sheila Smith-PP and their comparison to homologous elements found in other species of *Rickettsia* and *Orientia*.[64] To investigate their variability in *R. rickettsii*, we selected several VNTR sites with a size of repeat 6 nt or longer located in different regions of the chromosome as representative targets for study. Five of 12 sites selected were in coding regions, and the others were found in IGR. Four sites were found to exhibit polymorphisms in the size of amplicons encompassing the TR sites in different isolates as determined by variation in the relative electrophoretic mobility in 1 or 2% agarose gel and confirmed by direct sequencing of homologous amplicons of all the isolates. Respectively, 4 sites were shown to contain variable numbers of TR (VNTR sites), and the analysis of their concatenated sequences clustered all isolates studied into 6 groups (18 genotypes) that correlate with the specific tick vector from which the isolates were obtained or where these ticks are prevalent (human and animal isolates). The largest group comprised the isolates associated with *D. variabilis*, which included isolates from Virginia, Maryland, Ohio, Oklahoma, and North Carolina. Homologous sites of Iowa isolate were analyzed in silico [CP000766], since its DNA was not available for experimental confirmation. Three TR amplicons of Iowa differed in TR copy number compared to isolate Sheila Smith: (1) increase of mobility in 1 amplicon due to predicted absence of two 7 nt repeats compared to three 7 nt repeats in Sheila Smith isolate; (2) lack of 39 nt in the complex amplicon derived from the coding sequence of the actin-binding protein RicKA gene that contains repeated sequences encoding poly –P motifs and variations in isolates of *R. rickettsii* presented by 15 different genotypes; (3) surprisingly, 1 of the TR sites (encoding for a hypothetical protein with ankyrin-like repeats RR1030), which contained 8 copies of 84 almost identical nucleotides in all isolates studied, had only 1 repeat in Iowa isolate. Two VNTR sites, respectively found in IGR and exhibiting unique genotypes in Hlp#2 and 364D isolates, are identical in all other isolates of *R. rickettsii* including the Iowa isolate. Consequently, we confirmed the grouping of Iowa isolate as typical of other isolates associated with *D. variabilis* but with 1 new unique VNTR type due to gene RR1030.

Our VNTR typing system was used in molecular epidemiology to demonstrate the unique lineage of *R. rickettsii* isolates associated with *R. sanguineus* in Arizona,[5] distinguish unique genotype of *R. rickettsii* found in *R. sanguineus* in southern California,[7] and demonstrate that *R. rickettsii* circulating in Panama share the same *ric*KA VNTR genotype as isolates found in Central and Southern America and previously associated with *A. cajennense*.[10]

Typing Based on Variations in Sequences of Intergenic Regions

Our results reporting on differences in intergenic regions (IGR typing) among 35 isolates of *R. rickettsii* of human, tick, and animal origin have been published in detail[49] (Table 2). The groupings obtained with 6 variable sites correlated well with the previous genotyping system targeting the presence and distribution of tandem repeats (TR) (Table 3). Seven genotypes of *R. rickettsii* in 4 primary groups could be distinguished: isolates from Montana, isolates associated with *R. sanguineus* ticks and human infections in Arizona, other isolates from the USA where *D. variabilis* is thought to be the primary vector, and the isolates primarily associated with *Amblyomma* ticks from Central and South America. Iowa was identical to 6 isolates comprising a slightly divergent group of *D. variabilis* isolates including 84JG, Hino, OSU 83-13-4, OS 84-21C, 76RC, and Hauke. In addition, isolate Hlp#2, which is considered to be a nonpathogenic isolate of *R. rickettsii* and closely related serotype 364D, exhibited the most diversity from the other isolates compared, and these 2 isolates also differ significantly from each other.

Typing Based on Variations in Deletion/Insertion Sites

Analysis of the genome sequences of the cloned isolates Sheila Smith-PP [NZ_AADJ00000000] and Iowa [CP000766] identified 143 insertion/deletion sites (INDELS) ranging from 1 to 10,585 bp for the 2 genomes and 492 SNPs.[61] Only a third of INDELS (47) were within predicted coding regions, of which 23 were in isolate Sheila Smith-PP compared to Iowa, and 24 in Iowa compared to Sheila Smith-PP. Detailed analysis of these sites showed important gene alterations, including SNPs and deletions in ompA sequence, that may affect invasiveness of Iowa isolate, a defect similar but not the same as previously described for *R. peacockii*,[66,67] while deletions in the actin-binding protein RicKA gene did not alter its ability for intracellular movement and cell-to-cell spread.

As part of a more comprehensive analysis, 14 INDEL sites differing between isolates

TABLE 3. Preliminary Typing of *R. rickettsii*-like Isolates Based on INDEL Sites Found between Sheila Smith-PP and Iowa (I)

Isolate	Tick*	Total number of sites examined	Number of S-like sites	Number of I-like sites	Percentage of S-like sites
Bitterroot	DA	14	14	0	100
LHC	DA	14	13	1	93
Morgan	H-DA	13	13	0	100
Price T	DA	14	2	12	14
Sheila Smith	H-DA	14	14	0	100
Brazil	H-AC	14	12	2	86
Colombia	H-AC	14	11	3	79
Costa Rica	H-AC	14	12	2	86
Panama	H-AC	13	10	3	77
Hlp#2	HL	14	12	2	86
364D	DO	14	10	4	71
AZ3	H-RS	13	1	12	8
AZ4	H-RS	14	2	12	14
AZ5	RS	10	1	9	10
AZ6	H-RS	14	2	12	14
AZ8	RS	14	2	12	14
AZ9	RS	14	2	12	14
76RC	H-DV	14	2	12	14
78RL	H-DV	13	2	11	15
80JC	H-DV	14	1	13	7
81WA	H-DV	14	1	13	7
84JG	H-DV	14	2	12	7
BSF Di6	DV	14	2	12	7
BSF MP40	DV	12	1	11	8
BSF Rab1	DV	14	1	13	7
Coleman	H-DV	14	1	13	7
Duffey	H-DV	14	2	12	14
Hino	H-DV	12	1	11	8
Hauke	H-DV	13	2	11	15
OSU 83–13-4	DV	13	1	12	8
OSU 84–21C	DV	14	2	12	14
OSU 85-Lu1	DV	13	1	12	8
Snead	H-DV	14	2	12	14
Stewart	H-DV	14	2	12	14
Sutkiewicz	H-DV	13	2	11	15
Von Schlemmer	H-DV	12	0	12	0

*Presumed or known tick vector: DA, *Dermacentor andersoni*, AC = *Amblyomma cajennense*, HL = *Haemaphysalis leporispalustris*, DO = *D. occidentalis*, RS = *R. sanguineus*, DV = *D. variabilis*. H indicates isolates of human origin.

Iowa and Sheila Smith-PP were examined for their occurrence in other isolates of *R. rickettsii* by comparing the electrophoretic mobility of amplicons encompassing the INDEL sites (Table 3). Eleven genotypes were found. Most isolates from Montana associated with *D. andersoni* had genotypes most similar to those found in isolate Sheila Smith-PP, while the *D. variabilis*-associated isolates had INDEL patterns more similar to those determined for Iowa isolate. Isolates from Arizona shared its INDEL genotype with the most common *D. variabilis* isolate genotype, the same as found for the atypical PriceT isolate from

TABLE 4. Summary of 3 Genetic Typing Tools Applied to Collection of *R. rickettsii*-like Isolates

| Typing tool | Number of genotypes detected in isolates associated with | | | | | | |
	D. andersoni	*D. variabilis*	*R. sanguineus*	*A. cajennense*	*H. leporispalustris*	*D. occidentalis*	Totals
[Isolates]	[6]*	[21]	[8]	[4]	[1]	[1]	[40]
VNTR	4	10[§§]	1	3[¶]	1	1	18
IGR	5	3	1	2	1	1	9
INDEL	3[§]	5	1**	3	1	1	11
TOTAL	6	16	1	4	1	1	27

*Number of isolates examined.
**DNA of only 6 isolates was included.
[§]DNA of only 5 isolates was included.
[¶]DNA of only 3 isolates was included.
[§§]DNA of only 18 isolates was included.

Montana, which had also clustered with the *D. variabilis* group based on both VNTR and IGR typing. Hlp#2 and 364D isolates each had unique distributions of S-like and I-like INDELs (not shown), giving percentages of S-like sites intermediate between Sheila Smith and *D. variabilis* isolates, a finding in complete agreement with previous VNTR and IGR analyses and again suggesting that these 2 isolates might be unique species of spotted fever group rickettsiae or distinct subspecies of *R. rickettsii*.[49] Two of the INDEL sites evaluated were predominantly like Sheila Smith in all isolates except Iowa and 2 and 3 *D. variabilis*-associated isolates, respectively, suggesting they may be phenotypically important sites.

Discussion

A comparative summary of the 3 different genetic typing systems is shown in Table 4. Even though each typing system is not completely independent because INDEL sites may also encompass some of the VNTR sites or deletions detected in IGR, good agreement was found between all 3 of them. With the exception of PriceT strain, independently of genetic sites evaluated, each typing system separated isolates based on their association with a specific tick vector or its known geographic distribution region (human and animal isolates). Whether the Price strain is representative of a second type of

R. rickettsii isolate found less frequently in *D. andersoni* ticks than Sheila Smith type or whether Montana Sheila Smith-like isolates are representative of isolates from *D. andersoni* outside of Montana is unknown. Morgan had exactly the same genotype as Bitterroot despite its putative North Carolina origin and *D. variabilis* association, so it, like PriceT, likely became mislabeled during its laboratory passage. Additional isolates of *R. rickettsii* from the Rocky Mountain states are needed to resolve this question.

The greater resemblance of isolates from *R. sanguineus* and from Central and South America to the Montana isolates was clear using VNTR and IGR typing systems with the isolates from *Rhipicephalus* exhibiting the least divergence from the Montana *D. andersoni* isolates. However, INDEL typing placed the Arizona *Rhipicephalus* isolates with *D. variabilis* isolates and the Central and South America isolates more closely to Montana *D. andersoni* isolates. However, the Central/South American isolates were not homogeneous. Whether distinct subpopulations in the *D. variabilis* and Central/South America groups can be defined and whether all isolates of *R. rickettsii* from *Rhipicephalus* will be identical (the Arizona isolates were all from the same very small area in that state) regardless of their place of origin are presently unknown.

Because complex interactions underlie the pathogenesis of *R. rickettsii in vivo*, it is difficult to define the causality of individual events, which occur in infected vertebrate hosts and humans. Several microbial factors are likely to contribute to the varied ability of *R. rickettsii* to cause cellular injury *in vitro*, and many of them may also contribute importantly to its virulence for vertebrate hosts and may be due to the variable genetic markers identified in our studies. Since circulation of *R. rickettsii* in nature includes both vertical transstadial and transovarial transmission with tick vectors and horizontal passages through vertebrate hosts, it is plausible that isolates of different virulence differ because they were isolated during different phases of a normal cycle of physiological adaptation to their vertebrate hosts. Characterization of isolate differences in rickettsial gene expression that occur immediately after tick-to-human or tick-to-animal transitions may require development of more complex experimental systems than the straightforward genetic analysis performed here.

With a larger set of genetic markers and more representative set of isolates of *R. rickettsii*, it may be possible to estimate when isolation between different populations of this species occurred and how much gene flow occurs between these different populations. Sites that appear to be more variable within a geographic population may be useful for detecting mutation rates *in vitro* as well as for molecular epidemiological investigations. It is important to assess how much of the genetic variation of *R. rickettsii* is due to long-extant geographic isolation or biological barriers between populations and how much is due to evolutionary selection of phenotypic variants (neutral vs. natural selection). Finally, how much of the biologically relevant selection results in changes contributing to variations in human virulence and its immediate and long-term clinical manifestations? The genetic markers described here were obtained on a relatively large collection of the *R. rickettsii* isolates; however, it will be necessary to obtain more isolates to provide stronger evidences for genotypic variations among *R. rickettsii* circulating in different areas and probably to delineate its ancestral traits. Rickettsial

evolution probably largely reflects its adaptation to its invertebrate hosts and therefore is congruent to the phylogeny of its tick vectors. On the other hand, while a few isolates of *R. rickettsii* clearly cause detrimental effects on its tick vector in a laboratory setting,[38] it is not clear if this is true of all genetic stocks of *R. rickettsii*[50] or in all species of ticks it infects. This is an important question to define as it probably reflects the relative importance of vertical and horizontal mechanisms for sustaining populations of this agent in nature. Most experimental data accumulated to date have used a very narrow spectrum of reference isolates of *R. rickettsii*, and were blithely extrapolated to other isolates without independent evaluation or comparison. High throughput evaluation of biological and physiological characteristics of distinct genotypes of isolates of *R. rickettsii*, including both highly passaged reference isolates and low passage isolates, should allow for improved understanding of these issues.

Acknowledgments

We thank Sandor Karpathy, Kimetha Slater, Matt Erdman, Josef Limor, Cecilia Kato, Lauren Robinson, Frankie White, and Ryan Klemt for their contribution to the genotyping of isolates of *Rickettsia rickettsii*, Anup Madan for his work determining the genome sequence of *R. rickettsii* strain Sheila Smith-PP, and David J. Silverman, Lisa Domotor, and Nina Tioleco for their contribution to the cell culture experiments.

Conflicts of Interest

The authors declare no conflicts of interest.

References

1. Chapman, A.S. *et al*. 2006. Rocky Mountain spotted fever in the United States, 1997–2002. *Vector Borne Zoonotic Dis.* **6:** 170–178.
2. Bustamante, M.E., G. Varela & C.O. Mariotte. 1946. Estudios de fiebre manchada en Mexico: fiebre

manchada en la Laguna. *Rev. Inst. Salubr. Enferm. Trop.* **7:** 39–49.

3. Bustamante, M.E. & G. Varela. 1947. Estudios de fiebre manchada en Mexico: papel del *Rhipicephalus sanguineus* en la transmission de la fiebre manchada en la Republica Mexicana. *Rev. Inst. Salubr. Enferm. Trop.* **8:** 139–141.

4. Demma, L.J. *et al.* 2005. Rocky Mountain spotted fever from an unexpected tick vector in Arizona. *N. Engl. J. Med.* **353:** 587–594.

5. Eremeeva, M.E. *et al.* 2006. Molecular typing of novel *Rickettsia rickettsii* isolates from Arizona. *Ann. N. Y. Acad. Sci.* **1078:** 573–577.

6. Garrison, L.E., R. Kelly, W.L. Nicholson & M.E. Eremeeva. 2007. Tick surveillance notes: *Rickettsia rickettsii* in *Rhipicephalus sanguineus* ticks from Gordon County. *Georgia Epidemiol. Rep.* **23:** 1–2.

7. Wikswo, M.E., R. Hu, M.E. Metzger & M.E. Eremeeva. 2007. Detection of *Rickettsia rickettsii* and *Bartonella henselae* in *Rhipicephalus sanguineus* ticks from California. *J. Med. Entomol.* **44:** 158–162.

8. Zavala-Castro, J.E. *et al.* 2006. Fatal human infection with *Rickettsia rickettsii*, Yucatán, Mexico. *Emerg. Infect. Dis.* **12:** 672–674.

9. Acosta, J. *et al.* 2006. Outbreak of fatal Rocky Mountain spotted fever in Necocli, Antioqia, Colombia. Abstract 142. *20th Meeting of the American Society for Rickettsiology in conjunction with the 5th International Conference on Bartonella as Emerging Pathogen.*

10. Estripeaut, D. *et al.* 2007. Rocky Mountain spotted fever, Panama. *Emerg. Infect. Dis.* **13:** 1763–1765.

11. Fuentes, L.G. 1979. 1st case of Rocky Mountain fever in Costa Rica. *Central America Rev. Latinoam. Microbiol.* **21:** 167–172.

12. Galvao, M.A. *et al.* 2003. Fatal spotted fever rickettsiosis, Minas Gerais, Brazil. *Emerg. Infect. Dis.* **9:** 1402–1405.

13. Hidalgo, M. *et al.* 2007. Rocky Mountain spotted fever, Colombia. *Emerg. Infect. Dis.* **13:** 1058–60.

14. Patino, L., A. Afanador & J.H. Paul. 1937. A spotted fever in Tobia, Colombia. *Am. J. Trop. Med. Hyg.* **17:** 639–653.

15. Paddock, C.D. *et al.* 2008. Rocky Mountain spotted fever in Argentina. *Am. J. Trop. Med. Hyg.* **78:** 687–692.

16. de Rodaniche, E.C. 1954. Natural infection of the tick, *Amblyomma cajennense*, with *Rickettsia rickettsii* in Panama. *Am. J. Trop. Med. Hyg.* **2:** 696–699.

17. Guedes, E. *et al.* 2005. Detection of *Rickettsia rickettsii* in the tick *Amblyomma cajennense* in a new Brazilian spotted fever-endemic area in the state of Minas Gerais. *Mem. Inst. Oswaldo Cruz* **100:** 841–845.

18. Pinter, A. & M.B. Labruna. 2006. Isolation of *Rickettsia rickettsii* and *Rickettsia bellii* in cell culture from the tick *Amblyomma aureolatum* in Brazil. *Ann. N. Y. Acad. Sci.* **1078:** 523–529.

19. Chapman, A.S. *et al.* 2006. Diagnosis and management of tickborne rickettsial diseases: Rocky Mountain spotted fever, ehrlichioses, and anaplasmosis–United States: a practical guide for physicians and other health-care and public health professionals. *MMWR Recomm. Rep.* **55:** 1–27.

20. Walker, D.H. 1988. Pathology and pathogenesis of vasculotropic rickettsioses. *Biology of Rickettsial Diseases.* D.H. Walker, Ed.: 115–138. CRC Press, Inc. Boca Raton, FL.

21. Kirkland, K.B. *et al.* 1993. Rocky Mountain spotted fever complicated by gangrene: report of six cases and review. *Clin. Infect. Dis.* **16:** 629–634.

22. Helmick, C.G., K.W. Bernard & L.J. D'Angelo. 1984. Rocky Mountain spotted fever: clinical, laboratory, and epidemiological features of 262 cases. *J. Infect. Dis.* **150:** 480–488.

23. Sexton, D.J. & G.R. Corey. 1992. Rocky Mountain "spotless" and "almost spotless" fever: a wolf in sheep's clothing. *Clin. Infect. Dis.* **15:** 439–448.

24. Conlon, P.J. *et al.* 1996. Predictors of prognosis and risk of acute renal failure in patients with Rocky Mountain spotted fever. *Am. J. Med.* **101:** 621–626.

25. Kirkland, K.B., W.E. Wilkinson & D.J. Sexton. 1995. Therapeutic delay and mortality in cases of Rocky Mountain spotted fever. *Clin. Infect. Dis.* **20:** 1118–1121.

26. Harden, V.A. 1990. The beginnings of scientific investigations. *Rocky Mountain Spotted Fever. History of a Twentieth-Century Disease.* V.A. Harden, Ed.: 23–46. The John Hopkins University Press. Baltimore and London.

27. Paddock, C.D. *et al.* 2008. *Rickettsia parkeri* rickettsiosis and its clinical distinction from Rocky Mountain spotted fever. *Clin Infect Dis.* **47:** 1188–1196.

28. Fiebre maculosa. www.cve.saude.sp.gov.br/htm/zoo/fm_i8503.htm (accessed on October 28, 2008).

29. Surto de Febre Maculosa no municipio de Petropolis-RJ. Ministerio da Saude Secretaria de Vigilancia em Saude. (http://portal.saude.gov.br/portal/arquivos/pdf/nota_maculosa_corrigida.pdf) (accessed on October 28, 2008).

30. Fishbein, D.B., M.G. Frontini, R. Giles & L.L. Vernon. 1990. Fatal cases of Rocky Mountain spotted fever in the United States, 1981–1988. *Ann. N. Y. Acad. Sci.* **590:** 246–247.

31. Centers for Disease Control and Prevention. 2000. Consequences of delayed diagnosis of Rocky Mountain spotted fever in children – West Virginia, Michigan, Tennessee, and Oklahoma, May-July 2000. *MMWR* **49:** 887–891.

32. Hattwick, M.A. *et al.* 1978. Fatal Rocky Mountain spotted fever. *J. Am. Med. Assoc.* **240:** 1499–1503.

33. Pike, R.M. 1965. Continuing importance of laboratory-acquired infections. *Am. J. Publ. Health* **55:** 190–199.

34. Saslaw, S. & H.N. Carlisle. 1966. Aerosol infection of monkeys with *Rickettsia rickettsii*. *Bacteriol. Rev.* **30:** 636–645.

35. Walker, D.H., H.K. Hawkins & P. Hudson. 1983. Fulminant Rocky Mountain spotted fever. Its pathologic characteristics associated with glucose-6-phosphate dehydrogenase deficiency. *Arch. Pathol. Lab. Med.* **107:** 121–125.

36. Burgdorfer, W. 1975. A review of Rocky Mountain spotted fever (tick-borne typhus), its agents, and its tick vectors in the United States. *J. Med. Entomol.* **12:** 269–278.

37. Burgdorfer, W. & L.P. Brinton. 1975. Mechanisms of transovarial infection of spotted fever rickettsiae in ticks. *Ann. N. Y. Acad. Sci.* **266:** 61–72.

38. Niebylski, M.L., M.G. Peacock & T.G. Schwan. 1999. Lethal effect of *Rickettsia rickettsii* on its tick vector (*Dermacentor andersoni*). *Appl. Environ. Microbiol.* **65:** 773–778.

39. Anacker, R.L. *et al.* 1984. Biochemical and immunochemical analysis of *Rickettsia rickettsii* strains of various degrees of virulence. *Infect. Immun.* **44:** 559–564.

40. Anacker, R.L., R.H. List, R.E. Mann & D.L. Wiedbrauk. 1986. Antigenic heterogeneity in high- and low-virulence strains of *Rickettsia rickettsii* revealed by monoclonal antibodies. *Infect. Immun.* **51:** 653–660.

41. Anacker, R.L., R.E. Mann & C. Gonzales. 1987. Reactivity of monoclonal antibodies to *Rickettsia rickettsii* with spotted fever and typhus group rickettsiae. *J. Clin. Microbiol.* **25:** 167–171.

42. Philip, R.N. *et al.* 1978. Serologic typing of rickettsiae of the spotted fever group by microimmunfluorescence. *J. Immunol.* **121:** 1961–1968.

43. Parker, R.R. *et al.* 1951. Isolation and characterization of Rocky Mountain spotted fever rickettsiae from the rabbit tick *Haemaphysalis leporis-palustris* Packard. Public Health Rep. **66:** 455–463.

44. Cox, H.R. 1941. Cultivation of rickettsiae of the Rocky Mountain spotted fever, typhus and Q fever groups in the embryonic tissues of developing chicks. *Science* **94:** 399–403.

45. Hackstadt, T., R. Messer, W. Cieplak & M.G. Peacock. 1992. Evidence for proteolytic clevage of the 120-kilodalton outer membrane protein of rickettsiae: identification of an avirulent mutant deficient in processing. *Infect. Immun.* **60:** 159–165.

46. Eremeeva, M.E., G.A. Dasch & D.J. Silverman. 2001. Quantitative analyses of variations in the injury of endothelial cells elicited by 11 isolates of *Rickettsia rickettsii*. *J. Clin. Lab. Immunol.* **8:** 788–796.

47. Price, W.H. 1953. The epidemiology of Rocky Mountain spotted fever: I. The characterization of strain virulence of *Rickettsia rickettsii*. *Am. J. Hyg.* **58:** 248–268.

48. Price, W.H. 1954. The epidemiology of Rocky Mountain spotted fever: II. Studies on the biological survival mechanism of *Rickettsia rickettsii*. *Am. J. Hyg.* **60:** 292–319.

49. Karpathy, S.E., G.A. Dasch & M.E. Eremeeva. 2007. Molecular typing of *Rickettsia rickettsii* isolates using DNA sequencing of variable intergenic regions. *J. Clin. Microbiol.* **45:** 2545–2253.

50. Todd, W.J., W. Burgdorfer & G.P. Wray. 1981. Ultrastructural analysis of *Rickettsia rickettsii* in cultures of persistently infected vole cells. *Rickettsiae and Rickettsial Diseases*. W. Burgdorfer & R.L. Anacker, Eds. 255–265. Academic Press. New York, NY.

51. Matsumoto, M. *et al.* 1996. Deletion in the 190 kDa antigen gene repeat region of *Rickettsia rickettsii*. *Microb. Pathog.* **20:** 57–62.

52. Balraj, P., G. Vestris, D. Raoult & P. Renesto. 2008. Comparison of *R. conorii* growth and actin based motility within different cell lines, P047. *5th International Meeting on Rickettsiae and Rickettsial Diseases*. Marseille, France: ESCMID.

53. Eremeeva, M.E., N. Tioleco, D.J. Silverman & G.A. Dasch. 2004. Growth kinetics and cytopathic effects caused by different isolates of *Rickettsia conorii* in Vero and L929 cells, unpublished observations.

54. Spencer, H.R. & R.R. Parker. 1923. Rocky Mountain spotted fever: infectivity of fasting and recently fed ticks. *Public Health Rep.* **38:** 333–339.

55. Price, W.H. 1953. A quantitative analysis of the factors involved in the variations in virulence of rickettsiae. *Science* **118:** 49–52.

56. Gilford, J.H. & W.H. Price. 1968. Virulent-avirulent conversions of *Rickettsia rickettsii in vitro*. *Selected Papers on the Pathogenic Rickettsiae*. N. Hanon, Ed.: 285–290. Harvard University Press. Cambridge, MA.

57. Hayes, S.F. & W. Burgdorfer. 1982. Reactivation of *Rickettsia rickettsii* in *Dermacentor andersoni* ticks: an ultrastructural analysis. *Infect. Immun.* **37:** 779–785.

58. Eremeeva, M.E. *et al.* 2003. Genetic analysis of isolates of *Rickettsia rickettsii* that differ in virulence. *Ann. N. Y. Acad. Sci.* **990:** 717–722.

59. Regnery, R.L., C.L. Spruill & B.D. Plikaytis. 1991. Genotypic identification of rickettsiae and estimation of intraspecies sequence divergence for portions of two rickettsial genes. *J. Bacteriol.* **173:** 1576–1589.

60. Gilmore, R.D. & T. Hackstadt. 1991. DNA polymorphism in the conserved 190 kDa antigen gene repeat region among spotted fever group rickettsiae. *Biochim. Biophys. Acta* **1097:** 77–80.

61. Ellison, D.W. *et al.* 2008. Genomic comparison of virulent *Rickettsia rickettsii* Sheila Smith and avirulent *Rickettsia rickettsii* Iowa. *Infect. Immun.* **76:** 542–550.

62. Fournier, P.E. & D. Raoult. 2007. Identification of rickettsial isolates at the species level using multi-spacer typing. *BMC Microbiol.* **7:** 72.

63. Fournier, P.E., Y. Zhu, H. Ogata & D. Raoult. 2004. Use of highly variable intergenic spacer sequences for multispacer typing of *Rickettsia conorii* strains. *J. Clin. Microbiol.* **42:** 5757–5766.

64. Eremeeva, M.E. *et al.* 2005. New perspectives on rickettsial evolution from new genome sequences of *Rickettsia*, particularly *R. canadensis* and *Orientia tsutsugamushi*. *Ann. N. Y. Acad. Sci.* **1063:** 47–63.

65. McLeod, M.P. *et al.* 2004. Complete genome sequence of *Rickettsia typhi* and comparison with sequences of other rickettsiae. *J. Bacteriol.* **186:** 5842–5855.

66. Baldridge, G.D. *et al.* 2004. Sequence and expression analysis of the ompA gene of *Rickettsia peacockii*, an endosymbiont of the Rocky Mountain wood tick, *Dermacentor andersoni*. *Appl. Environ. Microbiol.* **70:** 6628–6636.

67. Simser, J.A., M.S. Rahman, S.M. Dreher-Lesnick & A.F. Azad. 2005. A novel and naturally occurring transposon, ISRpe1 in the *Rickettsia peacockii* genome disrupting the *rick*A gene involved in actin-based motility. *Mol. Microbiol.* **58:** 71–79.

68. Bell, E.J. & E.G. Pickens. 1953. A toxic substance associated with the rickettsias of the spotted fever group. *J. Immunol.* **70:** 461–472.

69. Bozeman, F.M., A. Shirai, J.W. Humphries & H.S. Fuller. 1967. Ecology of Rocky Mountain spotted fever. II. Natural infection of wild mammals and birds in Virginia and Maryland. *Am. J. Trop. Med. Hyg.* **16:** 48–59.

70. Burgdorfer, W. 1963. Investigation of "transovarial transmission" of *Rickettsia rickettsii* in the wood tick, *Dermacentor andersoni*. *Exp. Parasitol.* **14:** 152–159.

71. Bell, E.J. & H.G. Stoenner. 1960. Immunologic relationships among the spotted fever group of rickettsias determined by toxin neutralization tests in mice with convalescent animal serums. *J. Immunol.* **84:** 171–182.

72. Philip, R.N., R.S. Lane & E.A. Casper. 1981. Serotypes of tick-borne spotted fever group rickettsiae from western California. *Am. J. Trop. Med. Hyg.* **30:** 722–727.

73. Eremeeva, M.E., G.A. Dasch & D.J. Silverman. 2003. Evaluation of a PCR assay for quantitation of *Rickettsia rickettsii* and closely related spotted fever group rickettsiae. *J. Clin. Microbiol.* **41:** 5466–5472.

Note:

The detection of *Rickettsia rickettsii* in *Rhipicephalus sanguineus* from Rio de Janeiro State, Brazil was also reported in November, 2008 (NCBI accession number FJ356230).

Comparative Proteomic Analysis of Antibiotic-Sensitive and Insensitive Isolates of *Orientia tsutsugamushi*

Chien-Chung Chao,[a] Donita L. Garland,[b,*] Gregory A. Dasch,[c] and Wei-Mei Ching[a,d]

[a]*Viral and Rickettsial Diseases Department, Infectious Diseases Directorate, Naval Medical Research Center, Silver Spring, Maryland 20910, USA*

[b]*National Eye Institute, NIH, Bethesda, Maryland 20892, USA*

[c]*Rickettsial Zoonoses Branch, Centers for Disease Control and Prevention, Atlanta, Georgia 30333, USA*

[d]*Uniformed Service University of the Health Sciences, Bethesda, Maryland 20814, USA*

Scrub typhus, caused by infection with *Orientia tsutsugamushi*, is probably the most common severe rickettsial disease. Early diagnosis followed by treatment with antibiotics such as doxycycline or chloramphenicol usually quickly decreases fever in patients, and they often recover well from other symptoms of the disease. However, poorly responsive cases have been reported from northern Thailand and southern India. In order to identify protein factors that may be partially responsible for differential drug sensitivity of isolates of *Orientia*, we compared the protein profiles of doxycycline sensitive (Karp) versus (vs.) insensitive (AFSC4 and AFSC7) isolates. Tryptic peptides from both total water-soluble proteins and from protein spots separated by 2D-PAGE were analyzed using LC-MS/MS. The identity of each protein was established using the published genomic sequence of Boryong strain *O. tsutsugamushi*. The profiles of protein released into water from these isolates were quite different. There were 10 proteins detected only in AFSC4, 3 only in Karp, and 1 only in AFSC7. Additionally, there were 2 proteins not detected only in AFSC4, 4 not found only in Karp, and 3 not found only in AFSC-7. A comparison of 2D-PAGE protein profiles of drug sensitive strain versus (vs.) insensitive isolates has led to the identification of 14 differentially expressed or localized proteins, including elongation factor Ts and Tu, DNA-directed RNA polymerase α-subunit, ATP synthase β-subunit, and several hypothetical proteins. These data confirm the tremendous proteomic diversity of isolates of *Orientia* and suggest that drug insensitivity in this species may arise from multiple mechanisms.

Key words: *Orientia tsutsugamushi*; Proteomic; antibiotic sensitive

Introduction

Scrub typhus infection is caused by the obligately intracellular, gram-negative bacterium *Orientia tsutsugamushi*. It accounts for up to 23% of all febrile episodes in areas of the Asia-Pacific region where scrub typhus is endemic, and mortality can occur up to a third of cases if left untreated.[1,2] Symptoms may include pneumonitis, meningitis, rash, and headache. Differentiating scrub typhus from other acute febrile illness, such as leptospirosis, murine typhus, and malaria, can be difficult because of the similarities in signs and symptoms. The serodiagnosis of scrub typhus has been performed mainly by the methods of indirect immunofluorescent

Address for correspondence: Chien-Chung Chao, Ph.D., VRDD/IDD/NMRC, 503 Robert Grant Ave, RM3N71, Silver Spring, MD 20910. Voice: +301-319-7313; fax: +301-319-7451. chien-chung.chao@med.navy.mil
*Current address: Dr. Donita L. Garland, Scheie Eye Institute, FM Kirby Center for Molecular Ophthalmology, University of Pennsylvania, 306 Stellar Chance Labs, 422 Curie Boulevard, Philadelphia, PA. 19104–6100

Rickettsiology and Rickettsial Diseases-Fifth International Conference: Ann. N.Y. Acad. Sci. 1166: 27–37 (2009).
doi: 10.1111/j.1749-6632.2009.04525.x © 2009 New York Academy of Sciences.

assay (IFA) or the indirect immunoperoxidase (IIP) assay, which require the growth of rickettsiae in the embryonated eggs or cell culture.

Accurate diagnosis is very important because without appropriate antibiotic treatment a fatal course of disease is possible, especially if complicated by disseminated intravascular coagulation.[3] Before the age of antibiotic therapy, patients with scrub typhus had high mortality rates up to 50–60% with a clinical course ranging from 10 to 28 days and a protracted convalescence of up to 4 months.[4] Once accurately diagnosed, treatment with tetracycline class antibiotics resulted in dramatic recovery within 24 h. Doxycycline, a member of the tetracycline family, inhibits protein synthesis by blocking aminoacyl-tRNA binding at the A-site in the 30S ribosomal subunit.[5] Recent work has shown that patients in northern Thailand who were infected with *O. tsutsugamushi* responded poorly to appropriate antibiotic therapy.[5] Chloramphenicol or doxycycline treatments did not effectively clear fever or prevent death in mice infected with some isolates of *O. tsutsugamushi* from northern Thailand[6] and southern India.[7] Resistance to tetracyclines is typically associated with mobile genetic elements and falls into 3 classes: efflux pump, ribosomal protection, and enzymatic degradation.[5,8] Previous antibiotic sensitivity studies in tissue culture showed that 95% of L929 cells were infected by AFSC4 in the presence of 4 μg/mL doxycycline, 79% L929 cells were infected by AFSC7 in the presence of 16 μg/mL doxycycline, while less than 5% of L929 cells were infected by Karp in the presence of either 4 or 16 μg/mL doxycycline.[9] Experiments were also performed in the mouse challenge model by feeding mice infected with AFSC4 or Karp at 2 mg/kg/day doxycycline for 4, 6, 8, or 10 days. All mice survived subsequent Karp strain challenge, but only 20–60% mice survived AFSC4 challenge (Strickman D, unpublished data). These results indicate that these patient isolates from central Thailand are somewhat resistant to doxycycline *in vitro*, further suggesting the need to find alternative therapeutic treatments to doxycycline.

Gel electrophoresis and LC-MS/MS have made it possible to compare the global differential expression of proteins under various conditions. The availability of genomic DNA sequences and the development of computer software have allowed protein identification in a high-throughput fashion. Comparative proteomics of pathogenic bacteria has been shown to be very useful in elucidating potential vaccine candidates and diagnostic markers, as well as determining novel targets for drug design and the effects of these drugs on cellular physiology.[10]

In this report, we used LC-MS/MS and 2D gel electrophoresis to compare protein expression pattern of 3 isolates of *O. tsutsugamushi*. Among the 3 isolates, Karp, the classic prototype strain, is doxycycline sensitive, and AFSC4 and AFSC7 are doxycycline-insensitive isolates to different extents.[9] The genome sequence of Boryong strain was used to characterize and identify proteins in all 3 of these isolates, which differ significantly in GroESL, 56 kDa, and 22 kDa restriction fragment length polymorphism types and reactivity to antisera in Western blotting (Dasch, unpublished observations and Ref. 11).

Materials and Methods

Preparation of Samples and 2D Gel Electrophoresis

Renografin density gradient purified *O. tsutsugamushi* (500 μg) was suspended in 50 μl of water and kept frozen at $-80°C$ until use. The sample was centrifuged at 16,000 $\times$ g for 15 minutes, and supernatant was collected for further processing as described below. The pellet was lysed in 2D lysis buffer containing 9 M Urea (Acros, Pittsburgh, PA, USA), 4% 3-[(3-Cholamidopropyl)dimethylammonio]-1-propanesulfonate (CHAPS, Sigma-Aldrich, St. Louis, MO, USA) and 50 mM 1,4-dithiothreitol (DTT, Sigma-Aldrich). Protein concentration was then determined using the

Bradford method (Bio-Rad, Hercules, CA, USA). Total 200 μg of protein was subjected to isoelectric focusing at 20°C (18 cm IPG strips, nonlinear pH 3–10 gradient, Amersham Bioscience, Piscataway, NJ, USA) followed by SDS-PAGE on 20 × 25 cm gels with a 15–18% polyacrylamide gradient. Images of the gels stained with colloidal coomassie blue (Invitrogen, Carlsbad, CA, USA) were taken with a Molecular Dynamics' Personal Densitometer and stored as JPEG file for analysis with Progenesis software (Nonlinear Dynamics, Cary, NC, USA). The automatically generated spot detection, segmentation, and matching were checked manually. Experiments were repeated 2 more times to get triplicate data to be averaged for data analyses.

Reduction, Alkylation, and Digestion of Proteins for MS Analysis

Samples from Cell Pellet

Selected 2D gel spots were cut with razor blade and washed with wash buffer containing 50 mM ammonium bicarbonate (AmBic, Fluka, St Louis, MO, USA) and 50% acetonitrile (ACN, Burdick Jackson, Muskegon, MI, USA) until the stain was removed, then HPLC grade water (Burdick and Jackson), followed by neat ACN for drying. Reduction with 5 mM DTT (Sigma-Aldrich) was carried out at 60°C for 30 min., followed by adding a 3 molar ratio of iodoacetamide (IAA, Sigma-Aldrich) in the dark at room temperature for 30 min. All excess reagents were wash buffer twice before drying in neat ACN in SpeedVac. Approximately, 100–300 ng trypsin (Promega, Madison, WI, USA) was added to the dry and rehydrated with 100 mM AmBic (amount of trypsin used is dependent on estimated amounts of the protein present in the gel, usually 1:50 w/w). The samples were incubated at 37°C overnight. The digested peptide mixtures were extracted with 50 μL 5% formic acid (EM Science, Deerfield, IL, USA) in water/ACN in 3 cycles, and all extracts were combined. The combined liquids

were dried down in SpeedVac concentrator, dissolved in 20 μL of water containing 0.1% formic acid and used for LC-MS/MS analysis.

Samples from Supernatant

Supernatant collected from the original 16,000 × g centrifugation to separate the water-soluble components and cell pellet was analyzed for protein concentration. Equal amounts (100 μg) of proteins from supernatants of Karp strain (plaque purified) and 2 isolates (AFSC4 and AFSC7) were dried in SpeedVac and resuspended in 6M Guanidinine-HCl (Gn-HCl, pH 8.0, Sigma-Aldrich) at 0.5 mg/mL to completely unfold the proteins. The samples were reduced by DTT (10 μM/1 mg protein) at 37°C for $^1/_2$ h., alkylated by IAA for 30 min. at room temperature. Samples were then loaded into Millipore centricon (10 K molecular weight cutoff, Billerica, MA, USA) and centrifuged at 13,000 rpm to concentrate and exchange Gn-HCl with AmBic. The final concentration of Gn-HCl in the concentrated samples was lowered to less than 1/10 of the original concentration. The volume of each sample was adjusted to maintain 0.5 mg/mL protein concentration, and trypsin was added to achieve protein:trypsin = 50:1 for digestion, which was done at 37°C overnight. Digested samples were dried in SpeedVac and resuspended in 100 μL of water containing 0.1% formic acid. The samples were used for LC-MS analysis as described below.

LC/MS-MS Analysis

The digested proteins (peptides) were loaded onto a PicoFrit reverse phased (RP) column (New Objectives, MA, USA) and eluted with 0–65% ACN gradient containing 0.1% formic acid in 120 minutes. The eluted peptides were delivered into an ion trap mass spectrometer (ProteomeX, Thermo Electron, Waltham, MA, USA) with nanospray ionization for analysis of peptide sequence information. The mass spectrometer was set to automatically fragment (MS/MS) the top 3 most intense base

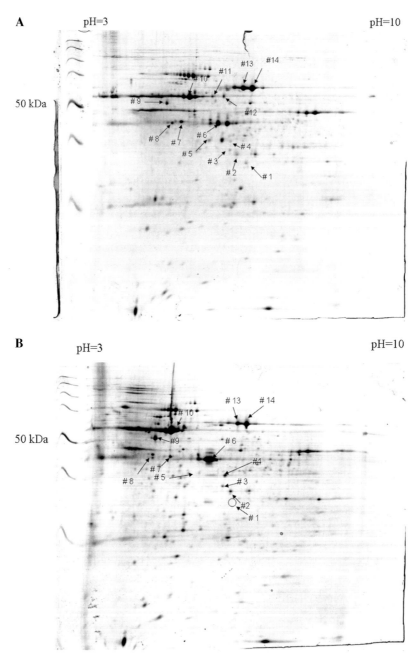

Figure 1. Representative images of 2D- PAGE of water-insoluble fraction. (**A**) 2D-PAGE image of Karp strain *O. tsutsugamushi*. Proteins with differential expression were indicated by arrows. (**B**) 2D-PAGE image of AFSC4 isolate. (**C**) 2D-PAGE image of AFSC7 isolate. Detail description of data analysis and experimental condition for 2D-PAGE are in Materials and Methods.

peaks obtained from full scan MS with dynamic exclusion. The chromatograms were reviewed for the efficiency of chromatographic separation. Once the chromatogram indicated good separation and interpretable mass spectra, BioWorks 3.2 (Thermo Electron) was launched for the analysis of MS/MS data using the genomic DNA sequence of *O. tsutsugamushi*

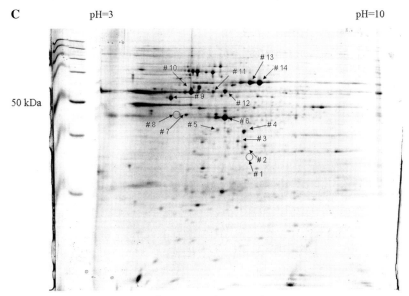

Figure 1. *Continued.*

Boryong strain. Only the best matched peptides were evaluated further as described below. Any of the best peptides can be considered as a positive identification if it successfully passes the following 3 criteria: charge state of a peptide vs. Xcor (1+ > 1.5, 2+ > 2.0 and 3+ > 2.5), delta Cn > 0.1 (delta Cn is a measurement for the dissimilarity between the best matched peptide and the 2nd best matched peptide), and peptide probability $<10^{-3}$ (an indication of an identification as a random match between the theoretical and experimental spectra). In order for a protein to be positively identified, it has to have at least 2 different peptides detected by LC-MS. If only 1 peptide was observed, this peptide has to be observed in at least 3 independent LC-MS analyses.[12]

Results and Discussion

In this study, equal amounts of proteins from each strain and isolates were used for all 2D-PAGE and LC-MS/MS analyses, and the annotated database of Boryong strain of *O. tsutsugamushi*[13] available in NCBI website (www.ncbi.nlm.nih.gov) was used for protein identification analysis. If a peptide does not

match with the sequences in the database, it can be due to highly divergent sequences found in different isolates, or the peptide is from host cells, or it is a fragment of a unique protein in other isolates, or errors in the annotation of sequence of Boryong or post-translational modifications of proteins. This study was performed based on the assumption that the variation in protein sequences of different strain or isolates was minimal so that the use of Boryong sequences would not significantly affect the ability to identify the same protein from other strain or isolates.

Comparison and Identification of Proteins on 2D Gels

Typical 2D gel images of each strain and isolates are shown in Figure 1 (panel A to C). It is evident that each strain and isolates shared similarity in the distribution of proteins and the relative intensity of major spots. A closer comparison of each image has shown different intensities for at least 14 different spots (Fig. 2, panel A and B). The volume for each spot on an averaged gel was calculated as the sum of the normalized volumes of a spot divided by the number of gels used to generate

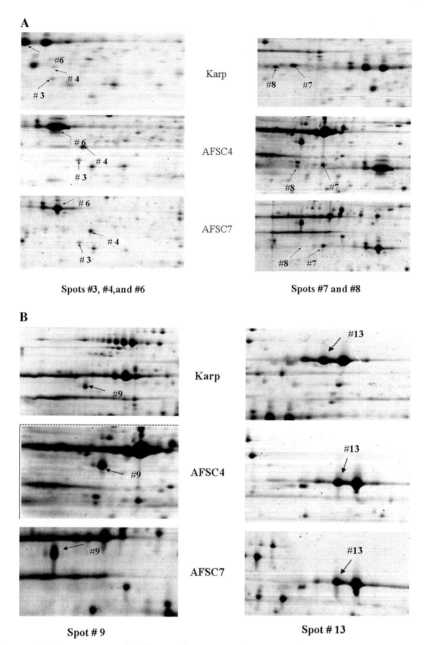

Figure 2. Comparison of differentially expressed protein of water-insoluble fractions by 2D-PAGE. (**A**) Protein spots 3, 4, 5, 7, and 8 are shown. The relative intensity of each spot can be compared. (**B**) Protein spots 9 and 13 are shown. The relative intensity of each spot can be compared. Proteins differentially expressed were determined and labeled as described in Materials and Methods.

the average. Of the 14 spots examined, only 9 of them were successfully identified using LC-MS (as described in Materials and Methods) so far. The average intensities of these 9 spots and names of proteins identified are shown in Table 1. One of the identified proteins, the 56-kDa protein (spot 9), which is the major outer membrane protein antigen, showed a decreased expression in the antibiotic-insensitive isolates. Two hypothetical proteins (spots 5 and 7) that did not belong to any cluster of orthologous group family (COGs) showed reduced expression in antibiotic-insensitive isolates relative to the Karp strain. The other 6 proteins were classified to 5 different COG functional categories. Two of the elongation factors belonging to the translation (COG: J) were identified. EF-Ts, which is a highly conserved protein, was only detected in Karp strain possibly due to lower abundance in the antibiotic-insensitive isolates. On the contrary, increased expression of EF-Tu was observed in antibiotic-insensitive isolates. EF-Ts is known to serve as the guanidine nucleotide exchange factor for EF-Tu, the enzyme that binds to the charged tRNA molecules and allows this complex to transiently enter the ribosome for translation. It has been demonstrated in *Streptomyces coelicolor* and *Streptomyces ramocissimus* that a single EF-Ts suffices for the recycling of multiple and divergent EF-Tu species.[14] One of the mechanisms for tetracycline resistance is the presence of ribosomal protection proteins. These proteins are known homologs of EF-Tu and EF-G[15,16] and are known to reduce the susceptibility of ribosomes to tetracyclines.[5] Therefore, the increased expression of EF-Tu in the antibiotic-insensitive AFSC4 and AFSC7 isolates may result in a reduced susceptibility of ribosomes to tetracyclines. The different trends in EF-Ts and EF-Tu expression between Karp and insensitive isolates of AFSC4 and AFSC7 indicated that amounts of EF-Ts is sufficient for recycling of EF-Tu as has been shown previously.[14] Alternatively, this may result in an overall slower rate of translation, also possibly diminishing the effect of doxycycline. This is consistent with the observations that other identified proteins that belonged to the following COGs, C (energy production and conversion), V (defense mechanism), and T (signal transduction mechanisms) all showed a decreased expression in antibiotic-insensitive isolates. Only the DNA-directed RNA polymerase α-subunit (transcription, COG: K) showed an increased expression in antibiotic-insensitive isolates. The overall effect of these changes is not clear, but it may result in an overall slow growth, which has been shown to affect the accumulation of antibiotics in *E. coli* and *Bacillus megaterium*.[17]

Comparison and Identification of Protein Released into Water Using LC-MS/MS

Proteins are present in the water fraction depleted of intact *O. tsutsugamushi* cells and envelopes. This fraction was collected and analyzed on 1D SDS-PAGE to compare the pattern of released proteins (Fig. 3). The resolution was not as good as the 2D-PAGE. The protein mixture in water was digested with trypsin then processed for LC-MS analysis. We were able to identify some peptides present in the mixture and consequently the proteins attributed to these identified peptides. Table 2 shows the comparison of differentially released proteins in 1 strain and 2 isolates based on their COGs. Proteins detected only in 1 isolates but absent in other 2 isolates or proteins not detected in 1 isolate but present in the other 2 strains were highlighted in lavender for AFSC4, in pink for AFSC7, and in blue for Karp as shown in Table 2. Cytoplasmic, periplasmic, and ribosomal proteins are present in the water- soluble fraction indicating that the osmotic shock released various proteins. Only few proteins were identified under all conditions, and they are all known abundant proteins, such as heat shock chaperonin protein 60 (GroEL), heat shock molecular chaperone protein (grpE), elongation factor EF-Ts (tsf), and EF-Tu (tuf). Both EF-Ts and EF-Tu were differentially expressed as determined by 2D-PAGE (Table 1). The majority of proteins were uniquely detected or not detected in 1 isolate, suggesting that profile of the released proteins due to a simple freeze and thaw in a hypotonic solution (i.e., water) is very different. There were a total of 14 proteins detected only in 1 isolate but not in the other 2 strains. Ten of them were found in AFSC4, 3 in Karp, and 1 in AFSC7. Similarly, among the 9 proteins that were not detected only in the 1 isolate, but were detected in the other 2 isolates, 4 were found in Karp, 3 in AFSC7,

TABLE 1. Identification of Differentially Expressed Proteins of *O. tsutsugamushi* by 2D-PAGE Analysis and LC-MS*

Spot #	Karp	AFSC4	AFSC7	Names of identified proteins
1	0.09	ND[a]	ND	Elongation factor Ts (EF-Ts, OTBS_1139, COG0264J)
2	0.18	0.13	0.21	Microcin C7 self immunity protein (mccF, OTBS_0277, COG1619V)
3	0.06	0.08	0.11	DNA-directed RNA polymerase α-subunit (rpoA, OTBS_0353, COG0202K)
4	0.14	0.29	0.33	Elongation factor Tu (EF-Tu, OTBS_0378, COG0050J)
5	0.21	0.03	0.09	Hypothetical protein (OTBS_0575)
6	1.97	1.37	1.00	Signal transduction histidine kinase, putative (htpK10, OTBS_0618, COG0642T)
7	0.94	0.28	0.38	Hypothetical protein (OTBS_1633)
8	0.59	0.19	ND	ATP synthase F1, β-subunit (atpD, OTBS_0738, COG0055C)
9	0.73	0.46	0.50	56-kDa protein antigen (OTBS_0601)

*Numbers represent the volume of individual spot on an averaged gel was calculated as the sum of the normalized volumes of a spot divided by the number of gels used to generate the average. Spots # 5, 7, and 9 do not have corresponding COG information available in the database.

[a]ND, Not detected.

and 2 in AFSC4. One of the proteins released into this fraction was an ankyrin protein, which is known to play an important role in protein-protein interactions. Since it has been shown that ankyrins are involved in cell survival,[18] it is plausible that the presence of this protein in the AFSC4 and AFSC7 isolates may interact with host protein to increase the survival of *O. tsutsugamushi* in the presence of antibiotics. The difference observed may be the real difference in protein release from freezing and thawing in water. Alternatively, it is possible that the difference may reflect the different amount of these proteins in the periplasmic and cytoplasmic space. Furthermore, the LC-MS/MS data only provided qualitative differences as detected or not detected, it did not rule out the possibility that those unidentified may be due to their lower abundance in 1 isolate. Attempt to further enrich membrane proteins and cytoplasmic proteins by fractionation are in progress. Preliminary studies using Na_2CO_3 to extract membrane proteins from Middleton isolate of *O. tsutsugamushi* found that the 56-kDa protein antigen, known to be a membrane protein, was only identified in this Na_2CO_3 extracted fraction and not in the water fraction. However, non-membrane proteins, such as heat shock chaperonin protein 60 were also present in this fraction, indicating a very inefficient

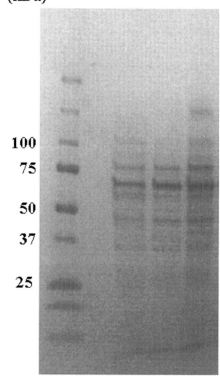

MW (kDa)

Figure 3. SDS-PAGE analysis of proteins released into water. Equal amounts (10 μg) of proteins from each isolate were analyzed using a 4–20% polyacrylamide gradient precast Tris-Glycine gel. Lane 1: AFSC7 isolate, lane 2: AFSC4 isolate and lane 3: Karp strain. The analysis was performed as described in Materials and Methods.

TABLE 2. LC-MS Identification of Proteins Released in Water

OTBS#	Name of identified proteins[a]	COG family #	ASFC4	ASFC7	Karp[b]
	COG: C, energy production and conversion				
0150	Succinyl-CoA synthetase, alpha chain (sucD)	0074C	+	+	+
0434	Thioredoxin (trxA)	0526OC	+	+	+
0151	Succinyl-CoA synthetase beta chain (sucC)	0045C	+	+	+
	COG:E, amino acid transport and metabolism				
1718	Aminopeptidase	0006E	+	+	+
	COG:F, nucleotide transport and metabolism				
0123	Hypothetical protein	0775F	−	−	+
	COG:J, translation				
0211	50S ribosomal protein L1 (rplA)	0081J	+	+	−
0209	50S ribosomal protein L7/L12 (rplL)	0222J	+	+	+
1802	50S ribosomal protein L25 (rplY)	1825J	+	−	−
0202	50S ribosomal protein L28 (rpmB)	0227J	+	−	−
0355	30S ribosomal protein S13 (rpsM)	0099J	+	−	−
0378	Translation elongation factor EF-Tu (tuf)	0050J	+	+	+
1139	Elongation factor EF-Ts (tsf)	0264J	+	+	+
1784	Elongation factor EF-G (fusA)	0480J	+	−	+
2158	Ribosome recycling factor (rrf)	0233J	−	−	+
1366	Glutamyl-tRNA(Gln) amidotransferase subunit C (gatC)	0721J	+	−	−
0947	Translation elongation factor P (ef-p)	0231J	+	−	+
1368	Glutamyl-tRNA(Gln) amidotransferase subunit B (gatB)	0064J	−	−	+
	COG:K, transcription				
1788	Cold shock-like protein (cspA)	1278K	+	+	+
0213	Transcription antitermination protein (nusG)	0250K	+	−	−
	COG:L, replication, recombination, and repair				
0440	Histone-like DNA-binding protein HU (hupA)	0776L	+	+	+
1237	Single-stranded DNA-binding protein (ssb)	0629L	+	+	+
1046	Exodeoxyribonuclease VII small subunit (xseB)	1722L	+	−	−
	COG:O, posttranslational modification, protein turnover, chaperone				
0917	Heat shock chaperonin protein 60 kD (groEL)	0459O	+	+	+
0704	Chaperone protein (dnaK)	0443O	+	+	+
0916	Heat shock chaperonin protein, 10 kD (groES)	0234O	+	+	−
0585	Putative peptidylprolyl isomerase (ppiC)	0760O	+	−	−
0261	Heat shock molecular chaperone protein (grpE)	0576O	+	+	+
1124	Thioredoxin peroxidase 1 (tdpX1)	0450O	+	−	+
0554	FKBP-type peptidyl-prolyl cis-trans isomerase (trigger factor, tig)	0544O	−	+	+
1710	Conserved hypothetical protein	0694O	−	+	+
1837	Periplasmic serine protease (htrA)-47 kDa	0265O	+	+	−
0556	Heat shock protein 90 (htpG)	0326O	−	+	
	COG:R, general function prediction only				
1133	Ankyrin repeat protein with 8 ankyrin repeats (ank1F1, 1A2)	0666R	+	+	−
	COG:S, Function unknown				
0860	Conserved hypothetical protein	3750S	+	+	+
	No COG				
0295	Transposase and inactivated derivative (tnE)	−	+	+	+
0999	Conserved hypothetical protein	−	+	−	−
0790	Hypothetical protein OTBS_0790	−	+	−	−
0782	Hypothetical protein OTBS_0782	−	+	−	−

[a]Names of identified proteins in bold, red, and blue are those identified by multiple peptides, by different single peptide, and by identical single peptide in 3 runs, respectively. Proteins highlighted in yellow are those also identified as differentially expressed by 2D-PAGE.

[b]Plus means identified, and minus means not identified. Highlighted "+" or "−" indicates the protein was uniquely identified or not identified.

fractionation (data not shown). Therefore, improvement is needed to extract membrane proteins in order to better characterize the proteome of *O. tsutsugamushi*, as fractionation is known to improve the number of identified proteins.

Taken together the results from both analyses, there seem to be 9 proteins with decreased expression and 6 proteins with increased expression in both drug-insensitive isolates relative to Karp strain. The 6 proteins that are increased could all be involved in survival of the isolates against antibiotics, even though some of them may be general survival factors, such as heat shock chaperonin protein (groES) and periplasmic serine protease (htrA). The 9 proteins with decreased expression included nucleotide transport and metabolism, ribosomal recycling factor, EF-Ts, and hypothetical proteins, etc. It is possible that the potential mechanisms for antibiotic resistance involve protective mechanisms such as survival and heat shock proteins and alterations in ribosomal and nucleotide mechanisms.

Summary

We have compared the 2D-PAGE of 1 strain and 2 isolates of *O. tsutsugamushi* and found 14 proteins were differentially expressed. Two of these proteins (EF-Ts and EF-Tu) were also identified in the hypotonic water fraction of freeze-thaw cells, suggesting that they are easily released. Attempt to fractionate membrane proteins using Na_2CO_3 was not very specific, but it did result in the extraction of the known outer membrane-associated protein, 56-kDa antigen. The study presented here is the first to investigate differentially expressed proteins in the antibiotic sensitive strain and insensitive isolates and provided the first look of the global protein profiles involved in the difference of drug sensitivity.

Acknowledgments

The authors wish to thank Ms. Kynita Winn for her help in 2D-PAGE analysis and Dr. Paul Graf for his review of the manuscript. This work was supported by Work Unit Number (WUN) 6000.RAD1.J.A0310. The opinions and assertions contained herein are the private ones of the authors and are not to be construed as official or as reflecting the views of the Department of the Navy, the naval service at large, the Department of Defense, the Centers for Disease Control and Prevention, the Department of Health and Human Services, or the U. S. Government. Authors C. C. Chao, G. A. Dasch, and W. M. Ching are employees of the U. S. Government. This work was prepared as part of official duties.

Conflicts of Interest

The authors declare no conflicts of interest.

References

1. Brown, G.W. *et al*. 1977. Scrub typhus: a common cause of illness in indigenous populations. *Trans. R. Soc. Trop. Med. Hyg.* **70:** 444–448.
2. Brown, G.W. *et al*. 1978. Single dose doxycycline therapy for scrub typhus. *Trans. R. Soc. Trop. Med. Hyg.* **72:** 412–416.
3. Yi, K.S. *et al*. 1993. Scrub typhus in Korea: importance of early clinical diagnosis in this newly recognized endemic area. *Mil Med.* **158:** 269–273.
4. Sukoaoihajyk, K. 1997. *Ann. Acad. Med. Singapore* **26:** 794–800.
5. Chopra, I. & M. Roberts. 2001. Tetracycline antibiotics: Mode of action, applications, molecular biology, and epidemiology of bacterial resistance. *Microbiol. Mol. Biol. Rev.* **65:** 232–260.
6. Watt, G. *et al*. 1996. Scrub typhus infections poorly responsive to antibiotics in northern Thailand. *The Lancet* **348:** 86–89.
7. Mathai, E. *et al*. 2003. Outbreak of scrub typhus in southern India during the cooler months. *Ann. N.Y. Acad. Sci.* **990:** 359–364.
8. Walsh, C. 2003. *Antibiotics: Actions, Origins, Resistance.* 335. American Society for Microbiology Press. Washington, DC.
9. Strickman, D. *et al*. 1995. *In vitro* effectiveness of azithromycin against doxycycline-resistant and – susceptible strains of *Rickettsia tsutsugamushi*, etiologic agent of scrub typhus. *Antimicro. Agents Chemother.* **39:** 2406–2410.

10. Cordwell, S.J., A.S. Nouwens & B.J. Walsh. 2001. Comparative proteomics of bacterial pathogens. *Proteomics* **1:** 461–72.

11. Dasch, G.A., D. Strickman, G. Watt & C. Eamsila. 1996. Measuring genetic variability in *Orientia tsutsugamushi* by PCR/RFLP analysis: a new approach to questions about its epidemiology, evolution, and ecology. *Rickettsiae and Rickettsial Diseases. Vth International Symposium.* J. Kazar, Ed.: 79–84. Slovak Academy of Sciences. Bratislava.

12. Chao, C-C. *et al.* 2004. Proteome analysis of Madrid E strain of *Rickettsia prowazekii*. *Proteomics* **4:** 1280–1292.

13. Cho, N.H. *et al.* 2007. The *Orientia tsutsugamushi* genome reveals massive proliferation of conjugative type IV secretion system and host-cell interaction genes. *Proc. Natl. Acad. Sci. USA* **104:** 7981–7986.

14. Hoogvliet, G., G.P. van Wezel & B. Kraal. 1999. Evidence that a single EF-Ts suffices for the recycling of multiple and divergent EF-Tu species in *Streptomyces coelicolor* A3(2) and *Streptomyces ramocissimus*. *Microbiology* **145:** 2293–2301.

15. Sanchez-Pescador, R., J.T. Brown, M. Roberts & M.S. Urdea. 1998. Homology of the TetM with translational elongation factors: implications for potential modes of tetM conferred tetracycline resistance. *Nucleic Acids Res.* **16:** 12–18.

16. Taylor, D.E. & A. Chau. 1996. Tetracycline resistance mediated by ribosomal protection. *Antimicrob. Agents. Chemother.* **40:** 1–5.

17. Muir, M.E., R.S. van Heeswyck & B.J. Wallace. 1984. Effect of growth rate on streptomycin accumulation by *Escherichia coli* and *Bacillus megaterium*. *J. Gen. Microbiol.* **130:** 2015–2022.

18. Miles, M.C. *et al.* 2005. Molecular and functional characterization of a novel splice variant of ANKHD1 that lacks the KH domain and its role in cell survival and apoptosis. *FEBS J.* **272:** 4091–4102.

Mitochondrial Porin VDAC 1 Seems to Be Functional in Rickettsial Cells

Victor V. Emelyanov

Institute of Cell and Molecular Biosciences, Newcastle University, Newcastle upon Tyne, United Kingdom

We have recently shown that *Rickettsia prowazekii* (typhus group rickettsiae) cells incorporate human mitochondrial porin VDAC1. Here, I report on the import of porin by rickettsiae of spotted fever group. It was shown that rickettsial cells of heavy band of Renografin density gradient, known as permeabilized rickettsiae, contain much more VDAC 1 compared to the cells of light band, that is, non-permeabilized rickettsiae. These data hint at a functionality of mitochondrial porin in rickettsial cells. The cells of *Rickettsia canadensis* were broken in French-press, and total membranes were fractionated on linear sucrose density gradient. In this way, previous data were confirmed that an outer rickettsial membrane does not contain porin, while fraction of intermediate density, which likely represents Bayer's adhesion zones, is enriched in VDAC 1. This is consistent with earlier results and their interpretation that imported porin seems to localize to contact sites between inner and outer rickettsial membranes. Based on well-known phylogenetic relationship of Rickettsiales and mitochondria, an evolutionary scenario for the origin of protein import machinery is proposed. A dependence of rickettsiae upon essential protein(s), destined to organelle, is also viewed as a nature of their obligate endosymbiotic lifestyle.

Key words: rickettsiae; mitochondria; common evolutionary origin; protein import; beta-barrel proteins; mitochondrial porin; obligate endosymbiosis

Introduction

Numerous phylogenetic data point to the order Rickettsiales of obligate endosymbiotic α-Proteobacteria as a taxonomic source of mitochondria.[1-11] Given that Rickettsiales is a very broad paraphyletic group of obligate intracellular bacteria,[4,11,12] origin of organelle from within this group could be suspected. It would also be not surprising if some actual resemblance between rickettsiae and mitochondria underlies merely phylogenetic relationship. Earlier on, I suggested that an establishment of the oxygen-respiring organelle has been preceded by a long-term evolutionary relationship between rickettsia-like endosymbiont and primitively amitochondriate host. It is clear that there is a huge abyss separating organelle from bacterium, that is, large amount of time had passed until the latter has been converted into mitochondrion. In view that acquisition of ATP/ADP carrier (AAC) and origin of protein import machinery are two pivotal evolutionary events that transformed bacterium to organelle, I hypothesized that during this long period of time, the last common ancestor of rickettsiae and mitochondria just invented both the AAC to feed host with ATP, derived from extremely efficient aerobic respiration, and a sort of pristine protein import machinery. The latter invention allowed, in particular, a functional gene transfer (*i.e.*, transfer at which encoded protein is returned back to symbiont, followed by a loss of this gene from its own genome) of some endosymbiont genes

Address for correspondence: Victor V. Emelyanov, Institute of Cell and Molecular Biosciences, Newcastle University, Framlington place, Newcastle upon Tyne, NE2 4HH, UK. Voice: (0044) 191-222-3481; fax: (0044) 191-222-7424. Victor.Emelyanov@ncl.ac.uk

Rickettsiology and Rickettsial Diseases-Fifth International Conference: Ann. N.Y. Acad. Sci. 1166: 38–48 (2009).
doi: 10.1111/j.1749-6632.2009.04513.x © 2009 New York Academy of Sciences.

to the host genome. This evolutionary process facilitated bacterial genome shrinkage and rendered a dependence of the endosymbiont upon the host an irreversible event—a prerequisite of endosymbiont taming.[2,4,5,10] As incorporation into outer membrane (OM) would be the simplest protein trafficking, a primitive endosymbiont's system could first be able to mediate this process; perhaps typically to biological events, and as though paradoxically—first the process, next the system. This means that very important process is first established by means of rather simple molecular machine, but once this process started and created new condition—sophisticated and complex machinery comes to an existence via normal evolutionary mechanism. It is indeed impossible that very complex protein import machinery of mitochondria has appeared suddenly, at once; also, it is equally unlikely that multiple components of this system have been acquired one-by-one is a stepwise manner.[10] After divergence of rickettsiae and organelle, the former would have perforce retained a primitive capacity for protein import, inherited from their common evolutionary past with mitochondria. Obviously, imported proteins have to be a subset of those imported by full-fledged organelles. This obligate dependence of rickettsiae on mitochondrial proteins was also viewed as a possible nature of their obligate intracellular symbiosis.[2,4]

Thus, hypothetical proteins imported by rickettsiae would be expected to be outer membrane proteins (*e.g.,* peripheral benzodiazepine receptor[4] or porin). Not to mention that these are beta-barrel proteins, whose import is assisted in mitochondria by Tob55/Sam50[13,14]—the only evolutionarily conserved membrane subunit of extremely complex mitochondrial translocase.[15,16] Recently, we have shown that *Rickettsia prowazekii* cells incorporate human mitochondrial porin VDAC 1.[17] Now, these data were extended to involve various species of rickettsiae and sucrose gradient separation of their membranes. Most important, the data presented show that

mitochondrial porin seems to be functional in rickettsial cells and localize to contact sites between inner membrane (IM) and OM.

Materials and Methods

Growth and Purification of Rickettsiae

Rickettsiae of Spotted Fever Group (SFGR) used in this study were *Rickettsia canadensis* (nonpathogenic species), *R. raoultii,* and *R. conorii* (all from collection of rickettsial cultures at Gamaleya Institute, Moscow). They were grown in cultured L929 mouse cells in DMEM medium, and an efficiency of the cell growth was monitored by light microscopy of small samples differentially stained by Gimenez method. When most of L929 cells became heavily infected, they were scratched from flasks with glass beads, suspended in SPG buffer (10 mM potassium phosphate pH 7.0, 218 mM sucrose, 5 mM glutamate K),[18] and subjected to ultrasound treatment. Unbroken cells and debris were pelleted at $1000 \times g$, and supernatant was centrifuged at $12,000 \times g$ for 20 min. at 4°C in Sorvall SS-34 angle rotor. Pellet (containing rickettsial cells) was resuspended in SPG, magnesium chloride was added to 5 mM, and suspension was kept for 10 min. on ice followed by centrifugation at $300 \times g$ for 10 min. to remove pellet. This procedure was reported to partially eliminate mitochondria.[19]

Supernatant was centrifuged at $12,000 \times g$, and pellet was resuspended in SPG and layered on discontinuous Renografin gradient composed of 2 ml 42%, 3.5 ml 36%, 3 ml 30%, and 2 ml 20% (w/v) Renografin[18] in SPG, and centrifuged in SW40 bucket rotor at 28,000 rpm during 1 h. at 4°C. On this gradient, rickettsiae are known to form two bands—the so-called heavy one (H-band) at 36/42% interphase and light (L) band at 30/36% interphase.[18] Material of H-band is known to contain mitochondria.[19] The cells of H-band were discarded, while those of L-band collected, resuspended in SPG at protein concentration 5 mg per ml, and frozen in liquid nitrogen.

Cell Fractionation Experiments

Most of cell fractionation experiments were carried out with non-pathogenic *R. canadensis.* Two different approaches were used to obtain membrane fractions. 0.8 ml of cell suspension after thawing were subjected to the so-called controlled osmotic shock followed by cold osmotic shock, as described in previous paper.[17] Rickettsial cells were pelleted and suspended in 0.4 ml of hyperosmotic buffer (3× TES, TES is 10 mM tris-HCl pH 7.8, 0.25 M sucrose and 1 mM EDTA), and upon addition of chicken lysozyme at 0.2 mg/ml, the suspension was either slowly or suddenly diluted with 2 volumes of cold water (controlled osmotic shock). This procedure is known to remove the pieces of OM from the cells, generating sphaeroplasts.[20] After pelleting the unbroken cells and sphaeroplasts, supernatant was ultracentrifuged to sediment OM fragments. Collected sphaeroplasts were resuspended in a small volume of TES and broken by rapid dilution with 20 volumes of cold water (cold osmotic shock).[21] Supernatant after removal of intact cells and unbroken sphaeroplasts represents a fraction of total membranes (TM), a mixture of IM and OM. TM were concentrated by ultracentrifugation to apply for detergent treatments and electrophoresis.

Otherwise, the cells of 2 ml suspension were broken in a French pressure cell at 10,000 Ib/cm^2, and procedure was repeated once more. Unbroken cells were removed by centrifugation at $12,000 \times g$ 15 min. at 4°C, and supernatant containing TM was centrifuged in a Type 70.1 Ti angle rotor of L8-60M Beckman Ultracentrifuge at $150,000 \times g$ 1 h. at 4°C. Pellet was resuspended in HE buffer (20 mM HEPES-KOH pH 7.4 and 2 mM EDTA) and recentrifuged as above. Final pellet was resuspended in 0.2 ml HE and layered on 4.5 ml of 20–52% continuous sucrose density gradient (w/v sucrose in HE) in SW65 polyallomer tube. Material was ultracentrifuged at 39,000 rpm ($145,000 \times g$) for 46 h. at 4°C. The tube was punctured by tube piercer, and fractions (∼0.1 ml each) were collected from the bottom. Each second fraction was analyzed by the Laemmli electrophoresis followed by either silver staining or Western blot analysis.

Protein concentration of whole cells and membrane fractions was measured by the Lowry method[22] in the presence of 2% SDS in samples.

SDS-electrophoresis and Immunoblotting

Electrophoresis in sodium dodecyl sulphate-polyacrylamide gels (SDS-PAG) was carried out according to Laemmli method.[23] Proteins were stained in gels by silver nitrate method, as described by Oakley and colleagues[24] Blotting onto PVDF membrane was carried out using semi-dry transfer apparatus. Standard TBS + 0.3% Tween-20 was used at each stage of membrane processing. Monoclonal antibodies (Mab) against human mitochondrial porin VDAC 1 and cytochrome *c* were the same as in previous work.[17] Immunoreactivity was detected using ECL system.

Treatments of R. Canadensis Whole Cells and Isolated TM

Whole cells and TM at protein concentration 5 and 2 mg per ml, respectively, were treated by non-ionic detergents, 0.3 M NaCl or proteinase K, followed by SDS-PAGE and Western blot analysis of insoluble material as described earlier.[17]

Results

Rickettsial Cells of Heavy Renografin Band Contain More Mitochondrial Porin Compared to Light Band

It is known that freshly harvested rickettsiae form mostly light band during purification

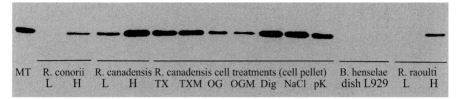

Figure 1. Western blot analysis of bacterial cells and mitochondria with anti-human VDAC 1 monoclonal antibody. MT, isolated mouse mitochondria; L and H, rickettsiae of light and heavy bands of Renografin gradient (H-band after second, and L-band after third gradient); TX, Triton X-100; TXM, TX + 5 mM MgCl$_2$; OG, octylglucoside; OGM, OG + 5 mM MgCl$_2$; Dig, digitonin; pK, proteinase K; *Bartonella henselae* cells grown on agar (dish) and in cultured mouse cells (L929).

on Renografin density gradient, which corresponds to a density 1.2 g/ml.[18] They can, however, split into L- and H-band (1.23 g/ml) depending on the diluent used and a treatment of rickettsial suspension. Ratio H-cells/L-cells can increase (*e.g.*, when using hypo-osmotic buffers). This ratio was also shown to depend upon a growth phase—stationary cells display shift to H-band. Hanson and colleagues have shown that material of H-band is represented by permeabilized cells that incorporated Renografin. By contrast, those of L-band keep permeability barrier, yet being potentially permeabilizable.[18]

It may be concluded from the data of Hanson et al. that rickettsial population is heterogeneous in a sense that a subpopulation can be easily permeabilized, while another subpopulation still remains to be relatively resistant to permeabilization. On discontinuous Renografin gradient, the cells thus display "quantum" behavior: those which included large amount of Renografin migrate at higher density zone, while the cells maintaining permeability barrier or incorporating low amount of Renografin migrate at lower density zone. In some experiments, the cells of L-band after first gradient were collected and submitted to "mild" shock, such as storage overnight at 4°C, quick dilution with SPG, or freezing-thawing. The suspension, diluted after shock 10 times with SPG, was centrifuged at 14,000 × *g* 20 min., and pelleted cells were again subjected to Renografin gradient centrifugation as above. The cells of both bands were then collected, and those of L-band

undergone once more to mild shock followed by gradient purification. Again, both bands were collected separately, the cells washed with SPG as above, and analyzed by electrophoresis and Western blotting. The results of Western blot analysis of rickettsial cells of H- and L-bands are shown in Figure 1. In is seen that after three consecutive Renografin gradients of L-cells, subjected to mild shock between centrifugations, they contain very little amount of porin.

Mitochondrial porin is not susceptible to proteinase K in the rickettsial cells (the cells of L-band after first gradient). Porin is weakly removed from the cells by 0.3 M NaCl and 1% (w/v) non-ionic detergents Triton X-100, octylglucoside or digitonin (Fig. 1).

The cells of *Bartonella henselae*, an α-Proteobacterium cultivable on axenic media, do not incorporate VDAC 1 when grown in L929 cells (Fig. 1). Figure 2 shows loading control (silver nitrate-stained PAG) of mitochondria and bacterial cells. As shown by Western blot analysis with Mab against mitochondrial cytochrome *c*, Renografin-purified rickettsiae of neither L nor H band are contaminated by mitochondria (Fig. 3).

Localization of Porin VDAC 1 in *R. canadensis* Cells

Cell fractionation experiments were performed essentially as described for gram-negative bacteria such as *Escherichia coli* and

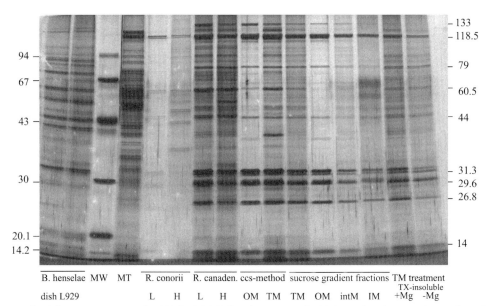

B. henselae MW MT   R. conorii   R. canaden. ccs-method sucrose gradient fractions TM treatment
                                                                                          TX-insoluble
dish L929   L   H   L   H   OM TM   TM   OM intM IM   +Mg -Mg

Figure 2. Silver nitrate-stained 10% SDS-PAG (loading control). MW, molecular weight markers (molecular masses in kDa are on the left margin); ccs-method, controlled osmotic shock/cold osmotic shock-method; intM, membrane fraction of intermediate density; TX-insoluble, material of TM insoluble in 0.5% Triton X-100 in the presence (+Mg) or absence (−Mg) of 5 mM $MgCl_2$. Molecular masses of *R. canadensis* OMPs in kDa are on the right margin.

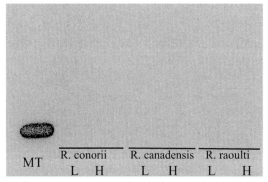

Figure 3. Western blot analysis of mitochondria and bacteria with Mab against mitochondrial cytochrome c.

Salmonella typhimurium.[20,21,25] Incorporation of human porin VDAC 1 in rickettsial membranes was first shown for relatively well-characterized *R. prowazekii,*[17] which belongs to typhus group rickettsiae (TGR). In that case, a combination of controlled osmotic shock and cold osmotic shock was used to fractionate the cells. First method is known to produce OM fraction, whereas the second one produces TM

(see above). Polypeptide composition of OM fraction proved to be essentially the same as described by other researchers using different methods, such as extrinsic iodination[26,27] and fractionation of total *R. prowazekii* membranes on sucrose density gradients.[28] The above crude OM fraction was shown to contain integral OM proteins (OMPs), but not mitochondrial porin, while fraction of TM contained a variety of minor proteins, OMPs and VDAC 1.[17] As porin is OMP in bacteria and organelles, it was suggested to localize to Bayer's adhesion zones, contact sites between IM and OM,[29] which may be retained in sphaeroplasts after controlled osmotic shock.

In the present work, method of consecutive osmotic shocks was applied to *R. canadensis* cells. Like for *R. prowazekii,* mitochondrial porin was shown to be present in total membranes, but not in OM fraction (Fig. 4). *R. canadensis* cells were also broken in French-press, and pelleted membranes were subjected to centrifugation in a linear sucrose density gradient. Proteins of various fractions were separated on 10%

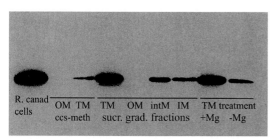

Figure 4. Western blot analysis of membrane fractions of *R. canadensis* with Mab against mitochondrial porin. For abbreviations see legend to Figure 2.

SDS-PAG followed by silver staining and Western blot analysis with anti-porin Mab. The fractions of heavy (no. 8 to 12), intermediate (16–19), and low (26–38) density were combined and electrophoresed as above with subsequent silver staining (Fig. 2) and immunoblotting for VDAC 1 (Fig. 4). Evidently, heavy gradient fraction is similar by polypeptide composition to OM fraction isolated during controlled osmotic shock (Fig. 2) and also lacks mitochondrial porin. In contrast, both the intermediate and light fractions contain porin (Fig. 4).

It may be concluded that OM of *R. canadensis*, poorly characterized species of SFGR, contains major polypeptides with molecular mass of 118.5, 31.3, 29.6, 26.8, and 14 kDa, and minor polypeptides of 133, 79, 60.5, and 44 kDa (Fig. 2). This polypeptide pattern appeared to be very similar to that of *R. prowazekii*.[17] In this regard, *R. canadensis* was earlier classified with TGR based on antigenic specificity.[12]

Like integral OMPs of gram-negative bacteria,[30] VDAC 1 is not solubilized upon treatment of total rickettsial membranes by Triton X-100 in the presence of magnesium ions and partially solubilized in the absence of Mg^{2+} (Fig. 4).

Discussion

Porins are essential proteins in gram-negative bacteria and organelles, which form channels in OM for transport of solutes. Pore size of bacterial porins typically allows penetration of molecules with molecular mass up to 600 Da.[31] Mitochondrial porins, voltage-dependent anion channels, are voltage-regulated gates—lowering trans-membrane potential induces slightly anion selective open state.[32] While bacterial porins are trimers, and each molecule forms channel,[31] mitochondrial porins function as monomers.[32,33] Mitochondria of different eukaryotes normally possess a variety of conserved porins, apparently originated via paralogous duplications, among which VDAC 1 is the major pore-forming protein.[34,35] There is, however, little porin homology across eukaryotic domain and no homology between mitochondrial porins and those of Proteobacteria, including α subdivision—a taxonomic source of mitochondria. Among salient features of bacterial and mitochondrial porins are similar molecular masses ∼33 kDa, abundance in bacteria and organelles, and extensive β-barrel structure.[31–33]

As typical gram-negative bacteria, rickettsiae are expected to possess porin(s). Complete genomes of several species of the genus *Rickettsia* are publicly available; however, it is impossible to predict robustly, using bioinformatics approach, which genome-encoded protein may be porin in view of its non-conserved nature. With respect to molecular mass and abundance, two major integral *R. prowazekii* OMPs of 31 kDa and 30 (in Breinl strain) kDa could be considered as candidates for porin. As to 30 kDa OMP, it was shown to be peptidyl-prolyl *cis/trans* isomerase (PPIase) forming mostly α-helices.[36] Major 31 kDa OMP of SFGR *R. rickettsii* was shown to be a carboxyl-terminal cleavage product of a large protein antigen precursor,[37] the β-barrel protein in *R. prowazekii*.[38] Because of high homology between these precursors,[37] it may be true for 31 kDa OMP of *R. prowazekii* as well. However, *in vitro* transport experiments in artificial liposomes are needed to conclude, whether or not this or any other OMP functions as porin.

On the other hand, both *R. prowazekii* (TGR) and SFGR were shown here and elsewhere[17] to incorporate mitochondrial porin VDAC 1.

Most important, permeabilized cells contain much more porin than intact cells (Fig. 1). It is thus suggested that imported mitochondrial porin is active in rickettsial cells and, in particular, induces permeability. As in the case of mitochondria,[15] VDAC 1 is insensitive in rickettsiae to externally added proteinase K (Fig. 1).

It should be pointed out that rickettsial membrane fractions were defined operationally, but not analytically in the present work. Indeed, treatment of gram-negative bacteria by lysozyme in isotonic buffer leads to removal of OM fragments.[20] Also, OM display higher density in sucrose gradients than IM.[25] In this regard, polypeptide composition of OM fractions obtained by two different methods is essentially the same (Fig. 2). In 1979, Smith and Winkler published data on separation of IM and OM of *R. prowazekii* by means of sucrose density gradients.[28] Using markers for both membranes, they have shown that the fraction of higher density contains pure OM, while one of lower density is represented by both IM and OM. They also observed a peak of intermediate density. By polypeptide composition, light fraction contained a variety of minor proteins and also integral OMPs. Smith and Winkler concluded that fraction of low density may contain contact sites between IM and OM.[28] Similar data were obtained during fractionation of *R. canadensis* cells (Fig. 2). My inference is that the fraction of intermediate density is enriched in Bayer's adhesion zones, whereas rather broad peak of low density consists of a mixture of OM, IM, and contact sites in a varying ratio. Maybe due to relative fluidity of rickettsial membranes,[39] this large fraction contains membranes of different origin stuck together. Obviously, OM fraction is apparently free of mitochondrial porin irrespective of isolation method used, while intermediate fraction is enriched in VDAC 1. These data hint at localization of porin not in OM, but in contact sites between IM and OM.[17]

Mitochondrial porin is known to localize not only in mitochondria, but also in other cell membranes.[34,40] While Renografin-purified rickettsiae do not contain mitochondria (Fig. 3), the question arises of whether they can be contaminated by cell membranes containing porin. It may be logically argued that it is not the case. Generally, two different possibilities should be considered. First, host membranes could stick to rickettsial cells. It would be, however, difficult to explain in this case, why during controlled osmotic shock only those patches of OM are removed from cell surface, which do not contain adhered cell membranes. Second, membrane vesicles of cellular origin could physically contaminate bacterial cells or membrane fractions. Were these vesicles small and non-sedimentable at low speed centrifugation, they would have been present in OM fraction obtained after controlled osmotic shock followed by low speed centrifugation; however, this fraction does not contain porin. On the other hand, were porin-containing host vesicles large, they would be co-sedimented with unbroken rickettsial cells and sphaeroplasts after cold osmotic shock and thus would not appear in supernatant (TM); however, this fraction does contain porin. Taken together, these data suggest that mitochondrial porin is indeed imported by rickettsiae from cytoplasm of host cell.

Phylogenetic analyses of small subunit[4,10] and large subunit[11] rRNAs, encoded by mitochondrial genomes, (these being thus true tracers for the origin of organelle per se) and chaperonin Cpn60,[2,4,10] encoded by nuclear genome, show that common ancestor of rickettsiae (families Rickettsiaceae and Anaplasmataceae) and mitochondria belonged to the group of rickettsia-like endosymbionts (family Holosporaceae), along with rickettsiae classified with the order Rickettsiales of obligate endosymbiotic α-Proteobacteria.[4] Based on these data, I earlier hypothesized that mitochondrial origin has been preceded by a long-term relationship of rickettsia-like bacterium with primitively amitochodriate host. During this relationship, endosymbiotic bacterium invented AAC and some primitive protein import system.[2,4] Phylogenetic analysis of AAC at both protein and gene level is consistent with this view, showing that bacterial-type AAC, which is also present in plastids and chlamydiae, may have first appeared in the family Holosporaceae.[41] During evolutionary conversion of endosymbiont to organelle, a gene encoding this IM protein with 12 trans-membrane domains could not be functionally transferred to the host genome, because of incompatibility of encoded hydrophobic protein with import. Thus, mitochondrial-type AAC has evolved as a member of mitochondrial carrier family (MCF) proteins with 6 trans-membrane domains in each of two identical importable subunits.[42] This hypothesis is at odds with a widespread opinion that mitochondrial ancestor has been a free-living α-Proteobacterium, which might neither produce ATP in excess nor consume ATP from milieu, hence, could not possess AAC.[3,43,44] Alternative view entertained here holds that mitochondrial progenitor and host did not evolve separately. Instead, they experienced co-evolution (*i.e.*, a consortium actually evolved). Long-term endosymbiotic relationship was mutualistic from the start—efficiently oxygen-respiring rickettsia-like bacterium delivered ATP to host in an exchange for reduced precursors of oxidative phosphorylation. In the course of long-term relationship, endosymbiotic bacterium has also acquired a primitive ability to import proteins from cytosol followed by a transfer of the genes, encoding these proteins, to the host genome. Functional transfer of essential endosymbiont genes has made an obligate dependence of endosymbiont upon host irreversible. A number of functionally transferred genes could be limited to those encoding OMPs, like porin and peripheral benzodiazepine receptor, whose import could involve a minimum number of participants.[4,17]

Recently, a new translocase of mitochondrial OM, called TOB (topogenesis of mitochondrial outer membrane beta-barrel proteins)[13] or SAM (sorting and assembly machinery),[14] was discovered, which mediates incorporation of beta-barrel proteins, such as porin and Tom40, into OM. Beta-barrel proteins first penetrate inter-membrane space through general import pore (Tom40) and bind to small TIM (translocase of IM) chaperones, which deliver them to TOB/SAM complex.[13,14,45] Final part of this process is thus reminiscent of export of OMPs in gram-negative bacteria, being obviously a relict of mitochondrial evolutionary past. In bacteria, incorporation of OMPs into OM is assisted by periplasmic chaperones SurA and Skp, which were shown to be functional analogs of small TIM proteins, but not homologs.[45] Among numerous membrane-associated subunits of mitochondrial translocases, only Sam50/Tob55—an essential protein in *Saccharomyces* and a key component of SAM/TOB system, was shown to be conserved protein partially homologous to bacterial Omp85.[13–16] These data suggest that rickettsiae may possess some primitive protein import mechanism for incorporation of beta-barrel proteins, such as porin, inherited from their last common ancestor with organelle. Contact sites between IM and OM of endosymbiotic bacterium are thought to be an evolutionary antecedent of those of mitochondria; notably, that porin localizes to these sites in mitochondria[35] and probably in rickettsiae. In organelle, they are suggested to be part of the so-called megachannel, or permeability transition pore (PTP). Along with porin and peripheral benzodiazepine receptor on outer side, megachannels also contain AAC and cyclophilin on inner side.[35,46] In this regard, rickettsiae also possess AAC, although of non-mitochondrial type (see above), and PPIase. The latter was shown to be major OMP in *R. prowazekii*, and differs from cyclophilin, belonging to different PPIase class.[36] Thus, evolutionary transformation of endosymbiont Bayer's adhesion zones into mitochondrial megachannels, actually a membrane heredity, might involve a replacement of rickettsial-type AAC and PPIase by non-related proteins of host origin. Among universally conserved components of mitochondrial protein import machinery are chaperones Cpn60 (GroEL) and Hsp70 (DnaK), phylogenetic analysis of which shows the closest relationship between Rickettsiales and mitochondria.[4,5,10] Curiously, aminopeptidase of *R. prowazekii* was recently described, substrate specificity of which overlaps with that of mitochondrial processing peptidase.[47] Thus, an appearance of sophisticated protein import machinery of mitochondria might be favored by such bacterial factors as chaperones, Omp85, and processing peptidase.

From an evolutionary perspective, it may be clear that rickettsiae can import a subset of proteins, imported by mitochondria, as a legacy of their common origin. Alternative view holds that import of mitochondrial porin by bacteria has no profound evolutionary connection. Specifically, regardless of whether mitochondrial porin is of endosymbiont or host origin, rickettsiae possessed porin once in their own evolutionary history. In this case, rickettsiae could have lost porin once they learned how to import it from host cytosol. This is, however, a less probable scenario for obvious reason. A trend of endosymbiotic bacteria to dispense with numerous metabolic capacities is apparent, given that these redundant pathways may be readily taken over by host. A loss of glycolysis and amino acid and nucleotide biosynthesis in rickettsiae[1,48] indeed represents drastic genome and metabolic reduction, so that loss of porin and maybe yet a few proteins would contribute a little to this reductive process. Not to mention that the latter would require specific import mechanism. Thus, evolutionary scenario seems more realistic. Very simple protein import machinery could originate in a group of rickettsia-like endosymbionts, based on pre-existing capacity provided by the above-mentioned factors, some of which could be initially involved in a protein export process. An ability of the last common ancestor of rickettsiae and mitochondria to import a few essential proteins (whose genes have been functionally transferred to the host genome) irreversibly forged endosymbiont and host. Further improvement of protein import machinery via normal evolutionary process has occurred during conversion of obligate intracellular bacterium into organelle. It will be interesting in this respect to know, whether bacteria of the family Holosporaceae, putative taxonomic source of both Rickettsiaceae and mitochondria, are able to import mitochondrial proteins (*e.g.*, porin). If so, it would lend additional support to the above-described scenario for the origin of protein import system.

Earlier on, I considered an obligate dependence of rickettsiae upon a subset of essential proteins, targeted to mitochondria, as a molecular basis of their obligate endosymbiotic lifestyle. According to this hypothesis, rickettsiae cannot grow in axenic media because their growth unavoidably depends on some essential proteins, which are synthesized by eukaryotic cell to serve in mitochondria.[4,5,10,11] Targeting of proteins to mitochondria is a complex process, involving cytosolic factors,[49] and this would seem to be true for rickettsiae too. Accordingly, rickettsial phospholipase activity manifests only during intimate contact with host cell,[50] thus allowing penetration of bacteria into living eukaryotic cell, capable to target proteins to mitochondria and, eventually, to bacteria.

Acknowledgments

I thank Oleg Mediannikov (Gamaleya Institute of Epidemiology and Microbiology, Moscow) and Mikhail Vyssokikh (Moscow State University) for propagation of bacteria and isolating mouse mitochondria, respectively. Thanks are also due to Irina Tarasevich, head of laboratory of rickettsial ecology (Gamaleya Institute), in which this work was accomplished.

Conflicts of Interest

The author declares no conflicts of interest.

References

1. Andersson, S.G. *et al.* 1998. The genome sequence of *Rickettsia prowazekii* and the origin of mitochondria. *Nature* **396:** 133–140.

2. Emelyanov, V.V. & B.V. Sinitsyn. 1999. A *groE*-based phylogenetic analysis shows the closest evolutionary relationship of mitochondria to obligate intracytoplasmic bacterium *Rickettsia prowazekii*. In *Rickettsiae and Rickettsial Diseases at the Turn of the Third Millennium.* D. Raoult & P. Brouqui, Eds.: 31–37. Elsevier. Paris.

3. Kurland, C.G. & S.G. Andersson. 2000. Origin and evolution of the mitochondrial proteome. *Microbiol. Mol. Biol. Rev.* **64:** 786–820.

4. Emelyanov, V.V. 2001. Evolutionary relationship of Rickettsiae and mitochondria. *FEBS Lett.* **501:** 11–18.

5. Emelyanov, V.V. 2003. Mitochondrial connection to the origin of the eukaryotic cell. *Eur. J. Biochem.* **270:** 1599–1618.

6. Emelyanov, V.V. 2003. Phylogenetic affinity of a *Giardia lamblia* cysteine desulfurase conforms to canonical pattern of mitochondrial ancestry. *FEMS Microbiol. Lett.* **226:** 257–266.

7. Emelyanov, V.V. 2003. Common evolutionary origin of mitochondrial and rickettsial respiratory chains. *Arch. Biochem. Biophys.* **420:** 130–141.

8. Wu, M. *et al.* 2004. Phylogenomics of the reproductive parasite Wolbachia pipientis wMel: a streamlined genome overrun by mobile genetic elements. *PLoS Biol.* **2:** E69.

9. Fitzpatrick, D.A., C.J. Creevey & J.O. McInerney. 2006. Genome phylogenies indicate a meaningful alpha-proteobacterial phylogeny and support a grouping of the mitochondria with the Rickettsiales. *Mol. Biol. Evol.* **23:** 74–85.

10. Emelyanov, V.V. 2007. Constantin Merezhkowsky and the Endokaryotic Hypothesis. In *Origin of Mitochondria and Hydrogenosomes.* W.F. Martin & M. Müller, Eds.: 201–237. Springer-Verlag. Berlin, Heidelberg.

11. Emelyanov, V.V. 2007. Holosporaceae, Rickettsiales, and mitochondrial origin: rickettsiae import mitochondrial porin. *Protistology* **5:** 26–27.

12. Drancourt, M. & D. Raoult. 1994. Taxonomic position of the rickettsiae: Current knowledge. *FEMS Microbiol. Rev.* **13:** 13–24.

13. Paschen, S.A. *et al.* 2003. Evolutionary conservation of biogenesis of beta-barrel membrane proteins. *Nature* **426:** 862–826.

14. Kozjak, V. *et al.* 2003. An essential role of Sam50 in the protein sorting and assembly machinery of the mitochondrial outer membrane. *J. Biol. Chem.* **278:** 48520–48523.

15. Gentle, I. *et al.* 2004. The Omp85 family of proteins is essential for outer membrane biogenesis in mitochondria and bacteria. *J. Cell Biol.* **164:** 19–24.

16. Gentle, I.E., L. Burri & T. Lithgow. 2005. Molecular architecture and function of the Omp85 family of proteins. *Mol. Microbiol.* **58:** 1216–1225.

17. Emelyanov, V.V. & M.Y. Vyssokikh. 2006. On the nature of obligate intracellular symbiosis of rickettsiae—*Rickettsia prowazekii* cells import mitochondrial porin. *Biochemistry (Moscow)* **71:** 730–735.

18. Hanson, B.A. *et al.* 1981. Some characteristics of heavy and light bands of *Rickettsia prowazekii* on Renografin gradients. *Infect. Immun.* **34:** 596–604.

19. Aniskovich, L.P. *et al.* 1989. Methods for purification of *Rickettsia prowazekii* separated from the host tissue: a step-by-step comparison. *Acta Virol.* **33:** 361–370.

20. Mizushima, S. & H. Yamada. 1975. Isolation and characterization of two outer membrane preparations from *Escherichia coli*. *Biochim. Biophys. Acta* **375:** 44–53.

21. Osborn, M.J. *et al.* 1972. Mechinism of assembly of the outer membrane of *Salmonella typhimurium*. Isolation and characterization of cytoplasmic and outer membrane. *J. Biol. Chem.* **247:** 3962–3972.

22. Lowry, O.H. *et al.* 1951. Protein measurement with the Folin-Phenol reagents. *J. Biol. Chem.* **193:** 265–275.

23. Laemmli, U. K. 1970. Cleavage of structural proteins during the assembly of the head of bacteriophage T4. *Nature* **227:** 680–685.

24. Oakley, B.R., D.R. Kirsch & N.R. Morris. 1980. A simplified ultrasensitive silver stain for detecting proteins in polyacrylamide gels. *Anal. Biochem.* **105:** 361–363.

25. Schnaitman, C.A. 1970. Protein composition of the cell wall and cytoplasmic membrane of *Escherichia coli*. *J. Bacteriol.* **104:** 890–901.

26. Osterman, J.V. & C.S. Eisemann. 1978. Surface proteins of typhus and spotted fever group rickettsiae. *Infect. Immun.* **21:** 866–873.

27. Smith, D.K. & H.H. Winkler. 1980. Radioiodination of an outer membrane protein in intact *Rickettsia prowazekii*. *Infect. Immun.* **29:** 831–834.

28. Smith, D.K. & H.H. Winkler. 1979. Separation of inner and outer membranes of *Rickettsia prowazeki* and characterization of their polypeptide compositions. *J. Bacteriol.* **137:** 963–971.

29. Bayer, M. E. 1974. Ultrastructure and organization of the bacterial envelope. *Ann. N. Y. Acad. Sci.* **235:** 6–28.

30. Schnaitman, C.A. 1971. Solubilization of the cytoplasmic membrane of *Escherichia coli* by Triton X-100. *J. Bacteriol.* **108:** 545–552.

31. Nikaido, H. 2003. Molecular basis of bacterial outer membrane permeability revisited. *Microbiol. Mol. Biol. Rev.* **67:** 593–651.

32. Benz, R. 1994. Permeation of hydrophilic solutes through mitochondrial outer membranes: review on mitochondrial porins. *Biochim. Biophys. Acta* **1197:** 167–196.

33. Mannella, C.A. 1996. Mitochondrial channels revisited. *J. Bioenerg. Biomembr.* **28:** 89–91.

34. Baker, M.A. *et al.* 2004. VDAC1 is a transplasma membrane NADH-ferricyanide reductase. *J. Biol. Chem.* **279:** 4811–4819.

35. Vyssokikh, M.Y. & D. Brdiczka. 2003. The function of complexes between the outer mitochondrial membrane pore (VDAC) and the adenine nucleotide translocase in regulation of energy metabolism and apoptosis. *Acta Biochim. Pol.* **50:** 389–404.

36. Emelyanov, V.V. & E.V. Loukianov. 2004. A 29.5 kDa heat-modifiable major outer membrane protein of *Rickettsia prowazekii*, putative virulence factor, is a peptidyl-prolyl *cis/trans* isomerase. *IUBMB Life* **56:** 215–219.

37. Hackstadt, T. *et al.* 1992. Evidence for proteolytic cleavage of the 120-kilodalton outer membrane protein of rickettsiae: identification of an avirulent mutant deficient in processing. *Infect. Immun.* **60:** 159–165.

38. Carl, M. *et al.* 1990. Characterization of the gene encoding the protective paracrystalline-surface-layer protein of *Rickettsia prowazekii*: presence of a truncated identical homolog in *Rickettsia typhi*. *Proc. Natl. Acad. Sci. USA* **87:** 8237–8241.

39. Winkler, H.H. & E.T. Miller. 1978. Phospholipid composition of *Rickettsia prowazeki* grown in chicken embryo yolk sacs. *J. Bacteriol.* **136:** 175–178.

40. Lawen, A. *et al.* 2005. Voltage-dependent anion-selective channel 1 (VDAC1)—a mitochondrial protein, rediscovered as a novel enzyme in the plasma membrane. *Int. J. Biochem. Cell Biol.* **37:** 277–282.

41. Emelyanov, V.V. 2007. Suggested mitochondrial ancestry of non-mitochondrial ATP/ADP carrier. *Mol. Biol. (Moscow)* **41:** 59–70.

42. Saraste, M. & J. E. Walker. 1982. Internal sequence repeats and the path of polypeptide in mitochondrial ADP/ATP translocase. *FEBS Lett.* **144:** 250–254.

43. Martin, W. & M. Müller. 1998. The hydrogen hypothesis for the first eukaryote. *Nature* **392:** 37–41.

44. Moreira, D. & P. Lopez-Garcia. 1998. Symbiosis between methanogenic archaea and delta-proteobacteria as the origin of eukaryotes: the syntrophic hypothesis. *J. Mol. Evol.* **47:** 517–530.

45. Alcock, F.H. *et al.* 2008. Conserved substrate binding by chaperones in the bacterial periplasm and the mitochondrial intermembrane space. *Biochem. J.* **409:** 377–387.

46. Juhaszova, M. *et al.* 2008. The identity and regulation of the mitochondrial permeability transition pore: where the known meets the unknown. *Ann. N. Y. Acad. Sci.* **1123:** 197–212.

47. Kitada, S. *et al.* 2007. A protein from a parasitic microorganism, *Rickettsia prowazekii*, can cleave the signal sequences of proteins targeting mitochondria. *J. Bacteriol.* **189:** 844–850.

48. Ogata, H. *et al.* 2001. Mechanisms of evolution in *Rickettsia conorii* and *R. prowazekii*. *Science* **293:** 2093–2098.

49. Hachiya, N. *et al.* 1995. Reconstitution of the initial steps of mitochondrial protein import. *Nature* **376:** 705–709.

50. Winkler, H.H. 1990. Rickettsia species (as organisms). *Annu. Rev. Microbiol.* **44:** 131–153.

Deciphering the Relationships between *Rickettsia conorii conorii* and *Rhipicephalus sanguineus* in the Ecology and Epidemiology of Mediterranean Spotted Fever

Philippe Parola, Cristina Socolovschi, and Didier Raoult

Unité de Recherche en Maladies Infectieuses et Tropicales Emergentes (URMITE), UMR CNRS-IRD 6236, WHO Collaborative Center for Rickettsial Diseases and Other Arthropod-Borne Bacterial Diseases, Marseilles, France

Mediterranean spotted fever is the most important tick-borne disease occurring in Southern Europe and North Africa. The first case of this life-threatening zoonosis was reported in 1910. In the 1930s, the role of the brown dog tick, *Rhipicephalus sanguineus*, and the causative agent, *Rickettsia conorii* were described. However, basic questions regarding the relationships between the rickettsia and its tick vector are still unresolved, and the life cycle of *R. conorii* is incompletely known. There is a lack of knowledge associated with the role of *Rh. sanguineus* in the maintenance and transmission of *R. conorii*. The infectious rate of *Rh. sanguineus* ticks with *R. conorii* has been found low every time it has been tested; usually lower that 1%. The deleterious impact of *R. conorii* on ticks has been suggested in experimental models as a potential reason to explain a low prevalence in nature. The long-recognized phenomenon known as reactivation has been suggested as a cause of negative effects – that is, the change in temperature and physiology of the tick host induces the agent to emerge from dormancy and attain infectivity with bad effects on ticks. However, naturally infected colonies of ticks have been maintained in laboratory conditions over several generations. We discuss here several aspects that have been recently studied to better understand *Rh. sanguineus*–*R. conorii* relationships, including comparison between the fitness of infected and non-infected ticks in laboratory conditions and the role of external factors such as temperature and starvation.

Key words: *Rhipicephalus sanguineus*; *Rickettsia conorii*; ticks – rickettsia

Spotted fever group (SFG) rickettsiae are obligatory intracellular gram-negative bacteria belonging to the genus *Rickettsia* within the order *Rickettsiales*, and are associated with arthropod vectors, mainly ticks.[1] These bacteria include human pathogens recognized since the beginning of the twentieth century, as well as many emerging pathogens with more than a dozen of new species or subspecies identified as emerging agents between 1984 and 2006.[2,3] Furthermore, many SFG rickettsiae have been isolated and detected only from ticks, and their pathogenicity in humans is still unknown.[4]

A Long-time Recognized but Poorly Understood Tick-rickettsia Association

Mediterranean spotted fever (MSF) is one of the oldest recognized vector-borne infectious diseases. The first cases were first described in Tunisia in 1909. As characteristic skin eruptions were popular rather than

Address for correspondence: Dr. Philippe Parola. Unité de Recherche en Maladies Infectieuses et Tropicales Emergentes (URMITE), UMR CNRS-IRD 6236, WHO Collaborative Center for Rickettsial Diseases and Other Arthropod-Borne Bacterial Diseases, Faculté de Médecine, 27 Bd Jean Moulin, 13385 Marseille Cedex 5, France. Voice: +33-04-91-32-43-75; fax: +33-04-91-38-77-72. philippe.parola@univmed.fr

Rickettsiology and Rickettsial Diseases-Fifth International Conference: Ann. N.Y. Acad. Sci. 1166: 49–54 (2009).
doi: 10.1111/j.1749-6632.2009.04518.x © 2009 New York Academy of Sciences.

macular, the disease was referred to as "bou-tonneuse" fever. The eschar at the site of the tick bite, the hallmark of rickettsial diseases, was described in Marseille in 1925 by Boinet and Pieri. Several years after the description of the first case by Conor, the researchers tried to identify the vector of disease. Olmer (1928) thought that the vector of disease was the brown dog tick, *Rhipicephalus sanguineus*. This hypothesis was supported by P. Durand and E. Conseil, when they inoculated humans with the crushed infected *Rh. sanguineus* ticks, and the patients contracted MSF. Brumpt described the infectious agent in tick samples and gave the name *Rickettsia conorii*, in honor of the work of Conor.[5,6] Recently, the nomenclature of the several strains recognized as belonging to the so-called *R. conorii* complex has been modified, and several species have been named, including *R. conorii* subsp. conorii subsp. nov. (type strain = Malish, ATCC VR-613), the agent of MSF.[7]

Although tick–rickettsia relationships were a focus of interest by many pioneering rickettsiologists, the life cycle of most tick-borne rickettsiae is poorly understood one century later. Particularly, basic questions remain regarding the brown dog tick *Rhipicephalus sanguineus* and its relationships with *R. conorii*. Indeed, *Rh. sanguineus* has become one of the most widespread ticks throughout the world because of its specialized feeding on domestic dogs. This tick is highly adapted to warm climates but also thrives in dog kennels, human homes, and even in cooler regions; thus, it has spread globally between 50°N and 35°S.[8] However, MSF due to *R. conorii* is known to be endemic in the Mediterranean area, including northern Africa and southern Europe. It has also been described in a few countries in sub-Saharan Africa, and few cases have also been sporadically reported in northern and central Europe, sometimes followed by the installation of a local focus of the disease, including in Belgium,[9] Switzerland,[10] and northern France,[11] where *Rh. sanguineus* can be imported with dogs and survive in peridomestic environments, providing acceptable mi-croclimatic conditions.[2] However, *R. conorii* infection has never been described in the USA, and more largely, in the Americas.

Do *Rhipicephalus sanguineus* Act as a Reservoir of *Rickettsia conorii*?

In the 1970s, it was generally accepted that most ticks associated with SFG rickettsiae were not only vectors, but also reservoirs for the bacteria. This would mean maintenance of rickettsiae relies on both transstadial transovarial efficient transmissions, and rickettsiae would have no effect on the reproductive fitness or viability of the tick host. However, even nowadays this has only been definitively demonstrated for a few rickettsia. In their review on transstadial and transovarial transmission of infectious agents in arthropods, Burgdorfer and Barma suggested that this phenomenom could exist. However, it is difficult to know when this appeared as a dogma for tick–rickettsia relationships, and it was written and rewritten in many reviews. Indeed, at that time (1966) and regarding *Rh. sanguineus–R. conorii* interactions, Burgdorfer and Barma reported works completed in the 1930s and published in the French publications.[12]

In 1932, Blanc and Caminopetros demonstrated that larvae, nymphs, adults, and duringwinter, unfed males and females could act as vectors of MSF.[13] It was also shown that when eggs or larvae obtained from infected *Rh. sanguineus* female were crushed and used to inoculated humans, the patients contracted MSF. These data suggest that transovarial transmission of the MSF agent occurs in ticks. However, we are unaware of any well-documented demonstration of transovarial transmission of *R. conorii* in *Rh. sanguineus*, the transovarial transmission (TOT) rate (the proportion of infected females giving rise to at least one positive egg or larva), or the filial infection rate (FIR) (proportion of infected eggs or larvae obtained from an infected female). It is not known if transovarial transmission of

R. conorii is maintained from generation to generation of *Rh sanguineus*. Finally, it should be remembered that in ancient experiments, the identification of some SFG rickettsiae is questionable. For example, it is now known that *Rh. sanguineus* are associated with other SFG rickettsiae such as *R. massiliae*[14] (which could have been misdiagnosed as *R. conorii* because of the lack of molecular species identification).

Interestingly in 2002, Santos and colleagues showed, using intracelomic inoculation of *R. conorii*, a negative effect on *Rh. sanguineus* nymphs, including death during molting or, soon after, hatching into adult instars, while the remaining 50% of infected adults showed severe malformations. Finally, in apparently healthy adults, time of engorgement was longer.[15] The inoculation method used could have lead to a decrease in tick survival, but the use of control groups suggested that *R. conorii* affects the survival of its tick vector, not the inoculation method. More recently, Matsumoto and colleagues reported a high mortality of *Rh. sanguineus* group ticks infected with *R. conorii* by several methods, including the use of a bacteremic rabbit model.[16] It has been speculated that reasons for this reduction in fitness include the geographic origin of the ticks, which came from Thailand where *R. conorii* has not been reported, or was associated with the pathogen load acquired during laboratory experiments.[16]

However, we have recently confirmed that the lethal effect of *R. conorii* on *Rh. sanguineus* ticks in an experimental model of infection was unrelated to the geographical origin of the ticks.[17] Similar results have been obtained by others.[18] It is possible that the number of rickettsiae in experimental ticks may not correspond to that of *R. conorii* acquired by ticks in nature. The markedly negative effects of *R. conorii* infection on the survival of *Rh. sanguineus* ticks suggest that these routes cannot be the major means for survival of the agent in nature. This could explain why the prevalence in nature of ticks infected by *R. conorii* is low (usually < 1%). For example, 2229 *Rh. sanguineus* ticks recently collected in Spain were tested for rickettsial agent, and *R. conorii* was not found.[19] It would be likely that vertebrate reservoirs play a more dominant role in the persistence of the agent than previously thought.

Other authors have demonstrated that spotted fever group rickettsiae may affect the longevity, fecundity, or molting success of ticks, including their usual vectors. For example, Burgdorfer and colleagues reported that in fifth generation ticks experimentally infected with *R. rickettsii*, the agent of Rocky Mountain spotted fever (RMSF), about 50% of repleted females died in one to two weeks, while surviving females oviposited poorly, and few eggs hatched. More recently, lethal effects from *R. rickettsii* were reported on *D. andersoni* ticks experimentally infected by *R. rickettsii*. Indeed, overall, 94.1% of nymphs infected as larvae by feeding on rickettsemic guinea pigs died during the molt into adults, and 88.3% of adult female ticks infected as nymphs died prior to feeding.[20] It was suggested that the lethal effect of *R. rickettsii* may explain the low prevalence of infected ticks in nature and affect its enzootic maintenance;[20] this maintenance and cycling being at least partially based on animal reservoirs including small mammals such as chipmunks, voles, ground squirrels, and rabbits.[20]

Recently, a total of 30 engorged females of *Rh. sanguineus* ticks were collected from 7 dogs—of patients who contracted MSF in Algeria in 2006. After they laid eggs, DNA was extracted, and one tick was found to be infected by *R. conorii*. The larvae, and all subsequent stages of this infected tick were placed on a New Zealand White rabbit (*Oryctolagus cuniculus*), which was used as the host for the blood meal, and specimens of all stages of the following generations were tested by PCR. We have shown vertical transmission of *R. conorii* in naturally infected *Rh. sanguineus* ticks over five generations. Furthermore, the TOT rate was 100%, and the FIR was up to 99% for the fourth generations of infected ticks. Also, *R. conorii* was detected in the ovaries of infected ticks, supporting the mechanism of transmission in infected *Rh. Sanguineus*.[21]

The vertical transmission rate (the product of the TOT and the FIR) has been shown as a population prevalence that is most useful for comparison with infection rates in nature. Therefore, the population of infected ticks in nature should be important. However, the prevalence in nature of ticks infected by *R. conorii* is low, as said above.[19]

Do Animal Reservoirs of *Rickettsia conorii* Exist?

The existence of animal reservoirs for *R. conorii*, as is the case for *R. rickettsii*, is suggested by several arguments: the low prevalence of infected ticks with *R. conorii* (for example, 2/207 in Greece and 0/120 in Spain, 3/288 in the Greek Islands,[22–25] and 0/123 in Chile [Raoult 2003, unpublished]), the possible but uncompletely explored deleterious impact of this bacterium on brown dog ticks, the narrow ecological niche inhabited by the bacterium, and the persistence of ticks infected in nature. Interestingly, the prevalence of *Rh. sanguineus* may vary from one specific setting to another within endemic areas. Early rickettsiologists such as D. and J. Olmer in southern France or Blanc and Caminopetros in Greece have shown that foci of MSF are usually small with low propensity for diffusion. For instance, several cases have been observed in one town over several years, while no cases were observed in a neighboring town only two kilometers away.[13] Similarly, focality has also been described for RMSF.[26]

A reservoir for *R. conorii* has not been definitively described. *Rickettsia* spp. seroprevalence in dogs (important hosts for *Rh. sanguineus*) is high (26–60%) in regions endemic for MSF, and proximity to seroreactive dogs has been suggested as a risk factor for MSF in humans.[27,28] However, *Rh. sanguineus* are also associated with other SFG rickettsiae, such as *R. massiliae*[14] that may induce cross-reacting antibodies in dogs.

In 1930, Durand infected two 6-week-old puppies with an emulsion of *Rh. sanguineus* ticks collected in Tunis, Tunisia, an endemic area for MSF.[29] No clinical symptoms were observed, but blood collected from the puppies, 10 days post-infection, caused typical symptoms of MSF when human subjects were inoculated. Thereafter, the blood of these subjects was used to inoculate new 6-week-old puppies but had no clinical consequences for the dogs. However, when their blood was obtained at day 10 and other human subjects were inoculated, typical symptoms of MSF were observed. Similar results were obtained using older dogs living in French areas where *Rh. sanguineus* had a low prevalence, but not with adult dogs living in areas where *Rh. sanguineus* was highly prevalent. Durand suggested at that time that non-immune dogs (puppies in endemic areas or dogs living outside endemic areas of MSF or, at least, *Rh. sanguineus*) might serve as reservoirs for what was presumed to be *R. conorii*.[29] Later in 1972, Kelly and colleagues showed that 5-to-7-month-old German Shepard dogs experimentally infected with a Zimbabwean strain of *R. conorii* presented no clinical signs, except pain, erythema, and edema at the inoculation site and regional adenopathy. No laboratory abnormalities were noticed. However, intermittent rickettsemia could be detected between day 2 and 10 post-infection.[30] Finally, three cases have been recently reported (supported by PCR, DNA sequencing, and seroconversion.[28]) in acutely ill febrile Yorkshire terrier dogs. Other animals have been found experimentally susceptible to *R. conorii*, such as hedgehogs, Swiss mice, Hartley guinea pigs, and *Spermophilus citellus* (*Citellus citellus*).[13,31] More interestingly, the role of the European rabbit *Oryctolagus cuniculus* in the epidemiology of MSF had been suggested by pioneering rickettsiologists. In 1932, the European rabbit *Oryctolagus cuniculus* was consider a possible reservoir.[32] In 1940, Violle and Joyeux isolated *R. conorii* by inoculation into guinea pigs of wild rabbit's blood, brain suspension, and crashed ticks, collected from these rabbits. Furthermore, in 1952, myxomatosis destroyed almost all the rabbits in southern France. Immediately thereafter, there was a spectacular drop in the incidence of MSF, and the reappearance of wild rabbits several years later was followed by an increased incidence of MSF. The role of rabbit tick and fleas, as well as that of small rodents such as *Pitymys duodecimcostatus* living in rabbits burrows, was suspected to be involved in the life cycle of *R. conorii*; however, this was never confirmed.[32]

Perspectives

Perspectives include determining if there is a difference of fitness and survival of ticks in nature and the analysis of the role of extrinsic factors such as stress and temperature. This should be explored in relation with the long-recognized phenomenon known as reactivation that remains poorly understood.

Reactivation may be a universal adaptation of tick-borne agents to the long periods of metabolic inactivity by their acarine hosts. By becoming dormant during the long transstadial phase and during host-seeking, the agent does not utilize scarce, stored resources and reduces any effect on fitness.[33] Interestingly, female *D. andersoni* ticks infected with *R. rickettsii* and incubated at 4°C demonstrate lower mortality than infected ticks at 21°C.[35] Once the tick attaches, the change in temperature and physiology of the tick host induces the agent to emerge from dormancy and attain infectivity. In nature, stress conditions encountered by rickettsiae within the tick include starvation and temperature shifts. In the laboratory, *R. rickettsii* in *D. andersoni* ticks loses its virulence for guinea pigs when the ticks are subjected to physiological stress, such as low environmental temperature or starvation.[20] However, subsequent exposure of these ticks to 37°C, for 24 to 48 hours, or the acquisition of a blood meal, may restore the original virulence of the bacteria. During tick blood-feeding, rickettsiae undergo various physiological changes and proliferate intensively during reactivation.

Similarly, we have recently compared the fitness and survival of several stages of uninfected *Rh. sanguineus* with specimen infected with *R. conorii*. Interestingly, engorged nymphs infected with *R. conorii* exposed during one month at low temperature (4°C) have a high mortality when they are transferred to 25°C (absence of molting), compared to uninfected ticks (unpublished). Because *Rh. sanguineus* overwinter as engorged nymphs, these preliminary results could lead to speculation that infected ticks would not pass the winter.

In conclusion, more work is needed to really decipher the relationship between *R. conorii* and its vector, *Rh. sanguineus*. It may be possible that some populations of *Rh. sanguineus* in natural small foci are better adapted to rickettsial infection. We need to definitely confirm the role of animal reservoirs in perpetuating *R. conorii*. Also, more investigations on *Rh. sanguineus–R. conorii* interactions are needed to understand the discrepancy between the efficient vertical transmission of the agent in naturally infected ticks and a low prevalence in nature.

Conflicts of Interest

The authors declare no conflicts of interest.

References

1. Parola, P. & D. Raoult. 2001. Ticks and tickborne bacterial diseases in humans: an emerging infectious threat. *Clin. Infect. Dis.* **32:** 897–928.
2. Parola, P., C. Paddock & D. Raoult. 2005. Tickborne rickettsioses around the world: emerging diseases challenging old concepts. *Clin. Microbiol. Rev.* **18:** 719–756.
3. Mediannikov, O., P. Parola & D. Raoult. 2007. Other tick-borne rickettsioses. In *Rickettsial Diseases*. D. Raoult & P. Parola, Eds.: 139–162. Informa Healthcare. New York.
4. Mediannikov, O., C. Paddock & P. Parola. 2007. Other rickettsiae of possible or undetermined pathogenicity. *Rickettsial diseases*. D. Raoult & P. Parola, Eds.: 163–177. Informa Healthcare. New York.
5. Brumpt, E. 1932. Longevité du virus de la fièvre boutonneuse (*Rickettsia conorii*, n. sp.) chez la tique *Rhipicephalus sanguineus*. *C R Soc Biol.* **110:** 1119.

6. Raoult, D. & V. Roux. 1997. Rickettsioses as paradigms of new or emerging infectious diseases. *Clin. Microbiol. Rev.* **10:** 694–719.

7. Zhu, Y. *et al*. 2005. Proposal to create subspecies of *Rickettsia conorii* based on multi-locus sequence typing and an emended description of *Rickettsia conorii*. *BMC Microbiol.* **5:** 1–11.

8. Estrada-Pena, A. *et al*. 2004. *Ticks of domestic animals in the Mediterranean region*. University of Zaragoza. Spain.

9. Lambert, M. *et al*. 1984. Mediterranean Spotted-Fever in Belgium. *Lancet.* **2:** 1038.

10. Peter, O. *et al*. 1984. *Rickettsia conorii* isolated from *Rhipicephalus sanguineus* introduced into Switzerland on a pet dog. *Z Parasitenkd.* **70:** 265–270.

11. Senneville, E. *et al*. 1991. *Rickettsia conorii* isolated from ticks introduced to northern France by a dog. *Lancet.* **337:** 676.

12. Burgdorfer, W. & M.G. Varma. 1967. Trans-stadial and transovarial development of disease agents in arthropods. *Annu. Rev. Entomol.* **12:** 376.

13. Blanc, G. & J. Caminopetros. 1932. Epidemiological and experimental studies on Boutonneuse fever done at the Pasteur Institute in Athens. *Arch. Inst. Pasteur. Tunis.* **XX:** 394.

14. Matsumoto, K. *et al*. 2005. Transmission of *Rickettsia massiliae* in the tick, *Rhipicephalus turanicus*. *Med. Vet. Entomol.* **19:** 263–270.

15. Santos, A.S. *et al*. 2002. Ultrastructural study of the infection process of *Rickettsia conorii* in the salivary glands of the vector tick *Rhipicephalus sanguineus*. *Vector Borne Zoonotic Dis.* **2:** 165–177.

16. Matsumoto, K. *et al*. 2005. Experimental infection models of ticks of the *Rhipicephalus sanguineus* group with *Rickettsia conorii*. *Vector Borne Zoonotic Dis.* **5:** 363–372.

17. Socolovschi, C. *et al*. 2009. Experimental infection of Rhipicephalus sanguineus with *Rickettsia conorii conorii*. *Clin. Microbiol. Infect.:* In press.

18. Levin, M.L. *et al*. 2008. Effects of *Rickettsia conorii* infection on survival of *Rhipicephalus sanguineus* ticks [abstract]. *Book of abstracts of the 5th International Meeting on Rickettsiae and Rickettsial Diseases.* **163:** 84.

19. Marquez, F.J. *et al*. 2008. Spotted fever group Rickettsia in brown dog ticks *Rhipicephalus sanguineus* in southwestern Spain. *Parasitol Res.*

20. Niebylski, M.L., M.G. Peacock & T.G. Schwan. 1999. Lethal effect of *Rickettsia rickettsii* on its tick vector (*Dermacentor andersoni*). *Appl. Environ. Microbiol.* **65:** 773–778.

21. Socolovschi, C. *et al*. 2009. Transmission of *Rickettsia conorii conorii* in naturally infected Rhipicephalus sanguineus. *Clin. Microbiol. Infect.:* In press.

22. Psaroulaki, A. *et al*. 2003. First isolation and identification of *Rickettsia conorii* from ticks collected in the region of Fokida in central Greece. *J. Clin. Microbiol.* **41:** 3317–3319.

23. Oteo, J.A. *et al*. 2006. Prevalence of spotted fever group Rickettsia species detected in ticks in La Rioja, Spain. *Ann. N. Y. Acad. Sci.* **1078:** 320–323.

24. Psaroulaki, A. *et al*. 2006. Ticks, tick-borne rickettsiae, and *Coxiella burnetii* in the Greek Island of Cephalonia. *Ann. N. Y. Acad. Sci.* **1078:** 389–99.

25. Bitam, I. *et al*. 2006. First molecular detection of *R. conorii*, *R. aeschlimannii*, and *R. massiliae* in ticks from Algeria. *Ann. N. Y. Acad. Sci.* **1078:** 368–372.

26. Jones, T.F. *et al*. 1999. Family cluster of Rocky Mountain spotted fever. *Clin. Infect. Dis.* **28:** 853–859.

27. Segura-Porta, F. *et al*. 1998. Prevalence of antibodies to spotted fever group rickettsiae in human beings and dogs from and endemic area of mediterranean spotted fever in Catalonia, Spain. *Eur. J. Epidemiol.* **14:** 395–398.

28. Solano-Gallego, L. *et al*. 2006. Febrile illness associated with *Rickettsia conorii* infection in dogs from Sicily. *Emerg. Infect Dis.* **12:** 1985–1988.

29. Durand, P. 1930. La fièvre boutonneuse en Tunisie. Le rôle du chien comme reservoir de virus dans la fièvre boutonneuse. *Tunisie Médicale* 239–251.

30. Kelly, P.J. *et al*. 1992. Experimental infection of dogs with a Zimbabwean strain of *Rickettsia conorii*. *J. Trop. Med. Hyg.* **95:** 322–326.

31. Ormsbee, R.A. 1979. A review: "Studies in *Pyroplasmosis hominis* ('spotted fever' or 'tick fever' of the Rocky Mountains)" by Louis B. Wison and William M. Chowning. *Rev. Infect. Dis.* **1:** 562.

32. Joyeux, C. & J. Pieri. 1932. Le lapin peut consituer un reservoir de virus pour la fièvre boutonneuse (exanthématique). *C. R. Acad. Sci.* **194:** 2342.

33. Telford, S.R. & P. Parola. 2007. Arthropods and Rickettsiae. In *Rickettsial Diseases*. D. Raoult & P. Parola, Eds.: 27–36. Informa Healthcare. New York.

Intracellular Life of *Coxiella burnetii* in Macrophages

An Update

Eric Ghigo, Lionel Pretat, Benoît Desnues, Christian Capo, Didier Raoult, and Jean-Louis Mege

URMITE CNRS UMR 6236 – IRD 3R198, Institut Fédératif de Recherche 48, Université de la Méditerranée, Marseille, France

Coxiella burnetii, the agent of Q fever, is an obligate intracellular bacterium that is considered a potential biological weapon of category B. *C. burnetii* survives within myeloid cells by subverting receptor-mediated phagocytosis and preventing phagosome maturation. The intracellular fate of *C. burnetii* also depends on the functional state of myeloid cells. This review describes the mechanisms used by *C. burnetii* to circumvent uptake and trafficking events, and the role of cytokines on *C. burnetii* survival in myeloid cells.

Key words: *Coxiella burnetii*; cytoskeleton; phagosome; endocytic pathway; cytokines

Introduction

Coxiella burnetii is the agent of Q fever, a worldwide zoonosis. After primary infection, about 60% of human beings are asymptomatic while 40% of individuals manifest clinical signs consisting of isolated fever, hepatitis, and pneumonia. The outcome of acute Q fever is usually favorable: it is due to protective immune response, as manifested by systemic cell-mediated responses and granuloma formation.[1] However, infection persists since *C. burnetii* DNA is still present in the host several months after acute Q fever.[2] In patients with valvulopathy and, to a lesser extent, in pregnant women and immunocompromised patients, acute infection may become chronic with endocarditis as the major clinical manifestation. Chronic Q fever is characterized by an inefficient protective response to *C. burnetii* infection, as demonstrated by defective cell-mediated response, the

lack of granulomas that are replaced by lymphocyte infiltration and necrosis foci, and high amounts of antibodies directed against *C. burnetii*. A long-term treatment consisting of the association of doxycycline with hydroxychloroquine improves the prognosis despite the persisting risk of relapses.[1]

C. burnetii is a small gram-negative bacterium that has been classified in the $\gamma-$ subdivision of *Proteobacteria* on the basis of the sequence of 16S rRNA. Essentially, domestic ruminants are infected by *C. burnetii*, but other hosts, including pets and arthropods, have been described. *C. burnetii* infection is usually asymptomatic in animals but induces abortions in livestock. As placenta is a major site of *C. burnetii* infection, *C. burnetii* shedding into the environment occurs mainly during parturition. The contamination by aerosols represents the main route of infection in animals and humans, and explains why persons at risk from Q fever include farmers, veterinarians, and slaughterhouse workers.[3] Aerosols may be used as a biological weapon because of the high infectivity of *C. burnetii*, the ability of producing large

Address for correspondence: URMITE, Faculté de Médecine, 27 Bld. Jean Moulin, 13385 Marseille Cedex 05, France. Voice: +33 4 91 32 45 86; fax: +33 4 91 38 77 72. Eric.Ghigo@univmed.fr

Rickettsiology and Rickettsial Diseases-Fifth International Conference: Ann. N.Y. Acad. Sci. 1166: 55–66 (2009).
doi: 10.1111/j.1749-6632.2009.04515.x © 2009 New York Academy of Sciences.

quantities and widespread availability of organisms, and environmental stability of *C. burnetii* through a sporulation-like mechanism.[4] *C. burnetii* has been already weaponized and likely used as a bioweapon during World War II.[5]

C. burnetii resides within myeloid cells,[6] and the adaptation of *C. burnetii* to this microenvironment is probably critical for the evolution of Q fever. Specifically, *C. burnetii* has developed a specific strategy to subvert the microbicidal activity of myeloid cells. The aim of this review is to describe the mechanisms used by *C. burnetii* to invade and survive within myeloid cells.

Virulence Factors of *C. burnetii*

The size of *C. burnetii* genome ranges from 1.5 to 2.4 Mb among different strains.[7] It has been tempting to relate genetic variability and *C. burnetii* virulence to specific plasmid regions since *C. burnetii* can harbor one of four plasmids, namely QpH1, QpRS, QpDG, QpDV or QpRS-like plasmid.[8] Plasmid types are associated with specific genomic groups. Isolates within genomic groups I, II, and III are derived from patients with acute Q fever, whereas isolates within genomic groups IV and V are derived from patients with chronic Q fever.[9,10] However, QpH1 plasmid has been found in genomic groups I, II, and III, and in strains inducing acute or chronic infections.[11] QpRS plasmid, found in the genomic group IV, has been associated with only strains responsible of chronic infection in patients.[3,11] These data lay the foundations of a controversial hypothesis in which plasmids and their associated genome encode pathotype-specific virulence factors.[12]

The genetic diversity and virulence of *C. burnetii* are also related to the expression of lipopolysaccharide (LPS) molecules. *C. burnetii* displays antigenic variations similar to the smooth-rough variation of enterobacteria. Phase I organisms are isolated from natural sources, and their full-length LPS (smooth form) is serologically defined as phase I. Serial passages in embryonated eggs or tissue culture lead to an irreversible modification of the LPS molecules, with decreased molecular weights culminating in the severely truncated LPS (rough form) of organisms, serologically defined as phase II LPS. Phase II organisms are considered as poorly virulent, and it has been demonstrated that their truncated rough-type LPS is caused by a genomic deletion.[3] Phase II LPS contains lipid A and some core sugars, but *O*-antigen sugars are missing. The lipids A from phase I and phase II *C. burnetii* display the same ionic species and fragmentation profiles, supporting the idea that these lipids A have very similar and probably identical structures.[13] Phase I LPS, but not phase II LPS, contains sugars such as L-virenose, dihydrohydroxystreptose, and galactosamine uronyl-α-(1,6)-glucosamine.[14] In addition, a third LPS has been identified as an intermediate-length LPS at the surface of the strain Nile Mile Crazy.[15] Large chromosomal deletions are found in phase II *C. burnetii* Nile Mile and Nile Mile Crazy.[16] These deletions eliminate open reading frames involved in the biosynthesis of *O*-antigen sugars, including the rare sugar virenose.[16]

The complete genome of *C. burnetii* (phase I Nine Mile RSA493) has been sequenced.[17] Genes encoding typical structures involved in adhesion to host cells, such as pili and adhesins, are lacking in *C. burnetii* genome. Several genes involved in adhesion, invasion, and detoxification have been identified. They encode proteins containing ankyrin repeats or RGD motif. It is interesting to note that the receptor of *C. burnetii* located on myeloid cells, the integrin $\alpha v\beta 3$, interacts with the RGD motif.[18] Other genes encode molecules similar to those involved in the uptake of *L. pneumophila* and enteropathogenic *Escherichia coli* by host cells and the cytoskeletal reorganization necessary to this uptake. These genes may account for the different levels of uptake of phase I and phase II organisms by macrophages (see below)[18] and the cytoskeleton rearrangement induced by phase I *C. burnetii*.[19] Other genes encode catalase, superoxide dismutase, and acid phosphatase, three enzymes that may permit *C. burnetii* to avoid the microbicidal activity of macrophages through the inhibition of reactive oxygen intermediates.[20,21] The gene encoding a peptidyl-polycis-trans-isomerase, similar to that expressed by *L. pneumophila*, may affect the production of cytokines[22] and, consequently, the replication of *C. burnetii* (see below). Finally, genes encoding components of a type IV secretion system (IcmT, IcmS, and IcmK), which are mechanistically related to the *Legionella* Dot/Icm apparatus,[23] could play a major role in the formation of *C. burnetii*-containing phagosome.[24,25]

Uptake of *C. burnetii* by Myeloid Cells

Phagocytosis, an ancestral defense mechanism against microbial infection, is essentially due to professional phagocytes (including myeloid cells) that normally ingest and degrade bacteria, virus, fungi, and protozoa. To discriminate between the multiple infectious agents they meet, myeloid cells possess a restricted number of phagocytic receptors. They include Fc receptors that recognize opsonized microorganisms, the complement receptor CR3 (CD11b/CD18) that recognizes opsonized and unopsonized organisms, the mannose receptor that recognizes conserved motifs on infectious agents, scavenger receptors that recognize diacyl lipids at the bacterium surface, and Toll-like receptors (TLRs) that recognize bacterial structures such as LPS, peptidoglycan, or flagellin.[26]

Integrin-dependent Phagocytosis of *C. burnetii*

Phagocytosis is a localized event that requires spatially and temporally restricted signals. Different bacterial pathogens have taken advantage of the properties of the phagocytic process to invade host cells. *C. burnetii* has developed a specific survival strategy based on subverted receptor-mediated phagocytosis[18] that may determine the evolution of Q fever. Phase I

C. burnetii organisms survive in human monocytes, whereas phase II variants are eliminated. The intracellular fate of *C. burnetii* is associated with different modes of *C. burnetii* entry. Indeed, phase I organisms are poorly internalized by monocytes, whereas phase II variants are efficiently ingested. The molecular mechanisms involved in the different efficiencies of bacterial uptake by monocytes have been elucidated. The uptake of phase II variants is mediated by $\alpha v \beta 3$ integrin and CR3, whereas the internalization of phase I organisms involves the engagement of $\alpha v \beta 3$ integrin, but not that of CR3. The phagocytic efficiency of CR3 depends on its activation through $\alpha v \beta 3$ integrin and CD47 (integrin-associated protein), a molecule physically and functionally associated with $\beta 3$ integrins, since macrophages from CD47-deficient mice are unable to ingest phase I bacteria through CR3. Phase I organisms prevent CR3 activation by interfering with its lectin sites[18] and, consequently, with conformational changes of the I domain and exposure of activation epitopes.[27] The inhibitory mechanism mediated by phase I bacteria do not target CD47, since they do not down-regulate the expression of CD47. They rather interfere with its cosignal activity, since the uptake of phase I and phase II organisms is similar in CD47-deficient macrophages.[18]

The inhibition of the cross talk between $\alpha v \beta 3$ integrin and CR3 induced by phase I organisms suggests that CR3 engagement is deleterious for *C. burnetii*. The role of CR3 in the microbicidal activity of myeloid cells likely depends on the nature of pathogens and their opsonization.[28] *Pseudomonas aeruginosa, Salmonella* sp., and *E. coli* are eliminated after CR3-mediated uptake, whereas *Bordetella* sp. avoid killing by taking advantage of CR3.[29] The aggregation substance of *Enterococcus faecalis* that interacts with CR3 increases bacterial uptake and prevents the microbicidal activity of macrophages.[30] In contrast, CR3 engagement does not affect the intracellular survival of *Mycobacterium tuberculosis*[31], and CR3 is not involved in the outcome of *M. tuberculosis* infection.[32]

Cytoskeleton Remodeling Induced by *C. burnetii*

C. burnetii virulence is associated with the cytoskeletal rearrangement of myeloid cells. In monocytes, phase I *C. burnetii* organisms stimulate morphologic changes consisting of membrane protrusions and polarized projections as determined by scanning electron microscopy.[19] They increase their content in filamentous actin (F-actin) and induce an intense and transient rearrangement of F-actin. As F-actin colocalizes with myosin in cell protrusions, morphological changes likely require actin polymerization and the tension of actin-myosin filaments. The contact between bacteria and monocytes is necessary to induce cytoskeleton reorganization: bacterial supernatants do not stimulate F-actin reorganization, and bacteria are in close apposition with F-actin protrusions. In contrast, phase II organisms do not induce any change in cell morphology, actin polymerization, and F-actin organization.

The efficiency of *C. burnetii* phagocytosis is dependent on the spatial distribution of CR3.[33] Indeed, CD11b and CD18 molecules, but not $\alpha v \beta 3$ integrin, are excluded from the protrusions induced by *C. burnetii* in THP-1 monocytes. Chemoattractants such as RANTES/CCL5 (Regulated on Activation Normal T cell Expressed and Secreted) increase *C. burnetii* uptake and restore CR3 localization in cell protrusions, suggesting that bacterial uptake and CR3 localization are related. The expression of HIV-1 Nef protein by THP-1 monocytes induces CR3 redistribution in *C. burnetii*-induced protrusions and also restores the *C. burnetii* uptake mediated by CR3. Moreover, CR3 redistribution and increased bacterial uptake in RANTES-stimulated monocytes and Nef-expressing monocytes are associated with inhibited *C. burnetii* replication. It is therefore likely that the survival strategy of *C. burnetii* involves limited engagement of CR3 through the manipulation of the actin cytoskeleton.

Finally, protein tyrosine kinases (PTK) downmodulate *C. burnetii* uptake by acting on actin cytoskeleton. Indeed, phase I bacteria induce early PTK activation and the tyrosine phosphorylation of several endogenous proteins, including Hck and Lyn, two Src-related kinases.[34] PTK activation reflects *C. burnetii* virulence, since phase II bacteria do not stimulate PTK. Tyrosine-phosphorylated molecules colocalize with F-actin inside cell protrusions induced by phase I *C. burnetii*, and PTK activity is increased in Triton X-100-insoluble fractions. PTK and Src kinase inhibitors block the formation of cell protrusions and F-actin remodeling induced by phase I *C. burnetii*. The pretreatment of monocytes with PTK inhibitors increases the uptake of phase I organisms, but not that of phase II organisms. It has been demonstrated that PTK activation also provides an uptake signal for several invasive bacterial pathogens, including *Listeria monocytogenes*, enteropathogenic *E. coli*, *Helicobacter pylori*, and *Campylobacter* spp.[35] Concerning the interaction of *C. burnetii* and monocytes, we can suppose that PTK activation results in membrane ruffling, which may limit the colocalization of CR3 with $\alpha v \beta 3$ integrin and phase I bacteria. Alternatively, PTK may target $\alpha v \beta 3$ integrin, thus interfering with the cross talk between $\alpha v \beta 3$ integrin, CR3, and actin cytoskeleton.[19,36] In contrast, some bacterial pathogens inhibit PTK and PTK-mediated microbicidal responses: a tyrosine phosphatase of *Yersinia* spp. and *Salmonella enterica* serovar Typhimurium disrupts actin cytoskeleton and regulates bacterial uptake.[35]

Toll-Like Receptors and *C. burnetii* Infection

The recognition of microbial molecules by TLRs initiates innate and adaptive immune responses. Among TLRs, TLR4 is involved in the recognition of gram-negative bacteria such as *E. coli* through recognition of prototypic LPS. TLR2 interacts with gram-positive bacteria following interaction with lipoproteins, proteoglycans, lipopeptides, or with LPS from *Porphyromonas gingivalis*.[37,38]

During the course of *C. burnetii* infection, TLR4 controls the bacterial uptake by macrophages.[39] Indeed, polymyxin B, which interferes with LPS binding, inhibits the uptake of phase I organisms without affecting the entry of phase II organisms. The uptake of phase I organisms is also reduced in TLR4-deficient macrophages, whereas the uptake of phase II organisms remains unaffected, and it has been demonstrated that it is also independent of TLR2.[39] Besides its role in the uptake of phase I *C. burnetii*, TLR4 is also involved in *C. burnetii*-induced F-actin remodeling, highlighting again the close relationship between *C. burnetii* uptake and cytoskeletal organization. The mechanism by which TLR4 and actin cytoskeleton are related remains hypothetical, even if the LPS-TLR complex is known to induce a transient F-actin remodeling in a p38- and ERK-dependent pathway.[40]

TLR4 controls the immune response against *C. burnetii* through granuloma formation and cytokine production. Indeed, *C. burnetii* infection results in sustained formation of granulomas in wild-type mice, indicative of a protective immune response, but granuloma formation is only transient in TLR4-deficient mice.[39] Altered granuloma formation may be due to changes in granuloma cell composition or impaired cytokine production.[41] It has been demonstrated that Interferon (IFN)-γ levels are decreased in TLR4-deficient mice as compared to wild-type mice.[39] Interleukin (IL)-10, known to impair the production of inflammatory type 1 cytokines, is also reduced in TLR4-deficient mice, suggesting that cytokines are involved in the defective formation of granulomas.

In contrast to early events of *C. burnetii* infection, TLR4 is dispensable for bacterial survival in macrophages and bacterial clearance *in vivo*.[39] Indeed, the survival of phase I *C. burnetii* is not affected in TLR4-deficient macrophages.[39] *In vivo* findings also show that *C. burnetii* infection of tissues and bacterial clearance are similar in wild-type and TLR4-deficient mice. Similarly to TLR4, TLR2 is involved in the inflammatory and immune responses to *C. burnetii*, but is not necessary for bacterial clearance.[42] These results may be explained by the observations of Zamboni and colleagues, since purified lipids A from phase I and phase II *C. burnetii* organisms fail to activate TLR2 and TLR4.[13] We can suppose that some functions induced by *C. burnetii* need TLR4 (and/or TLR2), whereas other functions are independent of TLR4 (and/or TLR2).

Immune Response to *C. burnetii* Infection

The immune control of *C. burnetii* infection appears to be T-cell dependent; however, it does not lead to complete *C. burnetii* eradication.[39] *C. burnetii* is found in apparently cured people but also in the dental pulp of cured guinea pigs. Nucleic acids from *C. burnetii* are also present in monocytes and bone marrow of individuals infected months or years earlier.[1] *In vivo, C. burnetii* infection leads to the formation of granulomas that depend on the ability of myeloid cells to migrate across the vascular endothelium. The center of a typical Q fever granuloma is composed of a lipid vacuola surrounded by a fibrinoid ring.[3] During the acute phase of Q fever, few, if any, isolated bacteria are found in granulomas. Granuloma formation is, at least in part, dependent on TLR4, since TLR4-deficient mice infected with *C. burnetii* display decreased numbers of granulomas.[39] Specific antibodies are produced in acute Q fever: IgG are mainly directed against phase II variants, whereas IgM are directed against both phase I and phase II bacteria.[3] In addition, monocytes from convalescent patients are able to eliminate *C. burnetii*.[39]

In contrast, chronic Q fever is characterized by an inefficient immune response.[1] *C. burnetii* organisms replicate despite high levels of specific antibodies (IgG, IgM, and IgA) directed against phase I and phase II *C. burnetii*. Lymphocyte counts and the CD4/CD8 ratio are decreased.[43] In contrast to acute Q fever, granulomas are lacking in chronic Q fever and infected tissues, including heart valves and liver, and aneurysms present large *C. burnetii*-containing vacuoles.[3] The formation of these large vacuoles seems to depend on specific antibodies.[44] In addition, monocytes are unable to kill *C. burnetii*[45] and migrate across the endothelium[7,46,47,50] in a IL-10-dependent manner (see below).

It has been recently reported that the polarization of macrophages governs their microbicidal activity against *C. burnetii*.[48] Hence, *C. burnetii* mainly induces the expression of M2 polarization-related genes, such as those encoding Transforming Growth Factor (TGF)-β1, IL-1 receptor antagonist (IL-1ra), CCL18, the mannose receptor, and arginase-1, even if organisms also induce the expression of genes encoding IL-6 and CXCL8, two cytokines associated with M1 program. In contrast, *C. burnetii* inhibits the expression of M1-associated genes such as those encoding Tumor Necrosis Factor (TNF), CD80, CCR7, and TLR2. The expression and the secretion of M1-associated molecules are related to the transductional data. *C. burnetii*-stimulated macrophages secrete high levels of TGF-β1 and CCL18, and express the mannose receptor and arginase-1, the latter being associated with the absence of nitric oxide release by macrophages. IL-6 and CXCL8 are poorly released by *C. burnetii*-stimulated macrophages.[48] It is likely that this atypical M2 activation program accounts for *C. burnetii* persistence in macrophages.

The engulfment of apoptotic cells by monocytes and macrophages likely plays a major role in *C. burnetii* persistence.[49] Indeed, patients with valvulopathy exhibit high levels of circulating apoptotic leukocytes, suggesting that the uptake of apoptotic cells by myeloid cells may be associated with chronic Q fever. The binding of myeloid cells to apoptotic cells, but not to necrotic cells, enhances *C. burnetii* replication and induces a M2 polarization, with some slight differences between monocytes and macrophages. Monocytes express high levels of IL-10, IL-6, and CD14, and TNF levels are low. Macrophages release high levels of TGF-β1

and express the mannose receptor. IL-10 and TGF-β1 neutralization by specific antibodies inhibits *C. burnetii* replication, suggesting that both cytokines are involved in bacterial replication. IFN-γ, which is associated with the control of *C. burnetii* infection, shifts monocytes and macrophages that have engulfed apoptotic cells toward a M1 program. These findings suggest that valvulopathy-associated leukocyte apoptosis is critical in the pathogenesis of Q fever endocarditis by deactivating immune cells and creating a favorable environment for pathogen persistence.[50]

IL-10 and Chronic *C. burnetii* Infection

IL-10, through the induction of an anergic state, is involved in bacterial persistence in hosts and the evolution of infectious diseases.[51] The primary infection by *C. burnetii* is generally asymptomatic; however, it may become chronic in patients with valvulopathy or immune disorders.[1] The chronic evolution of the disease is dependent on IL-10. Indeed, monocytes from patients with Q fever endocarditis and from patients with acute Q fever and valvulopathy overproduce IL-10.[52] The risk of chronic evolution of the disease is associated with IL-10 overproduction.[53] When macrophages from patients with chronic Q fever are treated with antibodies specific for IL-10, their antimicrobial properties are restored.[54] Finally, IL-10 alters leukocyte trafficking and, consequently, the formation of granulomas that is critical for protection against *C. burnetii*.[46,47]

An efficient animal model for chronic Q fever pathogenesis has been recently developed using transgenic mice that constitutively express IL-10 in the macrophage compartment.[55] Transgenic mice infected with *C. burnetii* through the intraperitoneal route exhibit sustained tissue infection and strong antibody response in contrast to wild-type mice; thus, bacterial persistence is IL-10-dependent as in chronic Q fever. The number of granulomas is low in spleen and liver of transgenic mice infected, as in patients with chronic Q fever. Macrophages from transgenic mice are unable to kill *C. burnetii*. *C. burnetii*-stimulated macrophages are characterized by a non-microbicidal transcriptional program consisting of increased expression of arginase-1, mannose receptor, and Ym1/2, in contrast to wild-type macrophages in which expression of inducible NO synthase and inflammatory cytokines are increased. In spleen and liver of transgenic mice infected with *C. burnetii*, the expression of arginase-1 is increased, while microbicidal pathway consisting of IL-12p40, IL-23p19, and inducible NO synthase is depressed. As humans are most commonly infected with *C. burnetii* through inhalation of parturient secretions from infected animals, wild-type and transgenic mice have also been infected by the intratracheal route. The constitutive overexpression of IL-10 dramatically increases lung infection. The pulmonary lesions consisting of mixed interstitial and mild alveolar mononuclear cell pneumonia are more pronounced in transgenic mice than in wild-type mice. Interestingly, these results emphasize the role of the route of inoculation in *C. burnetii* infection in mice as well as in humans. We can conclude from these observations that the overexpression of IL-10 in macrophages prevents anti-infectious competence of host, including the ability to mount granulomatous response and microbicidal pathway in tissues as observed in chronic Q fever patients.

Nature of the Phagosome Harboring *C. burnetii*

Phagosome Conversion

After internalization, bacteria are localized within a compartment (phagosome) that undergoes a series of fusion/fission events with different populations of endocytic organelles such as endosomes. The ultimate stage of these events is the phagolysosome, in which bacteria are destroyed. The first step of phagosome conversion is the intermingled fusion/fission with early endosomes. Phagosomes gain several markers, such as Early Endosome Antigen-1 (EEA1) and the small GTPase rab5. The early phagosomes gradually transform into a compartment that present features of late endosomes. Markers of late endosomes, such as the small GTPase rab7 and Lysosomal membrane-associated protein-1 (Lamp-1), progressively replace early endosomal markers.[56,57] Whereas, the pH of early phagosomes is around 6.0, the acquisition of vacuolar proton pump ATPase (V-H$^+$-ATPase) allows the intraphagosomal pH to reach an acidic pH around 4.0.[57] Finally, late phagosomes interact with lysosomes that contain hydrolytic enzymes such as cathepsin D, thus leading to the formation of phagolysosomes.[57]

Different pathogens have developed strategies to control their intracellular fate and enhance their survival within host cells. *Listeria*, *Shigella*, and *Rickettsia* escape from phagosomes to the cytosol, to avoid destruction in phagolysosomes.[35] Other pathogens interfere with normal biogenesis of phagolysosomes, thus leading to the formation of replicative vacuoles.[58] *Brucella abortus* interact with endoplasmic reticulum, but not with the classical endocytic network.[59] *Mycobacterium* phagosomes fuse with early endosomes, since they exchange material such as transferrin with early endosomes. However, they are unable to fuse with late endosomes, as revealed by a pH around 6.0 and the lack of rab7 and V-H$^+$-ATPase.[57,60] *Salmonella* resides in an atypical phagosome, which is neither a late nor an early phagosome. At late times of infection, membranes of the trans-Golgi network surround *Salmonella*-containing vacuoles, suggesting interactions with endocytic and biosynthetic pathways.[61]

Intracellular Trafficking of *C. burnetii*

C. burnetii is described to survive in an acidic vacuole.[6,62–64] The low pH of phagosomes harboring *C. burnetii* accounts for the relative inefficiency of antibiotic treatment in Q fever.[1] The intracellular life of *C. burnetii* has been considered as a model of bacterial survival without alteration of the phagosome conversion.[6] However, numerous studies have been performed with phase II *C. burnetii*[65–68] or with murine macrophage-like cells and fibroblasts, in which phase I and phase II organisms replicate.[6] Since phase I, but not phase II, *C. burnetii* organisms (RSA493) survive in human monocytes and macrophages, we have reevaluated the intracellular trafficking of *C. burnetii* in monocytes and macrophages.[69,70]

After uptake, phase I and phase II bacteria are localized within an early phagosome as revealed by the transient presence of EEA1 in *C. burnetii*-containing phagosomes. Later, *C. burnetii* phagosomes interact with late endosomes as demonstrated by their colocalization with Lamp-1, CD63, and mannose-6-phosphate receptor (M6PR). Moreover, *C. burnetii* virulence is not related to acidic pH of phagosomes, since the percentage of phagosomes that accumulate V-H$^+$-ATPase is similar for phase I and phase II organisms. Rab7, a small GTPase involved in phagosome conversion,[71] is acquired by phagosomes containing phase II organisms, whereas those containing phase I organisms acquire rab7 only in part.[69] The differences in rab7 acquisition may explain the defective fusion of phagosomes containing phase I *C. burnetii* with lysosomes (see below), since the amounts of rab proteins on the endocytic organelles are critical for the fusion process.[56,72] The partial acquisition of rab7 suggests that downstream fusion events are impaired. Cathepsin D, a lysosomal protease, does not accumulate in phagosomes containing phase I *C. burnetii*. The lack of cathepsin D colocalization with phase I organisms is not due to a delayed acquisition, but rather to a defective fusion of phagosomes with lysosomes, as evidenced with a lysosomotropic probe. The impaired acquisition of cathepsin D is related to bacterial virulence, since phase II organisms colocalize with cathepsin D. Taken together, these data show that the survival of virulent *C. burnetii* in myeloid cells is associated with altered conversion of phagosomes. This

hijacking strategy is reminiscent of the escape mechanism used by *Salmonella enterica*.[61] However, the involved molecular mechanisms are different: *C. burnetii* phagosomes acquire rab7 only in part, whereas *Salmonella* phagosomes recruit Lamp-1 in a rab7-dependent manner.[73] The fact that *C. burnetii* does not modify the early acquisition of EEA1 strengthens the hypothesis that the ability of rab7 to regulate vesicle traffic in late endocytosis[74,75] is altered in *C. burnetii* infection. It is likely that the survival strategy of *C. burnetii* in human monocytes and macrophages is based on the interference of rab7 recruitment at the surface of *C. burnetii*-containing phagosome, thus leading to the formation of a phagosome unable to interact with lysosomes.

Although debated,[76] TLRs may regulate phagosome maturation in macrophages.[77] As the survival of phase I *C. burnetii* is associated with impaired fusion of phagosomes with lysosomes in human monocytes, *C. burnetii* trafficking has been investigated in murine TLR4$^{-/-}$ macrophages. TLR4 does not control the maturation of *C. burnetii* phagosomes, since bacteria colocalize with Lamp-1 and cathepsin D.[39] These data suggest that the defective maturation of *C. burnetii* phagosome is related to TLR exclusion from the phagosome membrane.

Modulation of Intracellular Trafficking of *C. burnetii* by Cytokines

The concept that phagosome conversion and macrophage microbicidal activity are linked is lacking *in vitro* and *in vivo*. As cytokines are known to modulate macrophage microbicidal activity, we have taken advantage of the modulation of the microbicidal activity of macrophages by cytokines to test this concept. The activation of host cells by IFN-γ leads to the control of infection by numerous intracellular pathogens[78] including *C. burnetii*,[79,80] whereas IL-10 supports their intracellular replication.[81–83]

IFN-γ induces the killing of phase I *C. burnetii* by naive monocytes.[84] IFN-γ also affects the conversion of phagosomes containing phase I *C. burnetii*, since, in the presence of IFN-γ, *C. burnetii* phagosomes fuse with lysosomes as demonstrated by the acquisition of cathepsin D.[69] IFN-γ acts through two different mechanisms. Adding IFN-γ to *C. burnetii*-infected monocytes stimulates phagosome-lysosome fusion, but does not affect vacuolar pH. Surprisingly, the treatment of monocytes by IFN-γ prior *C. burnetii* infection induces the alkalinization of *C. burnetii* vacuoles independently of the V-H$^+$-ATPase exclusion,[69] whereas IFN-γ has been reported to decrease the pH of *Mycobacterium*-containing phagosomes[85] and to rescue phagosome conversion.[86] IFN-β also induces the alkalinization of the trans-Golgi network by inhibiting V-H$^+$-ATPase activity.[87] The mechanism of vesicle alkalinization mediated by IFN-γ- is still unknown. It has been shown that IFN-γ inhibits the remodeling of *Legionella*-harboring phagosomes into endoplasmic reticulum-derived vesicles.[78] The production of IFN-γ by patients with acute Q fever is likely sufficient to control *C. burnetii* infection through phagosome-lysosome fusion.[54,69]

IL-10 is overproduced during chronic Q fever.[52,53] Monocytes from patients with chronic Q fever are unable to kill *C. burnetii* and exhibit a defective phagosome conversion.[54] In contrast, monocytes from convalescent patients recovering from acute Q fever efficiently kill *C. burnetii* with a normal phagosome conversion. The microbicidal defect observed in monocytes from patients with chronic Q fever is not constitutive, since other pathogens such as *L. pneumophila* are eliminated by monocytes. It is related to the activity of the disease, since *C. burnetii* killing and phagosome-lysosome fusion are restored in patients who have recovered from Q fever endocarditis. Interestingly, *C. burnetii* killing by monocytes and phagosome conversion are modulated by IL-10. The neutralization by specific antibodies of IL-10 in monocytes from patients with chronic Q fever increases *C. burnetii* killing and rescues phagosome conversion to the levels found in cured patients. In contrast, adding recombinant IL-10 to monocytes from patients with cured Q fever endocarditis prevents *C. burnetii* killing and induces phagosome conversion blockage.[54] IL-10 is also known to decrease the expression of cathepsin D in monocytes from patients with inflammatory bowel disease[88] and affect fluid-phase and mannose receptor-mediated endocytosis in human primary macrophages.[89] Finally, the conversion of phagosomes containing mycobacteria is improved in macrophages isolated from IL-10 deficient mice.[90]

Concluding Remarks

The pathogenicity of *C. burnetii* organisms is related to their ability to persist within myeloid cells by circumventing immune host defense responses and hijacking phagosome conversion. The analysis of the bacterial factors and host cell receptors involved in the invasion process and the relationship between immune response and endocytic network may help to understand the downstream steps of *C. burnetii* infection.

Conflicts of Interest

The authors declare no conflicts of interest.

References

1. Raoult, D., T. Marrie & J. Mege. 2005. Natural history and pathophysiology of Q fever. *Lancet Infect. Dis.* **5:** 219–226.
2. Harris, R.J. *et al.* 2000. Long-term persistence of Coxiella burnetii in the host after primary Q fever. *Epidemiol. Infect.* **124:** 543–549.
3. Maurin, M. & D. Raoult. 1999. Q fever. *Clin. Microbiol. Rev.* **12:** 518–553.
4. Regis, E. 1999. *The Biology of Doom: The History of America's Secret Germ Warfare Project.* New York.
5. Madariaga, M.G. *et al.* 2003. Q fever: a biological weapon in your backyard. *Lancet Infect. Dis.* **3:** 709–721.
6. Baca, O.G., Y.P. Li & H. Kumar. 1994. Survival of the Q fever agent *Coxiella burnetii* in the phagolysosome. *Trends Microbiol.* **2:** 476–480.
7. Willems, H., C. Jager & G. Baljer. 1998. Physical and genetic map of the obligate intracellular bacterium *Coxiella burnetii. J. Bacteriol.* **180:** 3816–3822.

8. Beare, P.A. *et al*. 2006. Genetic diversity of the Q fever agent, Coxiella burnetii, assessed by microarray-based whole-genome comparisons. *J. Bacteriol.* **188:** 2309–2324.

9. Mallavia, L.P. 1991. Genetics of rickettsiae. *Eur. J. Epidemiol.* **7:** 213–221.

10. Valkova, D. & J. Kazar. 1995. A new plasmid (QpDV) common to Coxiella burnetii isolates associated with acute and chronic Q fever. *FEMS Microbiol. Lett.* **125:** 275–280.

11. Glazunova, O. *et al*. 2005. *Coxiella burnetii* genotyping. *Emerg. Infect. Dis.* **11:** 1211–1217.

12. Thiele, D. & H. Willems. 1994. Is plasmid based differentiation of Coxiella burnetii in 'acute' and 'chronic' isolates still valid? *Eur. J. Epidemiol.* **10:** 427–434.

13. Zamboni, D.S. *et al*. 2004. Stimulation of toll-like receptor 2 by Coxiella burnetii is required for macrophage production of pro-inflammatory cytokines and resistance to infection. *J. Biol. Chem.* **279:** 54405–54415.

14. Toman, R. *et al*. 2003. Structural properties of lipopolysaccharides from Coxiella burnetii strains Henzerling and S. *Ann. N. Y. Acad. Sci.* **990:** 563–567.

15. Hackstadt, T. *et al*. 1985. Lipopolysaccharide variation in Coxiella burnetti: intrastrain heterogeneity in structure and antigenicity. *Infect. Immun.* **48:** 359–365.

16. Thompson, H.A. *et al*. 2003. Do chromosomal deletions in the lipopolysaccharide biosynthetic regions explain all cases of phase variation in Coxiella burnetii strains? An update. *Ann. N. Y. Acad. Sci.* **990:** 664–670.

17. Seshadri, R. *et al*. 2003. Complete genome sequence of the Q-fever pathogen Coxiella burnetii. *Proc. Natl. Acad. Sci. U.S.A.* **100:** 5455–5460.

18. Capo, C. *et al*. 1999. Subversion of monocyte functions by *Coxiella burnetii*: impairment of the cross-talk between alphavbeta3 integrin and CR3. *J. Immunol.* **163:** 6078–6085.

19. Meconi, S. *et al*. 1998. *Coxiella burnetii* induces reorganization of the actin cytoskeleton in human monocytes. *Infect. Immun.* **66:** 5527–5533.

20. Baca, O.G. *et al*. 1993. Acid phosphatase activity in *Coxiella burnetii*: a possible virulence factor. *Infect. Immun.* **61:** 4232–4239.

21. Cianciotto, N.P. 2001. Pathogenicity of Legionella pneumophila. *Int. J. Med. Microbiol.* **291:** 331–343.

22. Baca, O.G. & L.P. Mallavia. 1997. The identification of virulence factors of *Coxiella burnetii*. In *Rickettsial infection and immunity*. B. Anderson, H.F. & M. Bendinelli, Eds.: 131–147. Plenum Press. New York, NY.

23. Segal, G. & H.A. Shuman. 1999. Possible origin of the Legionella pneumophila virulence genes and their relation to Coxiella burnetii. *Mol. Microbiol.* **33:** 669–670.

24. Zamboni, D.S. *et al*. 2003. Coxiella burnetii express type IV secretion system proteins that function similarly to components of the Legionella pneumophila Dot/Icm system. *Mol. Microbiol.* **49:** 965–976.

25. Zusman, T., G. Yerushalmi & G. Segal. 2003. Functional similarities between the icm/dot pathogenesis systems of Coxiella burnetii and Legionella pneumophila. *Infect. Immun.* **71:** 3714–3723.

26. Taylor, P.R. *et al*. 2005. Macrophage receptors and immune recognition. *Annu. Rev. Immunol.* **23:** 901–944.

27. Vetvicka, V., B.P. Thornton & G.D. Ross. 1996. Soluble beta-glucan polysaccharide binding to the lectin site of neutrophil or natural killer cell complement receptor type 3 (CD11b/CD18) generates a primed state of the receptor capable of mediating cytotoxicity of iC3b-opsonized target cells. *J. Clin. Invest.* **98:** 50–61.

28. Stuart, L.M. & R.A. Ezekowitz. 2005. Phagocytosis: elegant complexity. *Immunity* **22:** 539–550.

29. Agramonte-Hevia, J. *et al*. 2002. Gram-negative bacteria and phagocytic cell interaction mediated by complement receptor 3. *FEMS Immunol. Med. Microbiol.* **34:** 255–266.

30. Sussmuth, S.D. *et al*. 2000. Aggregation substance promotes adherence, phagocytosis, and intracellular survival of Enterococcus faecalis within human macrophages and suppresses respiratory burst. *Infect. Immun.* **68:** 4900–4906.

31. Hirsch, C.S. *et al*. 1994. Enhancement of intracellular growth of *Mycobacterium tuberculosis* in human monocytes by transforming growth factor-beta 1. *J. Infect. Dis.* **170:** 1229–1237.

32. Hu, C. *et al*. 2000. Mycobacterium tuberculosis infection in complement receptor 3-deficient mice. *J. Immunol.* **165:** 2596–2602.

33. Capo, C. *et al*. 2003. Coxiella burnetii avoids macrophage phagocytosis by interfering with spatial distribution of complement receptor 3. *J. Immunol.* **170:** 4217–4225.

34. Meconi, S. *et al*. 2001. Activation of protein tyrosine kinases by *Coxiella burnetii*: role in actin cytoskeleton reorganization and bacterial phagocytosis. *Infect. Immun.* **69:** 2520–2526.

35. Cossart, P. & P.J. Sansonetti. 2004. Bacterial invasion: the paradigms of enteroinvasive pathogens. *Science* **304:** 242–248.

36. Patil, S. *et al*. 1999. Identification of a talin-binding site in the integrin beta(3) subunit distinct from the NPLY regulatory motif of post-ligand binding functions. The talin n-terminal head domain interacts with the membrane-proximal region of the beta(3) cytoplasmic tail. *J. Biol. Chem.* **274:** 28575–28583.

37. Underhill, D.M. 2004. Toll-like receptors and microbes take aim at each other. *Curr. Opin. Immunol.* **16:** 483–487.

38. Medzhitov, R. 2001. Toll-like receptors and innate immunity. *Nat. Rev. Immunol.* **1:** 135–145.

39. Honstettre, A. *et al.* 2004. Lipopolysaccharide from Coxiella burnetii is involved in bacterial phagocytosis, filamentous actin reorganization, and inflammatory responses through Toll-like receptor 4. *J. Immunol.* **172:** 3695–3703.

40. West, M.A. *et al.* 2004. Enhanced dendritic cell antigen capture via toll-like receptor-induced actin remodeling. *Science* **305:** 1153–1157.

41. Abel, B. *et al.* 2002. Toll-like receptor 4 expression is required to control chronic Mycobacterium tuberculosis infection in mice. *J. Immunol.* **169:** 3155–3162.

42. Meghari, S. *et al.* 2005. TLR2 is necessary to inflammatory response in Coxiella burnetii infection. *Ann. N. Y. Acad. Sci.* **1063:** 161–166.

43. Sabatier, F. *et al.* 1997. CD4+ T-cell lymphopenia in Q fever endocarditis. *Clin. Diagn. Lab. Immunol.* **4:** 89–92.

44. Desnues, B. *et al.* 2008. Role of specific antibodies in Coxiella burnetii infection of macrophages. *C. M. I.* **in press**.

45. Dellacasagrande, J. *et al.* 2000. *Coxiella burnetii* survives in monocytes from patients with Q fever endocarditis: involvement of tumor necrosis factor. *Infect. Immun.* **68:** 160–164.

46. Meghari, S. *et al.* 2006. Deficient transendothelial migration of leukocytes in Q fever: the role played by interleukin-10. *J. Infect. Dis.* **194:** 365–369.

47. Meghari, S. *et al.* 2006. Coxiella burnetii stimulates production of RANTES and MCP-1 by mononuclear cells: modulation by adhesion to endothelial cells and its implication in Q fever. *Eur. Cytokine Netw.* **17:** 253–259.

48. Benoit, M. *et al.* 2008. *Coxiella burnetii*, the agent of Q fever, stimulates an atypical M2 activation program in human macrophages. *Eur. J. Immunol.*

49. Benoit, M. *et al.* 2008. The uptake of apoptotic cells drives Coxiella burnetii replication and macrophage polarization: a model for Q fever endocarditis. *PLoS Pathog.* **4:** e1000066.

50. Benoit, M., B. Desnues & J.L. Mege. 2008. Macrophage polarization in bacterial infections. *J. Immunol.* **181:** 3733–3739.

51. Mege, J.L. *et al.* 2006. The two faces of interleukin 10 in human infectious diseases. *Lancet Infect. Dis.* **6:** 557–569.

52. Capo, C. *et al.* 1996. Production of interleukin-10 and transforming growth factor beta by peripheral blood mononuclear cells in Q fever endocarditis. *Infect. Immun.* **64:** 4143–4147.

53. Honstettre, A. *et al.* 2003. Dysregulation of cytokines in acute Q fever: role of interleukin-10 and tumor necrosis factor in chronic evolution of Q fever. *J. Infect. Dis.* **187:** 956–962.

54. Ghigo, E. *et al.* 2004. Link between impaired maturation of phagosomes and defective Coxiella burnetii killing in patients with chronic Q fever. *J. Infect. Dis.* **190:** 1767–1772.

55. Meghari, S. *et al.* 2008. Persistent *Coxiella burnetii* Infection in Mice Overexpressing IL-10: An Efficient Model for Chronic Q Fever Pathogenesis. *PLoS Pathog.* **4:** e23.

56. Henry, R.M. *et al.* 2004. The uniformity of phagosome maturation in macrophages. *J. Cell Biol.* **164:** 185–194.

57. Scott, C.C., R.J. Botelho & S. Grinstein. 2003. Phagosome maturation: a few bugs in the system. *J. Membr. Biol.* **193:** 137–152.

58. Alonso, A. & F. Garcia-del Portillo. 2004. Hijacking of eukaryotic functions by intracellular bacterial pathogens. *Int. Microbiol.* **7:** 181–191.

59. Meresse, S. *et al.* 1999. Controlling the maturation of pathogen-containing vacuoles: a matter of life and death. *Nat. Cell Biol.* **1:** E183–188.

60. Rohde, K. *et al.* 2007. Mycobacterium tuberculosis and the environment within the phagosome. *Immunol. Rev.* **219:** 37–54.

61. Holden, D.W. 2002. Trafficking of the Salmonella vacuole in macrophages. *Traffic* **3:** 161–169.

62. Akporiaye, E.T. *et al.* 1983. Lysosomal response of a murine macrophage-like cell line persistently infected with *Coxiella burnetii*. *Infect. Immun.* **40:** 1155–1162.

63. Chen, S.Y. *et al.* 1990. Isolated *Coxiella burnetii* synthesizes DNA during acid activation in the absence of host cells. *J. Gen. Microbiol.* **136:** 89–96.

64. Hackstadt, T. & J.C. Williams. 1981. Biochemical stratagem for obligate parasitism of eukaryotic cells by *Coxiella burnetii*. *Proc. Natl. Acad. Sci. USA* **78:** 3240–3244.

65. Heinzen, R.A. *et al.* 1996. Differential interaction with endocytic and exocytic pathways distinguish parasitophorous vacuoles of *Coxiella burnetii* and *Chlamydia trachomatis*. *Infect. Immun.* **64:** 796–809.

66. Maurin, M. *et al.* 1992. Phagolysosomes of *Coxiella burnetii*-infected cell lines maintain an acidic pH during persistent infection. *Infect. Immun.* **60:** 5013–5016.

67. Howe, D. & L.P. Mallavia. 2000. *Coxiella burnetii* exhibits morphological change and delays phagolysosomal fusion after internalization by J774A.1 cells. *Infect. Immun.* **68:** 3815–3821.

68. Beron, W. *et al.* 2002. Coxiella burnetii localizes in a Rab7-labeled compartment with autophagic characteristics. *Infect. Immun.* **70:** 5816–5821.

69. Ghigo, E. *et al.* 2002. Coxiella burnetii survival in THP-1 monocytes involves the impairment of phagosome maturation: IFN-gamma mediates its restoration and bacterial killing. *J. Immunol.* **169:** 4488–4495.

70. Ghigo, E. *et al.* 2006. Intracellular life of *Coxiella burnetii* in macrophages : Insight into Q fever immunopathology. *Curr. Immunol. Rev.* **2:** 225–232.

71. Desjardins, M. *et al.* 1994. Molecular characterization of phagosomes. *J. Biol. Chem.* **269:** 32194–32200.

72. Rink, J. *et al.* 2005. Rab conversion as a mechanism of progression from early to late endosomes. *Cell* **122:** 735–749.

73. Meresse, S. *et al.* 1999. The rab7 GTPase controls the maturation of Salmonella typhimurium-containing vacuoles in HeLa cells. *Embo J.* **18:** 4394–4403.

74. Zerial, M. & H. McBride. 2001. Rab proteins as membrane organizers. *Nat. Rev. Mol. Cell Biol.* **2:** 107–117.

75. Bucci, C. *et al.* 2000. Rab7: a key to lysosome biogenesis. *Mol. Biol. Cell.* **11:** 467–480.

76. Yates, R.M. & D.G. Russell. 2005. Phagosome maturation proceeds independently of stimulation of toll-like receptors 2 and 4. *Immunity.* **23:** 409–417.

77. Blander, J.M. & R. Medzhitov. 2004. Regulation of phagosome maturation by signals from toll-like receptors. *Science* **304:** 1014–1018.

78. Santic, M., M. Molmeret & Y. Abu Kwaik. 2005. Maturation of the Legionella pneumophila-containing phagosome into a phagolysosome within gamma interferon-activated macrophages. *Infect. Immun.* **73:** 3166–3171.

79. Koster, F.T., J.C. Williams & J.S. Goodwin. 1985. Cellular immunity in Q fever: specific lymphocyte unresponsiveness in Q fever endocarditis. *J. Infect. Dis.* **152:** 1283–1289.

80. Izzo, A.A. & B.P. Marmion. 1993. Variation in interferon-gamma responses to *Coxiella burnetii* antigens with lymphocytes from vaccinated or naturally infected subjects. *Clin. Exp. Immunol.* **94:** 507–515.

81. Park, D.R. & S.J. Skerrett. 1996. IL-10 enhances the growth of *Legionella pneumophila* in human mononuclear phagocytes and reverses the protective effect of IFN-gamma: differential responses of blood monocytes and alveolar macrophages. *J. Immunol.* **157:** 2528–2538.

82. Blauer, F. *et al.* 1995. Modulation of the antilisterial activity of human blood-derived macrophages by activating and deactivating cytokines. *J. Interferon Cytokine Res.* **15:** 105–114.

83. Ghigo, E. *et al.* 2001. Interleukin-10 stimulates *Coxiella burnetii* replication in human monocytes through tumor necrosis factor down-modulation: Role in microbicidal defect of Q fever. *Infect. Immun.* **69:** 2345–2352.

84. Dellacasagrande, J. *et al.* 1999. IFN-gamma-mediated control of *Coxiella burnetii* survival in monocytes: the role of cell apoptosis and TNF. *J. Immunol.* **162:** 2259–2265.

85. Schaible, U.E. *et al.* 1998. Cytokine activation leads to acidification and increases maturation of *Mycobacterium avium*-containing phagosomes in murine macrophages. *J. Immunol.* **160:** 1290–1296.

86. Tsang, A.W. *et al.* 2000. Altered membrane trafficking in activated bone marrow-derived macrophages. *J. Leukoc. Biol.* **68:** 487–494.

87. Sidhu, G.S. *et al.* 1999. Role of vacuolar H(+)-ATPase in interferon-induced inhibition of viral glycoprotein transport. *J. Interferon Cytokine Res.* **19:** 1297–1303.

88. Lugering, N. *et al.* 1998. IL-10 synergizes with IL-4 and IL-13 in inhibiting lysosomal enzyme secretion by human monocytes and lamina propria mononuclear cells from patients with inflammatory bowel disease. *Dig. Dis. Sci.* **43:** 706–714.

89. Montaner, L.J. *et al.* 1999. Type 1 and type 2 cytokine regulation of macrophage endocytosis: differential activation by IL-4/IL-13 as opposed to IFN-gamma or IL-10. *J. Immunol.* **162:** 4606–4613.

90. Via, L.E. *et al.* 1998. Effects of cytokines on mycobacterial phagosome maturation. *J. Cell Sci.* **111:** 897–905.

Coxiella burnetii Glycomics and Proteomics—Tools for Linking Structure to Function

Rudolf Toman, Ludovit Skultety, and Robert Ihnatko

Laboratory for Diagnosis and Prevention of Rickettsial and Chlamydial Infections, Institute of Virology, Slovak Academy of Sciences, 845 05 Bratislava, Slovakia

Coxiella burnetii, the causative agent of Q fever, is an obligate intracellular bacterium and a highly infectious pathogen. The disease is a widespread zoonosis and is endemic throughout the world. An easy aerosol dissemination, environmental persistence, and high infectivity make the bacterium a serious threat for humans and animals. Lipopolysaccharide is considered one of the major factors of virulence expression and infection of the bacterium. Detailed glycomic studies enabled to better understand structural and functional peculiarities of this biopolymer and its role in pathogenesis and immunity of Q fever. Recent proteomic studies of *C. burnetii* have brought new approaches in accurate detection of the infectious agent and offered new insights into the inter- or intra-species relatedness. Thus, structure/function relationship studies are currently of utmost importance in the field. This paper will focus on glycomic and proteomic approaches providing information on unique glycan and protein species of the microorganism as the candidate molecules for the use in detection/diagnosis, therapy, and prophylaxis.

Key words: *Coxiella burnetii*; glycomics; proteomics; Q fever

Introduction

Coxiella burnetii is an obligate intracellular, highly pleomorphic bacterium. It is extremely infectious and causes Q fever, a zoonotic disease, which is capable of being transmitted from animals to humans.[1,2] In humans, the most common acute form of Q fever is manifested[1] as a self-limited febrile illness or pneumonia, or less frequently as hepatitis. Persistent infection in humans can lead to a chronic form of Q fever, which may be associated with a fatal endocarditis.[1] In animals, Q fever affects livestock and is associated with pneumonia and reproductive disorders in livestock, with abortion, stillbirth, placentitis, endometritis, and infertility.[2]

It is well known that lipopolysaccharides (LPSs) and proteins of *C. burnetii* are of particular biological, immunological, and medical significance. Glycomics and proteomics have already demonstrated their immense potential for getting significantly deeper insight into the functional interaction of LPSs and proteins and their roles not only in growth and development of the microorganism, but also in pathogenesis and immunity of Q fever. This review is an attempt to summarize the current knowledge in these fields.

Glycomics of C. Burnetii

Like other gram-negative bacteria, *C. burnetii* expresses at its surface various amphophilic macromolecules among which LPSs were shown to play a crucial role in host-pathogen interactions.[3] Upon serial laboratory

Address for correspondence: Rudolf Toman, Institute of Virology, Slovak Academy of Sciences, Dubravska cesta 9, 845 05 Bratislava, Slovak Republic. Voice: +421-2-59302418; fax: +421-2-54774284. virutoma@savba.sk

Rickettsiology and Rickettsial Diseases-Fifth International Conference: Ann. N.Y. Acad. Sci. 1166: 67–78 (2009).
doi: 10.1111/j.1749-6632.2009.04512.x © 2009 New York Academy of Sciences.

passages in yolk sacs of embryonated hen eggs, the bacterium undergoes a virulent (phase I) to avirulent (phase II) variation.[3] This is accompanied by modifications in both composition and structure of the LPS macromolecule.[3-5] In phase I, *C. burnetii* biosynthesizes smooth (S) LPS I with O-specific chain whereas in phase II, it synthesizes rough (R) LPS II.[4] This phase variation was assumed[6] to resemble in many aspects the well-known smooth-to-rough variation found with many gram-negative bacteria. It was proposed[7] that LPS I reduces gradually its O-polysaccharide chain during the phase variation and a deep (R) LPS II is present in the outer membrane of the *C. burnetii* cell in phase II. When mapping the O-antigen biosynthesis region in the phase II Nine Mile strain, a large group of the genes was deleted.[8,9] However, some phase II isolates contained no apparent deletions.[9]

LPS molecules extracted from any (S) strain of gram-negative bacteria are heterogeneous in size. They may include some (R) LPS and in some cases variously truncated LPS molecules.[10] Thus, it can be assumed that strains/isolates of gram-negative bacteria contain cell populations that may express multiple LPS structures. The similar phenomenon was also observed[5] in LPSs isolated during serial passage of *C. burnetii* in embryonated hen eggs. It was suggested that a redistribution of the existing LPS populations took place due to an increasing prevalence of those cells in the whole cell population that express LPS molecules with truncated O-chains and those being of (R) type. At present, however, the molecular mechanisms influencing LPS modifications during the *C. burnetii* phase variation remain unclear.

Further studies are necessary in this direction, and in addition, there is a need to better characterize the relatively poorly understood *C. burnetii* LPS I (see below) in relation to its various biological activities. In this connection, a more detailed knowledge of its chemical structure is required.

Chemical Composition and Structural Features of LPS I

It has been established[6,11,12] that LPS I contains, in addition to the sugar residues found in LPS II and some frequently occuring sugars, two unusual sugar units in its O-polysaccharide chain, namely virenose (Vir, 6-deoxy-3-C-methyl-D-gulopyranose) and dihydrohydroxystreptose (Strep, 3-C-[hydroxymethyl]-L-lyxofuranose). Both sugars have not been found in other enterobacterial LPSs and are considered unique biomarkers of *C. burnetii*. Recently, candidate genes that might be involved in the synthesis of Vir and Strep have been suggested[8,13] and their protein products NDP-hexose 3-C-methyltransferase TylCIII (CBU 0691) and methyltransferase FkbM family (CBU 0683) were identified by proteomic analysis.[14] In addition, a unique galactosaminuronyl-α-$(1 \rightarrow 6)$-glucosamine disaccharide was found[15] in the acid hydrolyzate of LPS I, but its location in the polymer chain was not established with certainty. The methylation-linkage analyses of two polysaccharide fractions of LPS I performed recently[16] revealed the presence of terminal Vir, Strep, and mannose (Man), 4-substituted Vir, 4-substituted Man, and 2,3- and 3,4-disubstituted D-*glycero*-D-*manno*-heptose (Hep). It could be anticipated from the previous studies[17] that two terminal Man, 2,3- and 3,4-disubstituted Hep were from the core region of LPS I and thus, other terminal and substituted sugars should be located in the O-polysaccharide chain. In previous works[6,11,12] it was suggested that Vir and Strep are located in terminal positions. However, these recent findings show that this is probably true only for Strep as Vir is also $(1 \rightarrow 4)$-linked.

The lipid A portion of LPS is linked to the core oligosaccharide mostly via 3-deoxy-D-*manno*-oct-2-ulosonic acid (Kdo) and serves as the hydrophobic anchor of LPS in the outer membrane.[18] It was suggested that lipid A, as the principal endotoxic component of LPS, plays a major role in the pathogenesis of

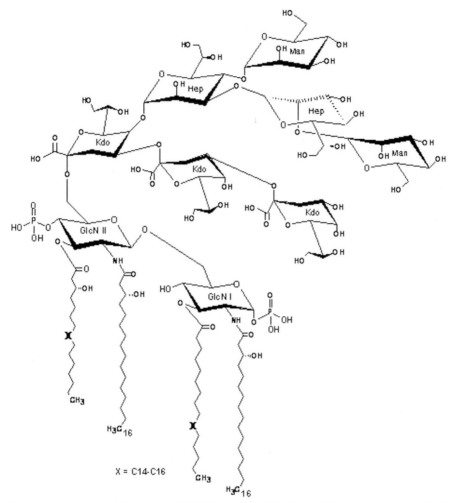

Figure 1. Structural features of LPS II from *Coxiella burnetii* in avirulent phase II. X is length of the acyl fatty acid chain. For abbreviations, see text.

bacterial infections and is an important contributor to massive inflammation, sepsis, and septic shock leading to fatalities in gram-negative bacteria infections.[18] It also promotes the activation of the innate immune system via induction of inflammatory cytokines released by human cells. We performed more detailed studies[19,20] on lipids A isolated from LPSs I of several strains of *C. burnetii* in virulent phase I. In the strain Priscilla, two major tetra-acylated molecular species were found[20] as the major components despite a considerable microheterogeneity of the lipid A. They shared the classical backbone of diphosphorylated glucosamine (GlcN) disaccharide, in which both reducing-end GlcN I and terminal GlcN II carried amide-linked iso-branched or normal (n) 3-hydroxyhexadecanoic fatty acids. One of the species had ester-linked n-hexadecanoic acids at both GlcNs while the other had ester-linked anteiso-branched pentadecanoic instead of n-hexadecanoic acid at GlcN II. In contrast with these studies, Zamboni and colleagues[21] proposed an asymmetrical structural model for the *C. burnetii* lipid A where a 3-acyloxyacyl chain, alternatively composed of 3-hydroxytetra- to hexadecanoic acids, is attached to the amide-linked 3-hydroxylated fatty acid at the N-2' of the GlcN II residue. However, our latest studies have shown (unpublished results) that lipids A isolated from LPS I and LPS II of the Nine Mile strain have similar structural features that resemble those published for the strain Priscilla.[20] This most recent chemical structure proposed for the lipid A is shown in Figure 1 as an integral part of the structural features of LPS II. It appears that like in other bacterial LPSs, lipid A represents the most conserved region of LPS of *C. burnetii*. Although the biochemical synthesis of lipid A is a highly conserved process, investigations of the lipid A structures of various bacteria and even the isolates of the same bacterium including *C. burnetii* show a noticeable diversity.[18] These differences can be attributed to the activities of enzymes, which are up- or down-regulated by environmental stresses or other extracellular factors and may modify the canonical lipid A molecule. Variation of the lipid A domain of LPS serves as one strategy utilized[18] by gram-negative bacteria to promote survival by providing resistance to components of the innate immune system and helping to evade recognition by Toll-like receptor 4 (TLR4).

The composition and structure of lipid A of *C. burnetii* differs considerably from those published[18] for the classical form of enterobacterial lipid A with high endotoxicity found; e.g., in *Escherichia coli* or *Neisseria meningitidis*. Thus, distinct structural features of the *C. burnetii* lipid A could be the reason for its reduced endotoxic potency in comparison with the enterobacterial lipids A. However, *C. burnetii* and its LPS have been shown to exhibit various immunomodulating activities despite their low endotoxic activity (see below). This fact can now be well understood by applying the previously presented conformational concept of endotoxicity,[22] a conical shape of the lipid A of *C. burnetii* and a sufficiently high inclination of the sugar backbone plane with respect to the membrane.[20]

Chemical Composition and Structural Features of LPS II

Both compositional and structural studies of LPS II produced a controversy in the past. This

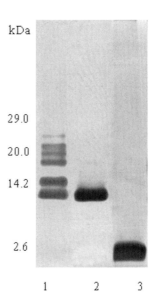

Figure 2. SDS-PAGE silver stain of LPSs of *C. burnetii*. LPS I, LPS Cr, and LPS II from lanes 1 to 3, respectively. For abbreviations, see text.

subject has been reviewed[4] by Toman recently. Man, Hep, and Kdo were found[17] to be the constituent sugars of the lipid A proximal region in a molar ratio 2: 2: 3 with the linkages depicted in Figure 1. As mentioned before, the structure of lipid A moiety reflects our recent findings in the field. The nonhydroxylated tetra- to hexadecanoic fatty acids are attached to O-3 of GlcN I while 3-hydroxytetra- to hexadecanoic fatty acids are linked to O-3′ of GlcN II. The two 3-hydroxyhexadecanoic acids are amide-linked to GlcN I and GlcN II, as suggested[20] previously.

Most recently, we have performed initial studies[23] on the chemical composition and structure of an LPS isolated from the *C. burnetii* strain Nine Mile, variant "Crazy" (Cr) that was together with the phase II variant investigated[8] in a considerable detail by the methods of molecular biology. In contrast to LPS I and LPS II, LPS Cr gave one band at about 14 kDa on SDS-PAGE (Fig. 2). Sugar analysis revealed the presence of Man, Glc, Hep, Strep, and GlcN in the molar ratio 3.1: 0.1: 1.0: 1.5: 1.2, respectively. No Vir was found. The matrix-assisted laser desorption/ionization mass spectrometry (MALDI-MS) analyses of lipid A indicated chemical structure similar to that found in LPS I and LPS II (Fig. 1). The truncated LPS II structure was shown to be a result of large chromosomal DNA deletions in the phase II cells of strain Nine Mile.[8] Deletions in the variant Cr were larger, extending on both ends beyond the phase II deletion junctions. However, both chemical composition and structural features of LPS Cr are more complex than those of LPS II. The reason for this discrepancy remains unknown.

Some Functional Characteristics of LPS

Phase variation of *C. burnetii* has a direct impact on the serological diagnosis of Q fever. During acute Q fever, *C. burnetii* induces antibodies against phase II (protein antigens), while in the later stages of the disease, and especially in its chronic form, the high titers of antibodies are directed against phase I (LPS I antigen).[1] Investigations focused on the immunoreactive proteins that might be involved in diagnosing Q fever are in progress.[24–27] Similarly, some work has already been performed[16] toward elucidation of interaction of phase I antibodies with the LPS I antigen. A remarkable decrease in the serological activity of the O-polysaccharide antigen was observed when terminal Vir and Strep were selectively removed from its chain.[16] At present, however, it is not known with certainty whether the immunoreactive epitopes are located only at both sugars in terminal positions or also at those Vir residues located in the O-polysaccharide backbone.

The unique *C. burnetii* biomarkers Vir and Strep could be used in the future for rapid, sensitive, and unambiguous detection of *C. burnetii* and differentiation of its isolates/variants. Thus, a monoclonal antibody (IgG2b subclass) has been generated that is highly specific for the presence of Vir in the *C. burnetii* LPS.[28]

Tumor necrosis factor-α (TNF-α) is a pivotal cytokine in inflammation and is considered to be a main endogenous mediator of septic shock. It is a protein with a molecular mass of 17 kDa and is produced mainly by mononuclear phagocytes following induction with an LPS.[29] It has been found that TNF-α overproduction is involved[30] in the survival of *C. burnetii* inside the patient monocytes and may be related to specific inflammatory syndrome of Q fever endocarditis consisting of an increase in circulating TNF-α without variations in cytokine antagonist.[31] Although LPS I and LPS II are weak endotoxins, their ability to induce TNF-α has been reported.[20,30] It appears that the TNF-α production does not directly reflect the virulence of *C. burnetii* since avirulent bacteria were also shown to induce[32] TNF-α. In fact, avirulent bacteria in phase II were even more potent than virulent organisms at stimulating TNF-α production.[30] Since lipids A in LPS I and LPS II have similar chemical structures, there must be another reason for this phenomenon. It could be possible that presence or absence of the O-specific chain in these LPSs might play a role. One can also hypothesize that the overproduction of TNF-α stimulated by avirulent *C. burnetii* can be related to the increase in bacterial binding to monocytes since the interaction of avirulent variants with monocytes was much more efficient than that of virulent organisms.[33] Most recently, the strain-specific differences in the induction of TNF-α have been reported.[34] Using the bioassay system, the highest TNF-α production was observed with both the whole cells and LPSs of the *C. burnetii* strains Scurry and Priscilla. The former strain was suggested to be associated with chronic Q fever, and similarity of both strains has been supported by the recent multiple locus variable number tandem repeats analysis of the *C. burnetii* strains using the unweighted pair-group method, in which both strains were shown to be genetically very close.[35] In contrast, previous SDS-PAGE and immunoblot analyses of their LPSs indicated that these LPSs might be structurally and antigenically distinct.[36]

The development of protective immune response against *C. burnetii* requires coordination of the innate and adaptive immune responses. Toll-like receptors (TLRs) are essential for the recognition of distinct pathogen-associated molecular patterns.[37] TLR4 appears to be highly specific, and its interaction with an LPS initiates intracellular signal transduction across the cell membrane.[18] In contrast, TLR2 seems to be very promiscuous, responding to multiple bacterial products, including lipoproteins, lipoteichoic acid, and peptidoglycans.[38–40] It has been reported recently that LPSs of some bacterial species failed to activate TLR4 and that these bacteria activated host cells through a TLR2-dependent mechanism.[41–43] In the initial studies, Honstettre and colleagues[44] demonstrated that TLR4 was involved in the recognition of *C. burnetii* LPS, initial activation of macrophages, and inflammatory response associated with the *C. burnetii* infection. It was shown[21] later, however, that a purified lipid A from *C. burnetii* antagonized activation of TLR4 by the highly endotoxic lipids A from *Escherichia coli* and *Bordetella pertussis*, and by the *E. coli* LPS. A similar competitive inhibition of LPS activation of TLR4-dependent responses was reported for other lipids A, such as those isolated from *Rhodobacter sphaeroides* and lipid IV_A.[45] Since the chemical structure of the *C. burnetii* lipid A differs[20,21] considerably from those reported[18] for the classical enterobacterial lipids A that activate TLR4 but not TLR2, it was suggested[21] that stimulation of TLR2 by *C. burnetii* is required for macrophage production of pro-inflammatory cytokines and resistance to infection. Nevertheless, TLR2 stimulation by the *C. burnetii* LPS, either by LPS I or LPS II could not be proved unambiguously. From recent studies[46] in the field, it appears that both TLR2 and TLR4 are required for granuloma formation in *C. burnetii* infection. It is likely that TLR4 is involved in initial responses and TLR2 is implicated in sustained responses. Thus, a synergistic action of both TLRs has been suggested as they stimulate the same signal transduction pathways. A more detailed role of LPS I and LPS II in these events remains to be elucidated.

Proteomics of *C. burnetii*

Proteins are one of the most important parts of living systems the proper function of which is essential for many physiological metabolic pathways of organisms and cells. In most cases, proteins either interact with other proteins with regulatory function or form large molecular complexes to carry out biological processes. Identification of these interacting proteins is a base toward understanding the functions of individual proteins that are an integral part the overall proteome of organisms. The extensive study of proteins, their structures, and functions is the main subject of proteomics. Introduction of MS into the proteomic studies has brought a considerable improvement in the detection and analysis of proteins or components of protein complexes, mainly for its speed and sensitivity. The complete sequencing of *C. burnetii* genome[47] (strain Nine Mile; RSA493) brought new opportunities to obtain information about the proteome of *C. burnetii*, and also provided a shift toward better understanding the mechanisms involved in pathogenesis of this bacterium. Compared with *C. burnetii* genome, the information of which encodes more than 2000 coding sequences, the proteomic studies have identified about 200 nonredundant protein species in each phase I and II of *C. burnetii*. Thus, presently only a small percentage of entire proteome of *C. burnetii* is unraveled.

Since the magnitude of protein species abundance within bacterial cell may differ by 7 to 10 orders of magnitude, the relatively low abundant proteins are probably most masked by more abundant ones; e.g., housekeeping and structural ones. This makes it a little difficult to relate results of proteome profiling to the biology of the system. In order to gain a better understanding of the inner workings of the bacterium, initial pre-fractionation is needed to detect the low copy number proteins in the cells.

The initial studies[14,48] were focused on the identification of proteins of *C. burnetii* strain Nine Mile (in virulent phase I and II) that were resolved by 2-dimensional electrophoresis (2-DE) and liquid chromatography. Using peptide mass fingerprinting and various MALDI-, electrospray ionization (ESI) tandem mass spectrometry (MS/MS) approaches, about 200 products of the *C. burnetii* open reading frames were identified in the whole cell lysates in each of both phases of *C. burnetii*. The function of each identified protein was then predicted, and extensive bioinformatic analyses were performed. Due to space limitations of this short review, we will focus only on some identified proteins with potential function in pathogenesis and live cycle of the bacterium.

The Tol proteins are located in the cell envelope of gram-negative bacteria and are probably involved in the integration of some outer membrane components such as porins or LPSs.[49–51] In *E. coli*, the TolB was also found cross-linked to the outer membrane peptidoglycan-associated proteins such as Lpp and OmpA.[52] The Tol-Pal protein complex probably links the peptidoglycan to the outer membrane, and in this way, it efficiently stabilizes the cell envelope integrity.[53] The Tol-Pal system is formed by TolQ, TolR, and TolA proteins located in the inner membrane, the periplasmic TolB, and the outer membrane Pal lipoprotein. The experiments using Tol-Pal mutants revealed that any defect in the Tol-Pal proteins or in the major lipoprotein Lpp causes a loss of the outer membrane integrity leading to hypersensitivity to drugs and detergents, periplasmic leakage, and outer membrane vesicle formation.[51,54,55] The TolB precursor (CBU_0090) and the Tol system periplasmic component (CBU_0092) were found in both phases of *C. burnetii*,[14,48] and thus a similar function of Tol-Pal system as that mentioned above could be expected in pathogenesis of *C. burnetii*.

In bacterial resistance, the outer membrane of gram-negative bacterium provides only a weak barrier. The bacteria need additional mechanisms to pump out toxins to achieve resistance. In this process, the protein pumps belonging to the resistance-nodulation-division family together with the outer membrane channels are highly efficient.[56] The AcrB pump of *E. coli* can serve as an example in forming a complex with AcrA and the outer membrane channel TolC. This complex eliminates some antibiotics, detergents, and various disinfectants from the inside of bacteria.[57–60] The AcrB/AcrD/AcrF transporter family protein (CBU_0804) was found in *C. burnetii*.[14]

As the proliferation of *C. burnetii* is executed within the harsh environmental condition of phagolysosome, the bacterium expresses proteins with the capacity to protect itself from the proteolytic attack. Several proteins with such a function were identified in proteomic studies[14,48] until now. Thus, the protective function of superoxide dismutase (CBU_1708) against hyperoxides has been well documented[61,62] earlier. The AhpC/Tsa family protein (CBU_1706) and peroxiredoxins (as the bacterioferritin comigratory protein, CBU_0963) are similarly highly effective antioxidant defense proteins[63] catalyzing the reduction of hydrogen peroxide, organic hyperoxides, and peroxonitrites, which are the reactive oxygen species often present within the phagolysosomal environment. Additional proteins like the stringent starvation protein A (CBU_1747), which is a highly conserved transcription factor among gram-negative bacteria and is essential for acid tolerance,[64,65] and two proteins CBU_1983 and CBU_1916 that belong to the universal stress protein A superfamily are being upregulated by a wide variety of stress conditions; e.g., nutrient starvation or exposure to oxidants[66] were found in *C. burnetii*.[48]

In pathogenesis of *C. burnetii*, the proteins that are involved in the processes of pathogen entry into the host cells are of high importance. The enhanced entry proteins B and C (CBU_1137 and CBU_1136), and a Mip precursor (CBU_0630) have been identified[14,48] thus far. The peptidyl-prolyl cis-trans isomerase (PPIase) Mip exhibits PPIase-activity, the intact active site of which was shown to be essential for an early establishment and initiation

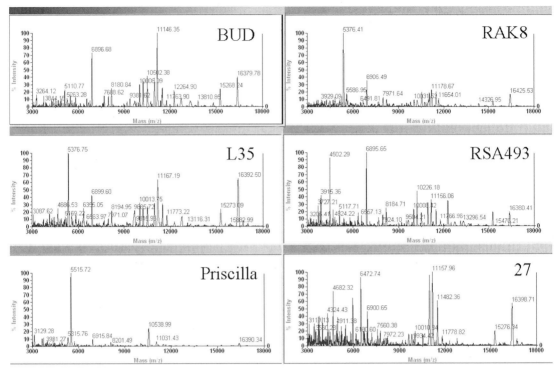

Figure 3. Representative linear MALDI- time of flight – MS profiles of the acetonitrile extracts of *C. burnetii* isolates BUD, RAK8, L35, RSA 493, Priscilla, and 27 acquired in the positive ion mode.

of intracellular infection of the closely related *Legionella pneumophila*.[67] Moreover, when the *C. burnetii* gene encoding Mip protein was cloned to *E. coli*, the overproduced *C. burnetii* protein also exhibited the PPIase activity.[68]

It has been shown[69] recently that *C. burnetii* expresses type IV secretion system proteins, the function of which is similar to the components of the *L. pneumophila* Dot/Icm system. The DotB protein (CBU_1645) as a secretion system IV component with the ATPase activity was found[48] in *C. burnetii*. It was suggested that it may play an important role in creating the specialized vacuole that supports replication of *C. burnetii*.[69] The turnover of peptidoglycan in a bacterium is highly controlled involving a complement of autolytic enzymes with specificity for either the carbohydrate or the peptide linkages of peptidoglycan. One major class of these autolysins represents N-acetylmuramoyl-L-alanine amidases that cleave the amide linkage between the stem peptides and the lactyl moiety of muramoyl residues. Therefore, the enzymatic function of *N*-acetylmuramoyl-L-alanine amidase (CBU_0379) will presumably play an important role in the process of peptidoglycan turnover in both cell phases of *C. burnetii*, although it has been found[48] in phase II cells thus far.

Analysis of the Developmental Forms of *C. Burnetii*

It is well known that *C. burnetii* undergoes a developmental cycle that generates the small-cell variants (SCV) and the replicative large cell variants (LCV). Both developmental forms were separated by 2-DE approach followed by MALDI-MS analysis.[70] Forty-eight proteins were differentially expressed in LCV when compared to SCV. Fifteen of them were analyzed by MS. Each of these proteins was involved in the cell division, RNA, and protein synthesis or processing. This result is in agreement with a well-known higher metabolic activity of LCV compared to SCV.

Detection of Specific Spectral Markers by Mass Spectrometry

Rapid and reliable detection, identification, and typing of bacterial species are necessary in response to natural or terrorist-caused outbreaks of infectious diseases and play crucial roles in diagnosis and efficient treatment. Various serological methods are currently used[1,2] for diagnosis of Q fever but ambiguous results have been obtained in several cases. Recently, diagnostic methods based on polymerase chain reaction have radically improved detection[2] of the infectious agent and diagnosing the disease. Implementation of mass spectrometry may also substantially contribute to a progress, especially in discrimination of *C. burnetii* strains/isolates. Currently, only few works have been focused on the determination and identification of specific *C. burnetii* biomarkers.[71–74] MALDI-MS analyses of intact bacterial cells and cell-free acetonitrile and trichloroacetic acid extracts have been applied to obtain characteristic and reproducible mass spectral fingerprints that contain unique biomarker profiles. This approach has recently been examined for typing of six *C. burnetii* isolates. In Figure 3, MS spectra of their acetonitrile extracts are depicted. Thus, it has been confirmed that the detection of specific spectral markers could be applied not only for detection of the bacterial pathogens, but also for their typing. These proteomic data might also be useful for some bacterial databases (MicrobeLynx, ProteinProfiler, Saramis) for rapid identification of the microbe.

In order to characterize specific *C. burnetii* proteins in a more detail, an ESI-MS/MS technique has been employed.[74] The MS/MS approach enabled identification of 63 distinct proteins in the acetonitrile extracts of *C. burnetii* strain RSA 493. Among them, 20 proteins that were observed in more than 3 out of 10 experiments were proposed as the *C. burnetii* biomarkers.

This paper reflects the authors' views on glycomic and proteomic studies on C. burnetii, providing information on unique glycan and protein species of the bacterium as the candidate molecules for the use in detection/diagnosis, therapy, and prophylaxis.

Acknowledgments

This work was supported in part by the Slovak Research and Development Agency, Slovak Republic, under the contract No. APVT-51-032804, and by grants No. 2/0127/09 and 2/0010/08 of the Scientific Grant Agency of Ministry of Education of the Slovak Republic and the Slovak Academy of Sciences.

Conflicts of Interest

The authors declare no conflicts of interest.

References

1. Marrie, T.J. & D. Raoult. 1997. Q fever – a review and issues for the next century. *J. Antimicrob. Agents* **8:** 145–161.
2. Arricau-Bouvery, N. & A. Rodolakis. 2005. Is Q fever an emerging or re-emerging zoonis? *Vet. Res.* **36:** 327–349.
3. Williams, J.C. & D.M. Waag. 1991. Antigens, virulence factors, and biological response modifiers of *Coxiella burnetii*: strategies for vaccine development. In *Q Fever: The Biology of Coxiella burnetii.* J.C. Williams & H.A. Thompson, Eds.: 175–222. CRC Press. Boca Raton, FL.
4. Toman, R. 1999. Lipopolysaccharides from virulent and low-virulent phases of *Coxiella burnetii*. In *Rickettsiae and Rickettsial Diseases at the Turn of the Third Millenium.* D. Raoult & P. Brouqui, Eds.: 84–91. Elsevier. Paris.
5. Ftacek, P., L. Skultety & R. Toman. 2000. Phase variation of *Coxiella burnetii* strain Priscilla: influence of this phenomenon on biochemical features of its lipopolysaccharide. *J. Endotoxin Res.* **6:** 369–376.
6. Mayer, H., J. Radziejewska-Lebrecht & S. Schramek. 1988. Chemical and immunochemical studies on lipopolysaccharides of *Coxiella burnetii* phase I and phase II. *Adv. Exp. Med. Biol.* **228:** 577–591.
7. Diaz, Q.M. & M. Lukacova. 1998. Immunological consequences of *Coxiella burnetii* phase variation. *Acta Virol.* **42:** 181–185.
8. Hoover, T.A. *et al.* 2002. Chromosomal DNA deletions explain phenotypic characteristics of two

antigenic variants, phase II and RSA 514 (Crazy), of the *Coxiella burnetii* Nine Mile strain. *Infect. Immun.* **70**: 6726–6733.

9. Denison, A.M., R.F. Massung & H.A. Thompson. 2007. Analysis of the O-antigen biosynthesis regions of phase II isolates of *C. burnetii. FEMS Microbiol. Lett.* **267**: 102–107.

10. Keenleyside, W. J. & C. Whitfield. 1999. Genetics and biosynthesis of lipopolysaccharide O-antigens. In *Endotoxin in Health and Disease.* H. Brade, S.M. Opal, S.N. Vogel & D.C. Morrison, Eds.: 331–358. Marcel Dekker. New York and Basel.

11. Skultety, L., R. Toman & V. Patoprsty. 1998. A comparative study of lipopolysaccharides from two *Coxiella burnetii* strains considered to be associated with acute and chronic Q fever. *Carbohyd. Polymers.* **35**: 189–194.

12. Toman, R. *et al.* 1998. NMR study of virenose and dihydrohydroxystreptose isolated from *Coxiella burnetii* phase I lipopolysaccharide. *Carbohyd. Res.* **306**: 291–296.

13. Thompson, H.A. *et al.* 2003. Do chromosomal deletions in the lipopolysaccharide biosynthetic regions explain all cases of phase variation in *Coxiella burnetii* strains? An update. *Ann. N.Y. Acad. Sci.* **990**: 664–670.

14. Skultety, L. *et al.* 2005. *Coxiella burnetii* whole cell lysate protein identification by mass spectrometry and tandem mass spectrometry. *Ann. N.Y. Acad. Sci.* **1063**: 115–122.

15. Amano, K. *et al.* 1987. Structure and biological relationships of *Coxiella burnetii* lipopolysaccharides. *J. Biol. Chem.* **262**: 4740–4747.

16. Vadovic, P. *et al.* 2005. Structural and functional characterization of the glycan antigens involved in immunobiology of Q fever. *Ann. N.Y. Acad. Sci.* **1063**: 149–153.

17. Toman, R. & L. Skultety. 1996. Structural study on a lipopolysaccharide from *Coxiella burnetii* strain Nine Mile in avirulent phase II. *Carbohydr. Res.* **283**: 175–185.

18. Alexander, C. & E.T. Rietschel. 2001. Bacterial lipopolysaccharides and innate immunity. *J. Endotoxin Res.* **7**: 167–202.

19. Toman, R. *et al.* 2003. Structural properties of lipopolysaccharides from *Coxiella burnetii* strains Henzerling and S. *Ann. N.Y. Acad. Sci.* **990**: 563–567.

20. Toman, R. *et al.* 2004. Physicochemical characterization of the endotoxins from *Coxiella burnetii* strain Priscilla in relation to their bioactivities. *BMC Biochem.* http://www.biomedcentral.com/1471-2091/5/1.

21. Zamboni, D.S. *et al.* 2004. Stimulation of toll-like receptor 2 by *Coxiella burnetii* is required for macrophage production of pro-inflammatory cytokines and resistance to infection. *J. Biol. Chem.* **279**: 54405–54415.

22. Seydel, U. *et al.* 1999. Biophysical view on the function and activity of endotoxins. In *Endotoxin in Health and Disease.* H. Brade, S.M. Opal, S.N. Vogel & D.C. Morrison, Eds.: 195–219. Marcel Dekker. New York and Basel.

23. Vadovic, P. *et al.* 2008. Structural studies of lipid A from the *Coxiella burnetii* strain Nine Mile, variant "Crazy". Presented at *5th International Meeting on Rickettsia and Rickettsial Diseases.* Marseille, France, May 18–20.

24. Zhang, G. *et al.* 2004. Identification and cloning of immunodominant antigens of *Coxiella burnetii.. Infect. Immun.* **72**: 844–852.

25. Zhang, G. *et al.* 2005. Identification and characterization of an immunodominant 28-kilodalton *Coxiella burnetii* outer membrane protein specific to isolates associated with acute disease. *Infect. Immun.* **73**: 1561–1567.

26. Beare, P.A. *et al.* 2008. Candidate Q fever serodiagnostic antigens revealed by immunoscreening a *Coxiella burnetii* protein microarray. *Clin. Vaccine Immunol.* **15**: 1771–1779.

27. Sekeyova, Z. *et al.* 2009. Identification of protein candidates for serodiagnosis of Q fever endocarditis by an immunoproteomic approach. *Eur. J. Clin. Microbiol. Infect. Dis.* **28**: 287–295.

28. Palkovicova, K. *et al.* 2008. A monoclonal antibody highly specific for lipopolysaccharides of *Coxiella burnetii* in virulent phase I. Presented at 5th *International Meeting on Rickettsia and Rickettsial Diseases.* Marseille, France, May 18–20.

29. Flebbe, L.M., S.K. Chapes & D.C. Morrison.1990. Activation of C3H/HeJ macrophage tumoricidal activity and cytokine release by R-chemotype lipopolysaccharide preparations. *J. Immunol.* **145**: 505–514.

30. Dellacasagrande, J. *et al.* 2000. $\alpha_v\beta_3$ Integrin and bacterial lipopolysaccharides are involved in *Coxiella burnetii*-stimulated production of tumor necrosis factor by human monocytes. *Infect. Immun.* **68**: 5673–5678.

31. Capo, C. *et al.* 1999. Circulating cytokine balance and activation markers of leucocytes in Q fever. *Clin. Exp. Immunol.* **115**: 120–123.

32. Tujulin, E. *et al.* 1999. Early cytokine induction in mouse P388D1 macrophages infected by *Coxiella burnetii. Vet. Immunol. Immunopathol.* **68**: 159–168.

33. Capo, C. *et al.* 1999. Subversion of monocyte functions by *Coxiella burnetii*: impairment of the cross-talk between alphavbeta3 integrin and CR3. *J. Immunol.* **163**: 6078–6085.

34. Kubes, M. *et al.* 2006. Induction of tumor necrosis factor alpha in murine macrophages with various strains of *Coxiella burnetii* and their lipopolysaccharides. *Acta Virol.* 50: 93–99.

35. Svraka, S. *et al*. 2006. Establishment of a genotyping scheme for *Coxiella burnetii. FEMS Microbiol. Lett.* **254:** 268–274.

36. Hackstadt, T. 1986. Antigenic variation in the phase I lipopolysaccharide of *Coxiella burnetii* isolates. *Infect. Immun.* **52:** 337–340.

37. Schnare, M. *et al*. 2001. Toll-like receptors control activation of adaptive immune responses. *Nat. Immunol.* **2:** 947–950.

38. Janeway, C.A. & R. Medzhitov. 2002. Innate imune recognition. *Annu. Rev. Immunol.* **20:** 197–216.

39. Takeda, K., T. Kaisho & S. Akira. 2003. Toll-like receptors. *Annu. Rev. Immunol.* **21:** 335–376.

40. Aliprantis, A.O. *et al*. 1999. Cell activation and apoptosis by bacterial lipoproteins through toll-like receptor-2. *Science* **285:** 736–739.

41. Darveau, R.P. *et al*. 2004. *Porphyromonas gingivalis* lipopolysaccharide contains multiple lipid A species that functionally interact with both toll-like receptors 2 and 4. *Infect. Immun.* **72:** 5041–5051.

42. Girard, R. *et al*. 2003. Lipopolysaccharides from *Legionella* and *Rhizobium* stimulate mouse bone marrow granulocytes via toll-like receptor 2. *J. Cell Sci.* **116:** 293–302.

43. Hirschfeld, M. *et al*. 2001. Signaling by toll-like receptor 2 and 4 agonists results in differential gene expression in murine macrophages. *Infect. Immun.* **69:** 1477–1482.

44. Honstettre, A. *et al*. 2004. Lipopolysaccharide from *Coxiella burnetii* is involved in bacterial phagocytosis, filamentous actin reorganization, and inflammatory responses through toll-like receptor 4. *J. Immunol.* **172:** 3695–3703.

45. Golenbock, D.T. *et al*. 1991. Lipid A-like molecules that antagonize the effects of endotoxins on human monocytes. *J. Biol. Chem.* **266:** 19490–19498.

46. Meghari, S. *et al*. 2005. TLR2 is necessary to inflammatory response in *Coxiella burnetii* infection. *Ann. N.Y. Acad. Sci.* **1063:** 161–166.

47. Seshadri, R. *et al*. 2003. Complete genome sequence of the Q-fever pathogen *Coxiella burnetii. Proc. Natl. Acad. Sci. U.S.A.* **100:** 5455–5460.

48. Samoilis, G. *et al*. 2007. Analysis of whole cell lysate from the intracellular bacterium *Coxiella burnetii* using two gel-based protein separation techniques. *J. Proteome Res.* **6:** 3032–3041.

49. Ray, M.C. *et al*. 2000. Identification by genetic suppression of *Escherichia coli* TolB residues important for TolB-Pal interaction. *J. Bacteriol.* **182:** 821–824.

50. Rigal, A. *et al*. 1997. The TolB protein interacts with the porins of *Escherichia coli. J. Bacteriol.* **179:** 7274–7279.

51. Lazzaroni, J.C. *et al*. 1999. The Tol proteins of *Escherichia coli* and their involvement in the uptake of biomolecules and outer membrane stability. *FEMS Microbiol. Lett.* **177:** 191–197.

52. Clavel, T. *et al*. 1998. TolB protein of *Escherichia coli* K-12 interacts with the outer membrane peptidoglycan-associated proteins Pal, Lpp and OmpA. *Mol. Microbiol.* **29:** 359–367.

53. Cascales, E. *et al*. 2002. Pal lipoprotein of *Escherichia coli* plays a major role in outer membrane integrity. *J. Bacteriol.* **184:** 754–759.

54. Cascales, E., M. Gavioli, J.N. Sturgis & R. Lloubes. 2000. Proton motive force drives the interaction of the inner membrane TolA and outer membrane Pal proteins in *Escherichia coli. Mol. Microbiol.* **38:** 904–915.

55. Bernadac, A., M. Gavioli, J.C. Lazzaroni, S. Raina & R. Lloubes. 1998. *Escherichia coli* Tol-Pal mutants form outer membrane vesicles. *J. Bacteriol.* **180:** 4872–4878.

56. Nikaido, H. 2001. Preventing drug access to targets: cell surface permeability barriers and active efflux in bacteria. *Semin. Cell Dev. Biol.* **12:** 215–223.

57. Tsukagoshi, N. & R. Aono. 2000. Entry into and release of solvents by *Escherichia coli* in an organic-aqueous two-liquid-phase system and substrate specificity of the AcrAB-TolC solvent-extruding pump. *J. Bacteriol.* **182:** 4803–4810.

58. Nikaido, H. 1998. Multiple antibiotic resistance and efflux. *Curr. Opin. Microbiol.* **1:** 516–523.

59. Poole, K. 2001. Multidrug resistance in gram-negative bacteria. *Curr. Opin. Microbiol.* **4:** 500–508.

60. Yu, E.W., J.R. Aires & H. Nikaido. 2003. AcrB multidrug efflux pump of *Escherichia coli*: composite substrate-binding cavity of exceptional flexibility generates its extremely wide substrate specificity. *J. Bacteriol.* **185:** 5657–5664.

61. Akporiaye, E.T. & O.G. Baca. 1983. Superoxide anion production and superoxide dismutase and catalase activities in *Coxiella burnetii. J. Bacteriol.* **154:** 520–523.

62. Heinzen, R.A., M.E. Frazier & L.P. Mallavia. 1992. *Coxiella burnetii* superoxide dismutase gene: cloning, sequencing, and expression in *Escherichia coli. Infect. Immun.* **60:** 3814–3823.

63. Poole, L.B. 2005. Bacterial defenses against oxidants: mechanistic features of cysteine-based peroxidases and their flavoprotein reductases. *Arch. Biochem. Biophys.* **433:** 240–254.

64. Hansen, A.M. *et al*. 2005. Structural basis for the function of stringent starvation protein A as a transcription factor. *J. Biol. Chem.* **280:** 17380–17391.

65. Hansen, A.M. *et al*. 2005. SspA is required for acid resistance in stationary phase by downregulation of H-NS in *Escherichia coli. Mol. Microbiol.* **56:** 719–734.

66. Kvint, K. *et al*. 2003. The bacterial universal stress protein: function and regulation. *Curr. Opin. Microbiol.* **6:** 140–145.

67. Helbig, J.H. *et al.* 2003. The PPIase active site of *Legionella pneumophila* Mip protein is involved in the infection of eukaryotic host cells. *Biol. Chem.* **384:** 125–137.

68. Mo, Y.Y., N.P. Cianciotto & L.P. Mallavia. 1995. Molecular cloning of a *Coxiella burnetii* gene encoding a macrophage infectivity potentiator (Mip) analogue. *Microbiology* **141:** 2861–2871.

69. Zamboni, D.S. *et al.* 2003. *Coxiella burnetii* expresses type IV secretion system proteins that function similarly to components of the *Legionella pneumophila* Dot/Icm system. *Mol. Microbiol.* **49:** 965–976.

70. Coleman, S.A. *et al.* 2007. Proteome and antigen profiling of *Coxiella burnetii* developmental forms. *Infect. Immun.* **75:** 290–298.

71. Shaw, E.I. *et al.* 2004. Identification of biomarkers of whole *Coxiella burnetii* phase I by MALDI-TOF mass spectrometry. *Anal. Chem.* **76:** 4017–4022.

72. Skultety, L. *et al.* 2007. Detection of specific spectral markers of *Coxiella burnetii* isolates by MALDI-TOF mass spectrometry. *Acta Virol.* **51:** 55–58.

73. Pierce, C.Y. *et al.* 2007. Strain and phase identification of the U.S. category B agent *Coxiella burnetii* by matrix assisted laser desorption/ionization time-of-flight mass spectrometry and multivariate pattern recognition. *Anal. Chim. Acta* **583:** 23–31.

74. Hernychova, L. *et al.* 2008. Detection and identification of *Coxiella burnetii* based on the mass spectrometric analyses of the extracted proteins. *Anal. Chem.* **80:** 7097–7104.

Q Fever during Pregnancy

A Cause of Poor Fetal and Maternal Outcome

Xavier Carcopino,[a,b] Didier Raoult,[b] Florence Bretelle,[a] Léon Boubli,[a] and Andreas Stein[b]

[a]*Service de Gynécologie Obstétrique, Hôpital Nord, Chemin des Bourrely, 13915 Cedex 20, Marseille, France*

[b]*Unité des Rickettsies, Unité Mixte de Recherche 6020, Université de la Méditerranée, Faculté de Médecine, 27 Boulevard Jean Moulin, 13385 Marseille Cedex 5, France*

Q fever is a worldwide zoonosis caused by *Coxiella burnetii*. Q fever may be present as an acute or a chronic infection and can be reactivated during subsequent pregnancies. Although its exact prevalence remains unknown, it is likely that the number of cases of Q fever in pregnant women is underestimated. During pregnancy, the illness is likely to be asymptomatic, and diagnosis is based on serology. Acute infection results in appearance of IgM and IgG antibodies mainly directed against the avirulent form of *C. burnetii* (phase II). Chronic Q fever results in particularly high level of IgG and IgA antibodies directed against both virulent (phase I) and avirulent (phase II) forms of the bacterium. Q fever may result in adverse pregnancy outcome, including spontaneous abortion, intrauterine growth retardation, oligoamnios, intrauterine fetal death (IUFD), and premature delivery. Obstetric complications occur significantly more often as *C. burnetii* infects the patient at an early stage of her pregnancy. Occurrence of IUFD is correlated with the presence of placental infection by *C. burnetii* and might be the consequence of direct infection of the fetus. The mother is exposed to the risk of chronic Q fever and endocarditis with potential fatal evolution. Long-term cotrimoxazole therapy prevents from placental infection, IUFD, and maternal chronic Q fever. Such treatment should be used to treat pregnant women with Q fever. Women with previous history of Q fever should have a regular serological follow up. Obstetricians' knowledge about Q fever must be improved.

Key words: *Coxiella burnetii*; pregnancy; Q fever; stillbirth; Trimethoprim-Sulfamethoxazole combination

Introduction

Query (Q) fever was named and first described by Derrick in 1937 after the outcome of nine cases of febrile illness among the employees of an abattoir in Brisbane.[1] It is a ubiquitous zoonosis caused by *Coxiella burnetii*, an obligate intracellular bacterium, almost simultaneously first isolated by Cox[2] and Burnet.[3,4]

Domestic animals and pets are the most frequent source of infection. Infected animals contaminate the environment by excreting the bacterium in milk and birth by-products, especially the placenta.[5] Humans may get infected after the inhalation of contaminated aerosols. Subclinical infection is common, and when symptomatic, the clinical presentation of Q fever is polymorphic and nonspecific. The disease may be acute, most often self-limited febrile illness possibly associated with pneumonia and/or hepatitis. Some patients will develop chronic Q fever, mostly represented by endocarditis.

Address for correspondence: Xavier Carcopino, M.D., Department of Obstetrics and Gynecology, Hôpital Nord, Chemin des Bourrely, 13915 Cedex 20, Marseille, France. Voice: +33 491964672. xcarco@free.fr

Financial support: none
Disclaimer: none

Rickettsiology and Rickettsial Diseases-Fifth International Conference: Ann. N.Y. Acad. Sci. 1166: 79–89 (2009).
doi: 10.1111/j.1749-6632.2009.04519.x © 2009 New York Academy of Sciences.

Q fever is endemic worldwide. Although the incidence of the disease varies between different geographic locations, epidemiological studies indicate that Q fever should be considered a public health problem in many countries, including France,[6,7] Spain,[8] Italy,[9] Switzerland,[10] the United Kingdom,[11] Germany,[12] Israel,[13] and Canada,[14] as well as in many countries where Q fever is prevalent but unrecognized because of poor surveillance of the disease. It is of interest to note that incidence of Q fever seems to be the highest in regions where there is medical or scientific interest in the disease.

Recently, knowledge of Q fever has greatly expanded. Clinical manifestations and the role of the host factor in the expression of acute Q fever and its evolution to chronic serologic profile is now better understood, and the benefit of prolonged combination of antibiotics for the treatment of Q fever endocarditis has been adopted.[15,16] Essential data on the expression of Q fever during pregnancy, its consequences, and treatment, has recently been published and the benefit of long-term cotrimoxazole therapy has been demonstrated.[6,17] Despite its potential severity in pregnant women, incidence of Q fever during pregnancy is likely to be underestimated, and the disease remains poorly known by obstetricians. The objective of this review is to report actual knowledge about Q fever during pregnancy.

Microbiology

C. burnetii is an obligate intracellular, small (0.3 to 10 μm) pleomorphic gram-negative coccobacillus.[15,18] It is characterized by a passive entry into hosts cells by phagocytosis, by survival in phagolysosomes where the low pH necessary for its metabolism is present (pH 4.5)[19,20] and by sporulation-like process conferring high resistance in the environment.[21]

One of the major characteristics of *C. burnetii* is its phase variation. This phenomenon is related to the appearance of lipopolysaccharide (LPS) mutants known to be the essential determinant of *C. burnetii*'s virulence.[22–25] Phase I is the natural phase isolated from humans or animals.[15,18] It is highly infectious, and a single bacterium may infect a human. In contrast, phase II is not very infectious and is obtained only in laboratories after serial passages in cell cultures or embryonated egg cultures.[15,18] Compared to phase I, phase II displays a truncated LPS and lacks some protein cell surface determinants.[26] LPS changes lead to different immunologic responses. During the acute phase of the disease, immunologic response is initially directed against phase II organisms.[18]

Epidemiology

Q fever is a ubiquitous zoonosis. Known reservoirs are mammals, but also birds, fishes, reptiles, amphibians and arthropods, and mostly ticks.[27–30] The most commonly identified sources of human infection are farm animals, especially cattle, goats, and sheep.[18] Pets, especially cats, have been described as an important reservoir and a potential source of Q fever outbreak in urban areas.[31–35]

Infected animals excrete *C. burnetii* in milk, urine, feces, and birth by-products; especially the placenta,[36–39] which can contain up to 10^9 organisms per gram of tissue.[40] One gram of infected placenta can therefore contain enough organisms to infect 100 million guinea pigs.[39] At the time of delivery, such infected placenta may contaminate the environment, and *C. burnetii* can survive in the soil for several months.[41]

Human infection mainly occurs following the inhalation of aerosols contaminated by particles coming from the amniotic fluid or the placenta of infected animals.[15,27,30] Therefore, people exposed to Q fever are mostly those living and/or working near farm animals. Because of the high resistance of *C. burnetii* in the environment, indirect human infection is also possible and may occur a few months to a few years after the excretion of *C. burnetii* by an infected animal.[42] Wind-borne spread is also possible, and contaminated particles might be disseminated over many kilometers.[7,43,44] Because of the excretion of *C. burnetii* in the milk, the ingestion of fresh milk or of unpasteurized milk products represents an alternative possible route of contamination.[45,46] Even if rare, interhuman transmission is possible. A case of Q fever occurring after contact with an infected pregnant woman at the time of her delivery has been reported.[47] Sexual transmission has been demonstrated in mice[48] and remains theoretically possible in humans.[49,50] Fetal infection, due to vertical transplacental contamination, is also possible.[47,51]

C. burnetii can persist in humans, being totally asymptomatic. Certain conditions such as pregnancy,[18] valvulopathy, anevrysm or vascular prosthesis, haemodialysis,[52] or any kind of immunosupression,[53,54] in particular AIDS[55] or organ transplant[56-58] might lead to the reactivation of the infection.

Cases of Q fever have been reported worldwide, except in New Zealand.[59-61] Because of the propagation mode of *C. burnetii*, the incidence of Q fever cases is known to vary according to seasons. In Europe, cases of acute Q fever are more frequent during spring and the beginning of summer.[7,46] Q fever concerns all age groups, but is more common in male than female, with a sex ratio of 2.5 to 1 in France.[16]

Because clinical symptoms of Q fever are variables and nonspecifics, its overall incidence is likely to be underestimated.[15,46,62] Diagnosis dramatically depends on the experience and the knowledge of doctors and on the availability of a reliable laboratory diagnosis. In the south of France, 5 to 8% of endocarditis is due to *C. burnetii*, and overall acute Q fever prevalence is of 50 cases per 100,000 inhabitants.[46] Seroepidemiological study demonstrated that 10 to 36% of blood donors worldwide possess anti-*C. burnetii* antibodies.[14,63-66] Worldwide seroprevalence of *C. burnetii* in pregnant women is poorly known. It has been evaluated to be of 3.8% in Canada[67] and 4.7% in Tanzania.[68] Incidence of Q fever during pregnancy would be of 1.3 per 1000 in the southeast of France.[69] In this area, the risk is particularly high in Martigues, where at least one delivery in 540 (0.19%) is affected.[70] In comparison, prevalence of Hbs antigen in French pregnant women is of 0.41%.[71]

Acute Q Fever

The clinical presentation of Q fever is polymorphic and nonspecific. After an incubation period ranging from 1 to 3 weeks,[15] acute Q fever generally presents as a self-limited febrile illness, possibly associated with pneumonia and/or hepatitis. In the absence of treatment, the fever will last for a median of 10 days (range, 5–57 days).[1] Q fever can also be asymptomatic[15,72,73] and is significantly more often asymptomatic in pregnant women than in the rest of the population.[6] This was demonstrated during a seroepidemiologic survey carried out after a large outbreak in the valley of Chamonix (French Alps). Among the 11 pregnant women diagnosed with Q fever, only one was symptomatic, while 48 out of the 54 nonpregnant women and 71 out of the 85 other patients were symptomatic ($P < 10^{-7}$ and $P < 10^{-6}$, respectively).[6] Blood testing may be abnormal. Leukocyte count is usually normal, but a thrombocytopenia and a moderate elevation of liver enzymes ranging from 2 to 10 times the normal value are quite evocative.[18] The mortality rate is low, varying from 1 to 2% in overall population.[46,74] Even if rare (<1%), myocarditis is one of the first causes of death[75] but has not yet been reported in a pregnant woman.

Chronic Q Fever

Chronic Q fever might occur a month to years after an acute illness[76] but may also occur directly without any previous acute episode.[5] Overall, approximately 5% of patients infected by *C. burnetii* will develop a chronic Q fever.[18] With reported rates ranging up to 52.8%,[17] pregnant women are particularly exposed to the risk of chronic form of the disease. It seems that the main risk factor for the chronic form of Q fever is the length of infection during pregnancy, and patients more often develop a chronic serologic profile when infected during their first trimester of pregnancy.[17,77]

Endocarditis represents the main complication of the chronic form. In global population, it occurs in 60 to 70% of cases of chronic Q fever[5,78] and supervenes mostly in patients with pre-existing cardiac valve defect and immunosuppressive illness.[5,54,79–81] The evolution is fatal in the absence of appropriate treatment.[82] At this stage, only one case of Q fever endocarditis during pregnancy has been reported in a woman with bioprosthetic aortic valve.[17] Endocarditis resulted in the maternofetal death at 27 weeks' gestation. Although diagnosis of Q fever endocarditis was done during the second trimester of the pregnancy, it was retrospectively assessed that this patient got infected before getting pregnant and probably developed endocarditis at that time. This evolution could be explained by the lack of an adapted immune response due to pregnancy and illustrates the potential severity of Q fever endocarditis in a pregnant woman. Moreover, this patient could not be given long-term cotrimoxazole therapy. This therapy was initially started but had to be stopped after 4 weeks because of drug-related hepatitis. At the time the cotrimoxazole was stopped, endocarditis dramatically aggravated, resulting in the maternofetal death just after an attempt for surgical bioprosthetic replacement.

Diagnostic Criteria

Serology

Diagnosis is exclusively based on serology,[18,78] with immunofluorescence being the reference method. Seroconversion usually occurs 2 to 3 weeks after the onset of illness. Thus, paired serum specimens 3 weeks apart are useful. Antigenic peculiarity of *C. burnetii* is extremely valuable for the serological differentiation between acute and chronic Q fever. Acute infection results in appearance of IgM and IgG antibodies mainly directed against the avirulent form of *C. burnetii* (phase II) when chronic Q fever results in particularly high levels of IgG and IgA antibodies directed against both virulent (phase I) and avirulent (phase II) forms of the bacterium.[15]

The choice for a threshold value is essential for the interpretation of serologic results and must consider the prevalence of the disease in the area. Positive and negative predictive values of such tests depend indeed on the prevalence of the disease. In Marseille, phase II IgG titers greater than 200 and IgM titers greater than 50 diagnose acute Q fever on a single serum with high sensibility and specificity of 100%.[15,18,83] Chronic Q fever is diagnosed on the basis of a phase I IgG titer greater than 800.[18] IgG and IgA titers are generally elevated, even if the IgA titer does not add anything to the diagnosis.[83] A Phase II IgG titer is lower or equal to the phase I titer, and IgM might be absent.[18] IgM is usually undetectable after 4 months but might persist for 12 months or more.[83,84]

Identification of *C. burnetii*

C. burnetii can be identified in tissue specimens by polymerase chain reaction (PCR).[18] Such technique allows the retrospective detection and quantification of *C. burnetii* from frozen samples or paraffin-embedded tissues.[85] PCR is highly sensible when used on samples such as placenta or fetal tissue. However, because only few copies of the organism are prevalent, PCR of blood specimens has a low sensibility and is currently inadequate for Q fever diagnosis. More sensitive nested PCR generates irreproducible results that may be caused by DNA contamination.

C. burnetii may be cultured only in biosafety level 3 laboratories because of its high infectivity.[5] Cell cultures are currently preferred to animal cultures, which cannot be considered reliable, because of exposing the personnel to

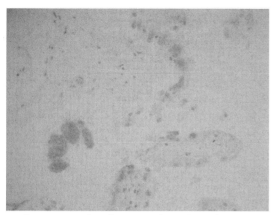

Figure 1. Identification of *Coxiella burnetii* in placental sample. Immunohistochemical detection of *Coxiella burnetii* in a placental sample from a patient with Q fever during pregnancy. Note the intracellular location of the bacteria as granular immunopositive material in macrophage cytoplasm (monoclonal mouse anti-*C. burnetii* antibody used at a dilution of 1:1000, hematoxylin counterstain, original magnification ×200).

a risk of contamination, cross-contamination of animals, and false-positive results. The shell vial assay with human embryonic fibroblasts is efficient with various specimens (blood, cerebrospinal fluid, tissue). The bacterium is identified 6 days later, by immunofluorescence (Fig. 1), Gimenez-staining, or PCR.[18]

Obstetrical Outcome

C. burnetii was shown to be present in placentas of naturally or experimentally infected animals,[86–88] in bovine amniotic fluid[89] and has been described as a cause of abortion, intrauterine growth retardation (IUGR), and premature delivery in sheep, goats, and mice.[40,86,90–94] In these studies, the etiologic role of *C. burnetii* was assessed by the animal serologic profiles and/or by the identification of the bacterium in placentas. In pregnant women, as in other mammals that become infected with *C. burnetii*, the bacteria will colonize and multiply in the uterus, placenta, and mammary glands. *C. burnetii* has also been identified in the placenta of infected pregnant women and in fetal viscera, demonstrating its transplacental transmission.[17,47,77,95]

At this stage, only 74 cases of Q fever during pregnancy have been reported.[6,17,40,47,51,70,77,95–108] In a series of 53 cases diagnosed and managed in our institution between 1991 and 2005, we recently appreciated the pathogenic role of *C. burnetii* in human pregnancy.[17] Analysis of these cases demonstrated Q fever as a significant cause of fetal morbidity and mortality. Thus, it can result in spontaneous abortion, IUGR, oligoamnios, stillbirth, or premature delivery, with such obstetrical complications being observed in 13.5%, 27%, 10.8%, 27%, and 27% of untreated patients, respectively.[17] To date, teratogenicity has never been associated with *C. burnetii* infection. Q fever does not necessarily lead to a poor fetal outcome, and from the patients we monitored only 18.9% of untreated pregnancies had a normal outcome and a healthy child at delivery.

The outcome of the pregnancy depends on the trimester of infection. Obstetrical complications are, therefore, significantly more frequent in patients who get infected during their first trimester of pregnancy compared with those who get infected later.[17] The pathogenetic mechanism for poor fetal outcome such as IUGR or prematurity may be placental insufficiency following vasculitis and vascular thrombosis.[70] Occurrence of STILLBIRTH is correlated with the presence of placental infection by *C. burnetii* (i.e., placentitis) and might be the consequence of direct infection of the fetus.[17]

Treatment

Being an obligatory intracellular bacterium, *C. burnetii* lives in acidic vacuoles, the phagolysosome, which may protect it from the bacteriocidal effects of antibiotics.[20] Several antibiotics have bacteriostatic effect on the organism, including tetracyclines, rifampin, cotrimoxazole, and fluoroquinolones.[109] Because chloroquine raises the pH in the phagolysosome, restoring the bacteriocidal effect of doxycycline, combination of doxycycline and chloroquine or OH-chloroquine is the only bacteriocidal regimen *in vitro*.[109,110]

In non-pregnant women with acute Q fever, oral administration of doxycycline 200 mg daily for 14 days is the treatment of choice.[5] Treatment of chronic Q fever requires prolonged courses of agents active against *C. burnetii*. Patients with Q fever endocarditis should be treated with combination of doxycycline (200 mg daily) and hydroxychloroquine (started at 600 mg daily) for a duration of 18 to 36 months.[110,111] The dose of hydroxychloroquine will be secondarily adjusted in order to obtain a level of 1 ± 0.2 mg/L.[5] Such treatment exposes patients to photosensitivity, and regular eye examination is required to detect intraretinal accumulation of the molecule.

Q fever treatment during pregnancy is a therapeutic challenge because both doxycycline and chloroquine are contra-indicated. Despite a theoretical risk of neonatal bilirubinemia when used just before delivery,[112] cotrimoxazole may be used but only has a bacteriostatic effect. Because a 3-week cotrimoxazole therapy did not prevent stillbirth,[47] Raoult and colleagues recommended the use of cotrimoxazole long-term therapy, defined as daily oral administration of combined 320 mg of trimethoprim and 1600 mg of sulfamethoxazole for at least 5 weeks and prolonged for the whole duration of pregnancy.[17,77] We have recently investigated the efficacy of long-term cotrimoxazole therapy in preventing maternofetal complications of Q fever. Our study provides the best current evidence about the value of treatment in order to prevent placentitis and stillbirth.[17] At this stage, no case of stillbirth has been reported in the 16 patients who received this therapy.[17] Long-term cotrimoxazole therapy also prevents the development of maternal chronic Q fever and the need for postpartum treatment.[17] Finally, although the efficacy of long-term cotrimoxazole to prevent endocarditis has not been proven, endocarditis was not diagnosed in any of the 16 patients who were given this therapy.[17]

Managing Q Fever during and After Delivery

As in other mammals, pregnant women who are infected with *C. burnetii* excrete the bacteria in birth by-products and milk. Delivery of a patient who has had Q fever during her pregnancy therefore exposes neonate, medical staff, and relatives to a risk of contamination and requires some precautions.[47] The delivery room should be kept closed and carefully decontaminated after use, all persons involved should wear a mask and gloves, and extreme care should be taken in the manipulation of the placenta. Finally, breastfeeding should not be recommended for women who have had Q fever during their pregnancy.

Patients' Follow-up and Subsequent Pregnancies

Q fever serology should be monitored in pregnant women with acute Q fever because of the possibility of developing chronic serologic profile.[77] After delivery, clinical and serological follow up of women who have had Q fever while being pregnant is required for possible evolution to chronic Q fever and endocarditis. In patients with postpartum "chronic" serologic profile, Raoult and colleagues recommend the use of the standard treatment of Q fever endocarditis (combination of doxycycline and hydroxychloroquine) to prevent the possible development of endocarditis, as may happen in mice.[86]

Reactivation of *C. burnetii* infection constitutes a potential risk for the fetus during the immunocompromised state of subsequent pregnancies. At the time they start a pregnancy, women with previous history of Q fever should be followed serologically on a monthly basis. A relapse should indicate a long-term cotrimoxazole therapy. However, we were involved in the follow up of 25 subsequent pregnancies in 19 patients with a history of infection by *C. burnetii* during their previous pregnancy. Only 6 of them required long-term cotrimoxazole therapy and all had normal evolution and outcome.[17]

Screening for Q Fever in Pregnant Women

Incidence of Q fever during pregnancy may be underestimated. Two major points support such hypothesis. First, *C. burnetii* infection during pregnancy is likely to be asymptomatic.[6] Second, the disease remains poorly known by physicians and especially obstetricians.[72] Diagnosis of Q fever should be considered in pregnant women suffering from nonspecific febrile illness, particularly in those with identified risk factors such as exposure to farm animals. Q fever serology is also indicated in pregnant women with fever associated with pneumonia, hepatitis, and severe thrombocytopenia, and in those undergoing recurrent miscarriage. Even if not being justified in global population, systematic serologic screening for Q fever should be considered in pregnant women living in endemic areas or exposed to farm animals and must be performed in any episode of Q fever outbreak. A pre-existing heart murmur, even minimal, exposes the patient to Q fever endocarditis,[53,79,81] which might be fatal during pregnancy. Finally, Q fever should be added to the etiological agents of intrauterine infections associated with fetal morbidity and mortality, which are grouped under the term TORCH for Toxoplasma, "others" (including Listeria, hepatitis B, and HIV), rubella, cytomegalovirus, and herpes. Q fever serology should therefore be part of the investigations performed in case of IUGR, oligoamnios, and stillbirth.

Prevention

As immunocompromised patients and those with known heart murmur, pregnant women should be excluded from high risk situations unless they are immune.[5] Contact with farm animals such as cattle, sheep, goats, and also parturient cats should be avoided. Q fever vaccines have been developed. A whole-cell vaccine (Q-Vax®) prepared from phase I organisms was licensed in Australia in 1989.[113] The main side effect of this vaccine is a possible severe local reaction at the injection site in those with previous immunity.[114] Pre-vaccination screening based on history, skin tests, and serology is therefore recommended. Q-Vax® efficacy has been previously demonstrated,[115] and a single 30 μg dose confers a minimum of 5 years immunity after 10 to 15 days.[114] Vaccination is recommended in risk occupations such as stockbreeder, abattoir employee, veterinarian, and laboratory staff working with animals infected by *C. burnetii*. Vaccination of those not directly exposed but with risk factors such as cardiac valve defect or immunocompromised status should also be considered.

Conclusion

Q fever may be present as an acute or a chronic infection and can be reactivated during subsequent pregnancies. Diagnosis is based on serology. During pregnancy, Q fever is a cause of morbidity and mortality, both for the mother and the fetus. It may result in severe fetal complications, including spontaneous abortion, IUGR, oligoamnios, stillbirth, and premature delivery. Obstetric complications occur significantly more often as *C. burnetii* infects the patient at an early stage of her pregnancy. The mother is exposed to the risk of chronic Q fever and endocarditis. Because it prevents from placentitis, stillbirth and maternal chronic Q fever, long-term cotrimoxazole therapy should be administered to all pregnant women with proven Q fever. Although its exact prevalence remains unknown, it is likely that the number of cases of Q fever in pregnant women is underestimated. Obstetricians' knowledge about Q fever must be improved.

Conflicts of Interest

The authors declare no conflicts of interest.

References

1. Derrick, E. 1937. "Q" fever, a new fever entity: clinical features, diagnosis and laboratory investigation. *Med. J. Aust.* **2:** 281–289.

2. Davis, G.E. & H.R. Cox. 1938. A filter-passing infectious agent isolated from ticks. I. Isolation from Dermacentor andersoni, reactions in animals, and filtration experiments. *Public Health Rep.* **54:** 2259–2267.

3. McDade, J.E. 1990. Historical aspects of Q fever. *Q Fever, the Disease.* T. Marrie, Ed.: 6–21. CRC Press. Boca Raton.

4. Burnet, M. & M. Freeman. 1937. Experimental studies on the virus of "Q" fever. *Med. J. Aust.* **2:** 299–305.

5. Parker, N.R., J.H. Barralet & A.M. Bell. 2006. Q Fever Lancet **367:** 679–688.

6. Tissot-Dupont, H. *et al.* 2007. Role of sex, age, previous valve lesion, and pregnancy in the clinical expression and outcome of Q fever after a large outbreak. *Clin. Infect Dis.* **44:** 232–237.

7. Tissot-Dupont, H. *et al.* 2004. Wind in November, Q fever in December. *Emerg. Infect. Dis.* **10:** 1264–1269.

8. de los Rios-Martin, R. *et al.* 2006. Q fever outbreak in an urban area following a school-farm visit. *Med. Clin. (Barc).* **126:** 573–575.

9. Starnini, G. *et al.* 2005. An outbreak of Q fever in a prison in Italy. *Epidemiol. Infect.* **133:** 377–380.

10. Dupuis, G. *et al.* 1987. An important outbreak of human Q fever in a Swiss Alpine valley. *Int. J. Epidemiol.* **16:** 282–287.

11. van Woerden, H.C. *et al.* 2004. Q fever outbreak in industrial setting. *Emerg. Infect. Dis.* **10:** 1282–1289.

12. Schneider, T. *et al.* 1993. A Q fever epidemic in Berlin. The epidemiological and clinical aspects. *Dtsch. Med. Wochenschr.* **118:** 689–695.

13. Oren, I. *et al.* 2005. An outbreak of Q fever in an urban area in Israel. *Eur J. Clin. Microbiol. Infect. Dis.* **24:** 338–341.

14. Marrie, T.J. 1988. Seroepidemiology of Q fever in New Brunswick and Manitoba. *Can. J. Microbiol.* **34:** 1043–1045.

15. Maurin, M. & D. Raoult. 1999. Q fever. *Clin. Microbiol. Rev.* **12:** 518–553.

16. Raoult, D. *et al.* 2000. Q fever 1985–1998. Clinical and epidemiologic features of 1,383 infections. *Medicine (Baltimore)* **79:** 109–123.

17. Carcopino, X. *et al.* 2007. Managing Q fever during pregnancy: the benefits of long-term cotrimoxazole therapy. *Clin. Infect Dis.* **45:** 548–555.

18. Fournier, P.E., T.J. Marrie & D. Raoult. 1998. Diagnosis of Q fever. *J. Clin. Microbiol.* **36:** 1823–1834.

19. Hackstadt, T. & J.C. Williams. 1981. Biochemical stratagem for obligate parasitism of eukaryotic cells by Coxiella burnetii. *Proc. Natl. Acad. Sci. USA* **78:** 3240–3244.

20. Maurin, M. *et al.* 1992. Phagolysosomes of Coxiella burnetii-infected cell lines maintain an acidic pH during persistent infection. *Infect Immun.* **60:** 5013–5016.

21. McCaul, T.F. 1991. The developmental cycle of Coxiella burnetii. In *Q Fever: The Biology of Coxiella Burnetii.* J. Williams & H.A. Thompson, Eds.: 224–258. CRC Press. Boca Raton.

22. Hackstadt, T. 1990. The role of lipopolysaccharides in the virulence of Coxiella burnetii. *Ann. N. Y. Acad. Sci.* **590:** 27–32.

23. Hackstadt, T. *et al.* 1985. Lipopolysaccharide variation in Coxiella burnetti: intrastrain heterogeneity in structure and antigenicity. *Infect Immun.* **48:** 359–365.

24. Hackstadt, T. 1986. Antigenic variation in the phase I lipopolysaccharide of Coxiella burnetii isolates. *Infect Immun.* **52:** 337–340.

25. Toman, R. & J. Kazar. 1991. Evidence for the structural heterogeneity of the polysaccharide component of Coxiella burnetii strain Nine Mile lipopolysaccharide. *Acta. Virol.* **35:** 531–537.

26. Amano, K. & J.C. Williams. 1984. Chemical and immunological characterization of lipopolysaccharides from phase I and phase II Coxiella burnetii. *J. Bacteriol.* **160:** 994–1002.

27. Hirai, K. & H. To. 1998. Advances in the understanding of Coxiella burnetii infection in Japan. *J. Vet. Med. Sci.* **60:** 781–790.

28. Lang, G. 1990. Coxiellosis (Q fever) in animals. *Q Fever, the Disease.* T. Marrie, Ed.: 23–48. CRC Press. Boca Raton.

29. Marrie, T.J., J. Embil & L. Yates. 1993. Seroepidemiology of Coxiella burnetii among wildlife in Nova Scotia. *Am. J. Trop. Med. Hyg.* **49:** 613–615.

30. Woldehiwet, Z. 2004. Q fever (coxiellosis): epidemiology and pathogenesis. *Res. Vet. Sci.* **77:** 93–100.

31. Higgins, D. & T.J. Marrie. 1990. Seroepidemiology of Q fever among cats in New Brunswick and Prince Edward Island. *Ann. N. Y. Acad. Sci.* **590:** 271–274.

32. Langley, J.M. *et al.* 1988. Poker player's pneumonia. An urban outbreak of Q fever following exposure to a parturient cat. *New Engl. J. Med.* **319:** 354–356.

33. Marrie, T.J. *et al.* 1988. Exposure to parturient cats: a risk factor for acquisition of Q fever in Maritime Canada. *J. Infect Dis.* **158:** 101–108.

34. Marrie, T.J. *et al.* 1988. An outbreak of Q fever probably due to contact with a parturient cat. *Chest* **93:** 98–103.

35. Morita, C. *et al.* 1994. Seroepidemiological survey of Coxiella burnetii in domestic cats in Japan. *Microbiol. Immunol.* **38:** 1001–1003.

36. Arricau Bouvery, N. *et al.* 2003. Experimental Coxiella burnetii infection in pregnant goats: excretion routes. *Vet. Res.* **34:** 423–433.

37. Berri, M. *et al.* 2001. Relationships between the shedding of Coxiella burnetii, clinical signs and serological responses of 34 sheep. *Vet. Rec.* **148:** 502–505.

38. Marrie, T. 1990. Epidemiology of Q fever. *Q Fever, the Disease.* T. Marrie, Ed.: 49–65. CRC Press. Boca Raton.

39. Stoker, M.G. & B.P. Marmion. 1955. The spread of Q fever from animals to man; the natural history of a rickettsial disease. *Bull World Health Organ* **13:** 781–806.

40. Babudieri, B. 1959. Q fever: a zoonosis. *Adv. Vet. Sci.* **5:** 81–102.

41. McCaul, T.F. & J.C. Williams. 1990. Localization of DNA in Coxiella burnetii by post-embedding immunoelectron microscopy. *Ann. N. Y. Acad. Sci.* **590:** 136–147.

42. Valero, F. *et al.* 1995. Pericardial effusion as the initial feature of Q fever. *Am. Heart J.* **130:** 1308–1309.

43. Hawker, J.I. *et al.* 1998. A large outbreak of Q fever in the West Midlands: windborne spread into a metropolitan area? *Commun Dis Public Health* **1:** 180–187.

44. Tissot-Dupont, H. *et al.* 1999. Hyperendemic focus of Q fever related to sheep and wind. *Am. J. Epidemiol.* **150:** 67–74.

45. Fishbein, D.B. & D. Raoult. 1992. A cluster of Coxiella burnetii infections associated with exposure to vaccinated goats and their unpasteurized dairy products. *Am. J. Trop. Med. Hyg.* **47:** 35–40.

46. Tissot Dupont, H. *et al.* 1992. Epidemiologic features and clinical presentation of acute Q fever in hospitalized patients: 323 French cases. *Am. J. Med.* **93:** 427–434.

47. Raoult, D. & A. Stein. 1994. Q fever during pregnancy–a risk for women, fetuses and obstetricians. *N. Engl. J. Med.* **330:** 371.

48. Kruszewska, D. & S. Tylewska-Wirzbanowska. 1992. Influence of Coxiella burnetii infection of male mice on their offspring. *Acta. Virol.* **36:** 79–82.

49. Milazzo, A. *et al.* 2001. Sexually transmitted Q fever. *Clin. Infect Dis.* **33:** 399–402.

50. Mann, J.S. *et al.* 1986. Q fever: person to person transmission within a family. *Thorax* **41:** 974–975.

51. Ludlam, H. *et al.* 1997. Q fever in pregnancy. *J. Infect.* **34:** 75–78.

52. Leonetti, F. *et al.* 1994. Chronic Q fever in hemodialysis patients. *Nephron* **67:** 231–233.

53. Raoult, D. 1990. Host factors in the severity of Q fever. *Ann. N. Y. Acad. Sci.* **590:** 33–38.

54. Raoult, D. *et al.* 1992. Acute and chronic Q fever in patients with cancer. *Clin. Infect Dis.* **14:** 127–130.

55. Heard, S.R., C.J. Ronalds & R.B. Heath. 1985. Coxiella burnetii infection in immunocompromised patients. *J. Infect.* **11:** 15–18.

56. Loudon, M.M. & E.N. Thompson. 1988. Severe combined immunodeficiency syndrome, tissue transplant, leukaemia, and Q fever. *Arch. Dis. Child.* **63:** 207–209.

57. Larsen, C.P. *et al.* 2006. Infection in renal transplantation: a case of acute Q fever. *Am. J. Kidney Dis.* **48:** 321–326.

58. Kanfer, E. *et al.* 1988. Q fever following bone marrow transplantation. *Bone Marrow Transplant* **3:** 165–166.

59. Kaplan, M.M. & P. Bertagna. 1955. The geographical distribution of Q fever. *Bull WHO* **13:** 829–860.

60. Hilbink, F. *et al.* 1993. Q fever is absent from New Zealand. *Int. J. Epidemiol.* **22:** 945–949.

61. Greenslade, E. *et al.* 2003. Has Coxiella burnetii (Q fever) been introduced into New Zealand? *Emerg. Infect. Dis.* **9:** 138–140.

62. Bartlett, J.G. 2000. Questions about Q fever. *Medicine (Baltimore)* **79:** 124–125.

63. Marrie, T.J. & L. Yates. 1990. Incidence of Q fever: pilot studies in two areas in Nova Scotia. *Ann. N. Y. Acad. Sci.* **590:** 275–280.

64. Marrie, T.J. *et al.* 1984. Seroepidemiology of Q fever in Nova Scotia and Prince Edward Island. *Can. J. Microbiol.* **30:** 129–134.

65. Blondeau, J. *et al.* 1990. Q fever in Sokoto, Nigeria. *Ann. N. Y. Acad. Sci.* **590:** 281–282.

66. Kelly, P.J. *et al.* 1993. Q fever in Zimbabwe. A review of the disease and the results of a serosurvey of humans, cattle, goats and dogs. *S. Afr. Med. J.* **83:** 21–25.

67. Langley, J.M. *et al.* 2003. Coxiella burnetii seropositivity in parturient women is associated with adverse pregnancy outcomes. *Am. J. Obstet. Gynecol.* **189:** 228–232.

68. Anstey, N.M. *et al.* 1997. Seroepidemiology of Rickettsia typhi, spotted fever group rickettsiae, and Coxiella burnetti infection in pregnant women from urban Tanzania. *Am. J. Trop. Med. Hyg.* **57:** 187–189.

69. Rey, D. *et al.* 2000. Seroprevalence of antibodies to Coxiella burnetti among pregnant women in South Eastern France. *Eur. J. Obstet. Gynecol. Reprod. Biol.* **93:** 151–156.

70. Stein, A. & D. Raoult. 1998. Q fever during pregnancy: a public health problem in southern France. *Clin. Infect Dis.* **27:** 592–596.

71. Denis, F., J.L. Tabaste & S. Ranger-Rogez. 1994. Prevalence of HBs Ag in about 21,500 pregnant women. Survey at twelve French University Hospitals. The Muticentric Study Group. *Pathol. Biol. (Paris)* **42:** 533–538.

72. Raoult, D. 2002. Q fever: still a mysterious disease. *Qjm* **95:** 491–492.

73. McQuiston, J.H. & J.E. Childs. 2002. Q fever in humans and animals in the United States. *Vector Borne Zoonotic Dis.* **2:** 179–191.

74. Kermode, M. *et al.* 2003. An economic evaluation of increased uptake in Q fever vaccination among meat and agricultural industry workers following implementation of the National Q Fever Management Program. *Aust. N. Z. J. Public Health* **27:** 390–398.

75. Fournier, P.E. *et al.* 2001. Myocarditis, a rare but severe manifestation of Q fever: report of 8 cases and review of the literature. *Clin. Infect Dis.* **32:** 1440–14407.

76. Fenollar, F. *et al.* 2001. Risks factors and prevention of Q fever endocarditis. *Clin. Infect Dis.* **33:** 312–316.

77. Raoult, D., F. Fenollar & A. Stein. 2002. Q fever during pregnancy: diagnosis, treatment, and follow-up. *Arch. Intern. Med.* **162:** 701–704.

78. Raoult, D. & T. Marrie. 1995. Q fever. *Clin. Infect Dis.* **20:** 489–495; quiz 496.

79. Tobin, M.J. *et al.* 1982. Q fever endocarditis. *Am. J. Med.* **72:** 396–400.

80. Raoult, D. *et al.* 1993. Q fever and HIV infection. *Aids.* **7:** 81–86.

81. Fenollar, F. *et al.* 2006. Endocarditis after acute Q fever in patients with previously undiagnosed valvulopathies. *Clin. Infect Dis.* **42:** 818–821.

82. Stein, A. & D. Raoult. 1995. Q fever endocarditis. *Eur. Heart J.* **16**(Suppl B): 19–23.

83. Dupont, H.T., X. Thirion & D. Raoult. 1994. Q fever serology: cutoff determination for microimmunofluorescence. *Clin. Diagn. Lab. Immunol.* **1:** 189–196.

84. Worswick, D. & B.P. Marmion. 1985. Antibody responses in acute and chronic Q fever and in subjects vaccinated against Q fever. *J. Med. Microbiol.* **19:** 281–296.

85. Stein, A. & D. Raoult. 1992. Detection of Coxiella burnetti by DNA amplification using polymerase chain reaction. *J. Clin. Microbiol.* **30:** 2462–2466.

86. Stein, A. *et al.* 2000. Repeated pregnancies in BALB/c mice infected with Coxiella burnetii cause disseminated infection, resulting in stillbirth and endocarditis. *J. Infect Dis.* **181:** 188–194.

87. Parker, R.R., E.J. Bell & D.B. Lackman. 1948. Experimental studies of Q fever in cattle: I. Observations on four heifers and two milk cows. *Am. J. Hyg.* **48:** 191–197.

88. Luoto, L. & R.J. Huebner. 1950. Q fever studies in southern California; IX. Isolation of Q fever organisms from parturient placenta; of naturally infected dairy cows. *Public Health Rep.* **65:** 541–544.

89. Abinanti, F.R. *et al.* 1953. Q fever studies. XVIII. Presence of Coxiella burnetii in the birth fluids of naturally infected sheep. *Am. J. Hyg.* **58:** 385–388.

90. Waldhalm, D.G. *et al.* 1978. Abortion associated with Coxiella burnetii infection in dairy goats. *J. Am. Vet. Med. Assoc.* **173:** 1580–1581.

91. Stoker, M.G. & J.F. Thompson. 1953. An explosive outbreak of Q fever. *Lancet* **1:** 137–139.

92. Stoenner, H.G. 1951. Experimental Q fever in cattle–epizootiologic aspects. *J. Am. Vet. Med. Assoc.* **118:** 170–174.

93. Palmer, N.C. *et al.* 1983. Placentitis and Abortion in Goats and Sheep in Ontario Caused by Coxiella burnetii. *Can. Vet. J.* **24:** 60–61.

94. Berri, M. *et al.* 2007. Goats may experience reproductive failures and shed Coxiella burnetii at two successive parturitions after a Q fever infection. *Res. Vet. Sci.* **83:** 47–52.

95. Kaplan, B. *et al.* 1995. An isolated case of Q-fever during pregnancy. *Acta. Obstet. Gynecol. Scand.* **74:** 848–849.

96. Gaburro, D. & A. Del Campo. 1956. Considerazioni epidemiologiche e cliniche su un' infezione de Coxiella burnetii in tre gemelle immature. *Mal. Inf. Parsit.* **8:** 384.

97. Tellez, A. *et al.* 1998. Q fever in pregnancy: case report after a 2-year follow-up. *J. Infect.* **37:** 79–81.

98. Syrucek, L., O. Sobeslavsky & I. Gutvirth. 1958. Isolation of Coxiella burneti from human placentas. *J. Hyg. Epidemiol. Microbiol. Immunol.* **2:** 29–35.

99. Riechman, N. *et al.* 1988. Chronic Q fever and severe thrombocytopenia in a pregnant woman. *Am. J. Med.* **85:** 253–254.

100. McGivern, D. *et al.* 1988. Concomitant zoonotic infections with ovine Chlamydia and 'Q' fever in pregnancy: clinical features, diagnosis, management and public health implications. Case report. *Br. J. Obstet. Gynaecol.* **95:** 294–298.

101. Marrie, T.J. 1993. Q fever in pregnancy: report of two cases. *Infect. Dis. Clin. Pract.* **2:** 207–209.

102. Jover-Diaz, F. *et al.* 2001. Q fever during pregnancy: an emerging cause of prematurity and abortion. *Infect Dis. Obstet. Gynecol.* **9:** 47–49.

103. Hellmeyer, L. *et al.* 2002. Q Fever in pregnancy: a case report and review of the literature. *Z Geburtshilfe Neonatol.* **206:** 193–198.

104. Friedland, J.S. *et al.* 1994. Q fever and intrauterine death. *Lancet* **343:** 288.

105. Ellis, M.E., C.C. Smith & M.A. Moffat. 1983. Chronic or fatal Q-fever infection: a review of 16

patients seen in North-East Scotland (1967–80). *Q. J. Med.* **52:** 54–66.

106. Dindinaud, G. *et al.* 1991. Q fever and fetal death in utero. Two cases. *J. Gynecol. Obstet. Biol. Reprod. (Paris)* **20:** 969–972.

107. Bental, T. *et al.* 1995. Chronic Q fever of pregnancy presenting as Coxiella burnetii placentitis: successful outcome following therapy with erythromycin and rifampin. *Clin. Infect Dis.* **21:** 1318–1321.

108. Wagstaff, D.F. *et al.* 1959. Q fever studies in Maryland. *Public Health Rep.* **80:** 1095–1099.

109. Raoult, D. 1993. Treatment of Q fever. *Antimicrob Agents Chemother.* **37:** 1733–1736.

110. Maurin, M. *et al.* 1992. Phagolysosomal alkalinization and the bactericidal effect of antibiotics: the Coxiella burnetii paradigm. *J. Infect Dis.* **166:** 1097–1102.

111. Raoult, D. *et al.* 1999. Treatment of Q fever endocarditis: comparison of 2 regimens containing doxycycline and ofloxacin or hydroxychloroquine. *Arch. Intern. Med.* **159:** 167–173.

112. Lim, W.S., J.T. Macfarlane & C.L. Colthorpe. 2003. Treatment of community-acquired lower respiratory tract infections during pregnancy. *Am. J. Respir. Med.* **2:** 221–233.

113. Marmion, B.P. *et al.* 1990. Vaccine prophylaxis of abattoir-associated Q fever: eight years' experience in Australian abattoirs. *Epidemiol. Infect.* **104:** 275–287.

114. Ormsbee, R. & B. Marmion. 1990. Prevention of Coxiella burnetii infection: vaccines and guidelines for those at risk. In *Q Fever, the Disease*. T.J. Marrie, Ed.: 226–248. CRC Press. Boca Raton.

115. Ackland, J.R., D.A. Worswick & B.P. Marmion. 1994. Vaccine prophylaxis of Q fever. A follow-up study of the efficacy of Q-Vax (CSL) 1985–1990. *Med. J. Aust.* **160:** 704–708.

Q Fever in Dairy Animals

Annie Rodolakis

INRA, UR 1282 Infectiologie Animale et Santé Publique, F-37380 Nouzilly

This review evaluates the threat to human health—with the shedding of *C. burnetii* in dairy animals with reproductive disorders or those without clinical signs. The review also discusses the diagnosis of Q fever in livestock and the possibility of *Coxiella*-free herds, and it reports the available methods for controlling Q fever. *C. burnetii* shedding seems to occur frequently in milk taken from asymptomatic dairy cows. The number of Coxiella shed in milk is generally low. The phase I vaccine prevented abortion and greatly decreased the shedding of *C. burnetii* in milk.

Key words: Q fever; *Coxiella burnetii*; dairy cattle; diagnosis; vaccine

Q fever is a widespread zoonosis caused by *Coxiella burnetii*. This intracellular gram-negative bacterium which can infect a wide range of susceptible hosts including farm animals, pets, wild mammals, and even non-mammalian species, such as domestic and wild birds, reptiles, and ticks. However, livestock is considered to be the major source for human infection. *C. burnetii* may induce reproductive disorders such as abortion, stillbirth, and delivery of weak and nonviable neonates in ruminants.[1] Metritis and infertility are frequently the main clinical signs of infection in cattle herds.[1,2] However, infection is frequently subclinical, and the prevalence of *Coxiella burnetii* in farm animals remains unclear because abortion rates are frequently low—other than in some herds of goats.

The *C. burnetii* Shedding in Dairy Herds

Herds with Reproductive Disorders

Infected females shed huge numbers of *Coxiella* into birth products[3–5] and smaller numbers in urine, feces, and milk. This shedding may persist over several months, particularly in vaginal mucus, feces, and milk, even in those of females with normal parturition.[6–8] None of these routes predominated over the others in 242 dairy cows from 31 herds in which abortions due to *C. burnetii* were reported.[9] In addition, most of the animals shedding the bacterium did so by only one route. By contrast, in 3 ovine flocks from the southwest of France, the ewes were found to shed the bacterium mostly in feces and vaginal mucus, with much lower levels of shedding in milk,[10] whereas vaginal mucus was found to be the major route for bacterial shedding in another flock from central France. Shedding into milk seems to be the most frequent route in goats. However, all three routes of shedding are observed in goats, as shown by a study in which goats were experimentally infected with 10^4 *C. burnetii* cells during gestation.[3,11] These differences in shedding patterns may account for the more frequent identification of sheep and goats than of cattle as the source of human Q fever. As *C. burnetii* is very stable in the environment, close contact with the herd is not required for infection.

Shedding in Herds without Clinical Signs

In asymptomatic herds, the cows shed *C. burnetii* almost exclusively in milk.[10] This shedding may persist for several months and may

Address for correspondence: Annie Rodolakis, INRA IASP311 37380 Nouzilly. Voice: +33-247-427-634; fax: +33-247-427-779. Annie.Rodolakis@tours.inra.fr

Rickettsiology and Rickettsial Diseases-Fifth International Conference: Ann. N.Y. Acad. Sci. 1166: 90–93 (2009).
doi: 10.1111/j.1749-6632.2009.04511.x © 2009 New York Academy of Sciences.

be continuous or intermittent. In some cases, the shedding of *C. burnetii* in milk is associated with chronic subclinical mastitis.[12]

C. burnetii shedding seems to be very frequent in milk from asymptomatic dairy cows, although its prevalence in France remains unknown. In the USA, 316 bulk tank milk samples from several herds displayed a very high prevalence (>94%) of shedding during a 3-year period.[8] By contrast, we tested bulk tank milk samples from more than 70 seropositive dairy sheep flocks by PCR. Negative results were obtained in all cases. These data suggest that *C. burnetii* shedding in milk is less widespread in ewes than in cows. These differences in shedding pattern may depend on host species or *C. burnetii* strain.

Impact of the Shedding of *C. Burnetii* in Milk on Disease Transmission

Contamination via the respiratory tract, through the inhalation of contaminated dust and spray from infected animals, is common.[13,14] Ingestion of contaminated untreated milk or dairy products appears to be a less efficient route of disease transmission to humans. It may lead to seroconversion and, perhaps in a few cases, to Q fever.[15,16] Consumption of dairy products (milk, cheese, and butter) is very rarely identified as a risk factor in epidemiological investigations of Q fever outbreaks. Few *Coxiella* cells are generally shed in milk, particularly in naturally infected cows, which do not shed the bacterium continuously. Experimentally infected ewes shed 100 to 1000 times less bacterial cells in milk than in vaginal mucus (unpublished data).

However, the kinetics of antibody production and *C. burnetii* shedding in herds of asymptomatic cattle shedding the bacterium are consistent with the circulation of *C. burnetii* within the herd. In addition, calves that have ingested infectious milk eliminate the bacterium in their urine and feces, thereby facilitating the spread of the infection in the environment.[17] Asymptomatic cattle herds must therefore be considered potential bacterial reservoirs capable of transmitting the disease. Nevertheless, *C. burnetii* shedding in milk presumably plays a lesser role in disease transmission than other routes of shedding, via birth products, vaginal mucus, and feces, for example, as these products may contaminate manure, which may contaminate the fields on which it is spread at some distance from the herd.

Diagnosis

Q fever diagnosis is generally undertaken only if abortions are observed. The detection of *C. burnetii* DNA in the placenta and vaginal mucus by PCR has radically changed the diagnosis of Q fever in veterinary medicine.[2,9,18] Several PCR kits are available and provide a specific, sensitive, and rapid tool for the detection of *C. burnetii* in various clinical samples. They can also be used to detect metritis caused by *C. burnetii*. The main limitation of conventional PCR techniques is that they cannot be used to determine the bacteriological load of the samples tested, whereas this assessment is essential to confirm that *C. burnetii* was truly responsible for the abortions observed, as the placenta and vaginal mucus of females producing healthy calves, kids, or lambs may be infected with fewer bacteria than those of females suffering abortions. Real-time PCR (Rt-PCR) kits are now available for such quantification. These tests may also be automated, decreasing the risk of sample contamination and saving time. Rt-PCR assays are now recognized as the most suitable tool for diagnosing abortion due to *C. burnetii* and for identifying animals shedding *Coxiella*.[9]

It is difficult to identify *Coxiella*-free herds. Bulk tank milk samples can be used to investigate the sanitary condition of dairy herds, by checking for the presence of *C. burnetii* by PCR and of antibodies by ELISA. There is no relationship between the antibody response and excretion. Most of the animals shedding *C. burnetii* in vaginal mucus, feces, or milk are seropositive or have antibodies in milk, but others remain seronegative despite excreting the bacterium.[7] This seronegative response is due to the antigen used in ELISA kits rather than a lack of antibody production. Thus, PCR and ELISA analyses must be repeated several times to ensure that they are efficient, and the ELISA should be carried out with an antigen isolated from ruminants. In herds with PCR-positive bulk tank milk, pools of 10 milk samples can be tested by PCR to identify animals shedding the bacterium. If these animals are few in number, they can be eliminated, and the other animals should be vaccinated with an efficient vaccine.

Disease Control

Particular care must be taken when introducing a new animal into a Q fever-free herd, but simply ensuring that the new animal is not infected is not sufficient, as Q fever is principally airborne, and direct contact with a female that has suffered abortion is not required for contamination.

During Q-fever outbreaks, the contamination of animals and the environment can be prevented or reduced by destroying placentas and fetuses, so as to prevent their ingestion by domestic or wild carnivores, which could disseminate the disease. If possible, births should be confined to a specific location that is disinfected without inducing aerosols.

Manure should be treated with lime, or 0.6% calcium cyanamide, before its spreading on fields. Manure should not be spread in windy conditions, as the wind may propagate the disease over large distances. However, the efficacy of disinfection procedures for preventing the spread of infection in ruminant and human populations remains unproven, particularly for contaminated manure. Efficacy has so far been tested only for the treatment of slurry.

Antibiotic treatment, consisting of two injections of tetracycline (20 mg/kg) during the last month of gestation is often used to reduce the number of abortions and the quantity of *C. burnetii* shed at parturition. The efficacy of this treatment has never been accurately assessed, but it has been shown that it does not entirely prevent abortion[7] or the shedding of *C. burnetii* at lambing.[19]

Only vaccination with an efficient vaccine can really control the disease in ruminants. The efficacy of two commercial vaccines—a phase I and a phase II vaccine—was compared in pregnant goats experimentally infected with a dose of *C. burnetii* sufficient to cause abortion or premature birth in 85% of the goats in the control group.[11] The phase I vaccine prevented abortion and drastically reduced the shedding of *C. burnetii* in the milk, vaginal mucus, and feces, reducing environmental contamination and thus, the risk of transmission to humans. By contrast, the phase II vaccine did not modify the course of the disease.

Therefore, the phase 1 vaccine has potential for the vaccination not only of infected flocks, but also of nearby uninfected flocks, to reduce the risk of disease dissemination.

In addition, studies of Coxiella infection among farm workers dealing with dairy cattle and individuals working in the milk processing industry, together with studies of the possible dangers of dairy products, would improve evaluations of the role of dairy ruminants in epidemiological aspects of Q fever.[2]

Conflicts of Interest

The author declares no conflicts of interest.

References

1. Lang, G.H. *et al.* 1994. Serological response in sheep vaccinated against Coxiella burnetii (Q fever). *Can. Vet. J.* **35:** 373–374.
2. To, H. *et al.* 1998. Prevalence of Coxiella burnetii infection in dairy cattle with reproductive disorders. *J. Vet. Med. Sci.* **60:** 859–861.
3. Arricau Bouvery, N. *et al.* 2003. Experimental *Coxiella burnetii* infection in pregnant goats: excretion routes. *Vet. Res.* **34:** 423–433.

4. Hatchette, T.F. *et al*. 2001. Goat-associated Q fever: a new disease in Newfoundland. *Emerg. Infect. Dis.* **7:** 413–419.

5. Masala, G. *et al*. 2004. Occurrence, distribution, and role in abortion of *Coxiella burnetii* in sheep and goats in Sardinia, Italy. *Vet. Microbiol.* **99:** 301–305.

6. To, H. *et al*. 1995. Isolation of *Coxiella burnetii* from dairy cattle and ticks, and some characteristics of the isolates in Japan. *Microbiol. Immunol.* **39:** 663–671.

7. Berri, M. *et al*. 2005. Spread of *Coxiella burnetii* infection in a flock of sheep after an episode of Q fever. *Vet. Rec.* **157:** 737–740.

8. Kim, S.G. *et al*. 2005. *Coxiella burnetii* in bulk tank milk samples, United States. *Emerg. Infect. Dis.* **11:** 619–621.

9. Guatteo, R. *et al*. 2006. Shedding routes of *Coxiella burnetii* in dairy cows: implications for detection and control. *Vet. Res.* **37:** 827–833.

10. Rodolakis, A. *et al*. 2007. Comparison of *Coxiella burnetii* shedding in milk of dairy bovine, caprine, and ovine herds. *J. Dairy Sci.* **90:** 5352–5360.

11. Arricau-Bouvery, N. *et al*. 2005. Effect of vaccination with phase I and phase II *Coxiella burnetii* vaccines in pregnant goats. *Vaccine* **23:** 4392–4402.

12. Barlow, J. *et al*. 2008. Association between *Coxiella burnetii* shedding in milk and subclinical mastitis. *Vet. Res.* **39:** 7.

13. Maurin, M. & D. Raoult. 1999. Q fever. *Clin. Microbiol. Rev.* **12:** 518–553.

14. Tissot-Dupont, H. *et al*. 2004. Wind in November, Q fever in December. *Emerg. Infect. Dis.* **10:** 1264–1269.

15. Benson, W.W. *et al*. 1963. Serologic analysis of a penitentiary group using raw milk from a Q fever infected herd. *Public Health Rep.* **78:** 707–710.

16. Fishbein, D.B. & D. Raoult. 1992. A cluster of *Coxiella burnetii* infections associated with exposure to vaccinated goats and their unpasteurized dairy products. *Am. J. Trop. Med. Hyg.* **47:** 35–40.

17. Lang, G.H. 1990. Coxiellosis (Q Fever) in animals. In *Q Fever: The Disease*. T. Marrie, Ed.: 23–48. CRC Press. Boca Raton, FL.

18. Berri, M. *et al*. 2000. The detection of *Coxiella burnetii* from ovine genital swabs, milk and fecal samples by the use of a single touchdown polymerase chain reaction. *Vet. Microbiol.* **72:** 285–293.

19. Arricau-Bouvery, N. & A. Rodolakis. 2005. Is Q fever an emerging or re-emerging zoonosis? *Vet. Res.* **36:** 327–349.

Advances in Rickettsia Pathogenicity

Premanand Balraj, Patricia Renesto, and Didier Raoult

*Unité des Rickettsies, URMITE IRD-CNRS 6236, Faculté de Médecine,
Marseille, France*

One century after the first description of rickettsiae as human pathogens, the rickettsiosis remained poorly understood diseases. These microorganisms are indeed characterized by a strictly intracellular location which has, for long, prohibited their detailed study. Within the last ten years, the completion of the genome sequences of several strains allowed gaining a better knowledge about the molecular mechanisms involved in rickettsia pathogenicity. Here, we summarized available data concerning the critical steps of rickettsia-host cell interactions that should contribute to tissue injury and diseases, that is, adhesion, phagosomal escape, motility, and intracellular survival of the bacteria.

Key words: actin-based motility; adhesins; phagosomal escape; PLD; rickettsia; T4SS

Introduction

One century elapsed since Ricketts provided the first experimental evidence for involvement of a transmissible microbe causing the Rocky Mountain spotted fever.[1] His investigations highlighted most of the major characteristics of the responsible infectious agent, including its intracellular nature and its arthropod transmission.[2] In honor to Ricketts's contribution to the description of a new class of pathogens that were not fulfilling the Koch's postulate, as uncultivable,[3] the genus *Rickettsia* was born. These gram-negative and rod-shaped bacterial species were divided in two main groups, the spotted fever group (SFG) and the typhus group (TG).[4] During the 80 years following their initial description, only a few rickettsiae were conclusively associated with human diseases.[4] The introduction of modern diagnostic tools including culture, PCR, and serological analysis[5] largely contributed to the recent expansion of rickettsia identification from human samples. This is exemplified by the fact that among the 20 pathogenic strains yet established, 13 new tick-borne rickettsiae were identified since 1991.[6] Significant progresses have also been achieved concerning both epidemiology[6] and genotyping.[7] In contrast, questions regarding the underlying mechanisms of their pathogenicity remained for long poorly understood.

The main steps of rickettsial infections can be depicted as follows: Rickettsiae are usually inoculated in human beings by arthropods that transmit bacteria through salivary secretion (ticks) or infected feces (flea and louse).[4] Indirect routes of transmission were also described, such as contamination of the eyes following crushing of ticks with the fingers and contamination of abraded skin by tick-borne rickettsiae excreted in tick feces.[6] In addition, *R. prowazekii* that is stable in dried louse feces can be transmitted through aerosols.[4] The risk of disease transmission results from a complex process that relies on various parameters including, for example, abundance of infected arthropod vectors, the prevalence of their infection rate, and increased attachment time (for tick-transmitted rickettsiosis).[4,6] Bacteria then invade human endothelial cells, via the process of induced phagocytosis,[8]

Address for correspondence: Pr Didier Raoult, Unité des Rickettsies, URMITE IRD-CNRS 6236, Faculté de Médecine, 27, Boulevard Jean Moulin, 13385 Marseille, France. Voice: +33-491-32-43-75; fax: +33-491-38-77-72. Didier.Raoult@medecine.univ-mrs.fr

Rickettsiology and Rickettsial Diseases-Fifth International Conference: Ann. N.Y. Acad. Sci. 1166: 94–105 (2009).
doi: 10.1111/j.1749-6632.2009.04517.x © 2009 New York Academy of Sciences.

and rapidly escape from the phagosome into the host cytoplasm[9] where they replicate. Historically, besides growth temperature and antigenicity, the actin-based motility was depicted as a major feature; allowing to differentiate SFG and TG rickettsiae. While actin polymerization promotes cell-to-cell spreading, TG rickettsiae that are devoid of motility replicate until the cell bursts. The clinical features mainly correspond to pulmonary and brain endothelial cell damages.[10]

The strictly intracellular location of bacteria from the *Rickettsia* genus has for long prohibited their study,[11] explaining that the detailed picture of their interaction with host cells was lacking. During the last few years, the completion of the genome sequence of several strains of rickettsiae,[12] starting from that of *R. prowazekii* (published in 1998),[13] allowed gaining a better understanding of the molecular mechanisms involved in tissue injury and disease caused by these pathogens. Based on the premise that differences or similarities in the ability of two microbes to promote disease is reflected in genomic sequence data, the comparison of two closely related genomes can theoretically allow the finding of differences that correlate with virulence. Therefore, due to the lack of non-pathogenic rickettsial mutants, the computational prediction and characterization of putative virulence factors is a hard task. In fact, to our knowledge, such a comparative analysis has been made possible only twice. Thus, identification of genes involved in the virulence of *R. rickettsii* was carried out from the genome sequences of the virulent strain *R. rickettsii* Sheila Smith and of *R. rickettsii* Iowa; the later being depicted as avirulent in a guinea pig model of infection.[14] Similarly, the comparative analysis of *R. prowazekii* Madrid E (avirulent) and BreinL (virulent) has been reported.[15–19] However, we have to keep in mind that the nonpathogenic phenotype of these strains has been established on experimental animal models, and extrapolation from such model studies to the human diseases is somewhere highly speculative.

Here, we review recent data concerning the main steps of such a bacteria-host cell interaction, namely adhesion, phagosomal escape, and motility. Most of the bacterial virulence factors are proteic compounds either secreted at the bacterial cell surface or released into the external environment. Gram-negative bacteria have developed only a small number of secretion systems by which such proteins pass through their outer membranes and exert their function. Rickettsial secretion system and putatively secreted virulence proteins will also be discussed. All these steps were depicted in Figure 1.

Rickettsial Ligands and Host Cell Receptors

A major constituent of the outer membrane of gram-negative bacteria is lipopolysaccharide, but in contrast to what was observed for several pathogens,[20] its role as rickettsial adhesin was discarded.[10,21] Because rickettsiae lost their ability to bind to host cells after heating or incubation with trypsin, involvement for a proteic ligand was suggested.[22] The proteins susceptible to play a role in binding and entry of the bacteria into their host cells are listed above.

Sca Family Proteins

It was long evidenced that rickettsiae were surrounded by a regularly arrayed surface structure (S-layer)[23] containing proteins able to elicit protective immune responses.[24,25] Prior to *rickettsial* genome sequencing, only two surface protein antigens (SPAs), namely rOmpA and rOmpB, were identified. Analysis of their amino acid sequence highlighted the presence of a conserved autotransporter β-barrel domain otherwise called autotransporter domain (AT) at their C-terminal end. Availability of *R. prowazekii* and *R. conorii* genomes[13,26] further allowed evidence of three additional genes encoding such an AT domain. These genes were annotated as "surface cell antigen" (*sca*) genes

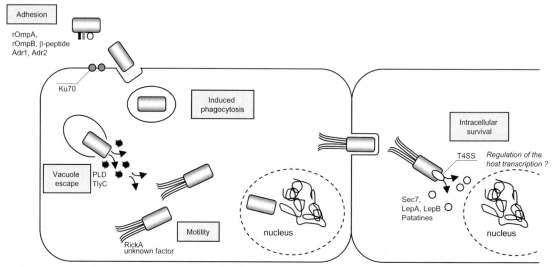

Figure 1. Schematic representation of rickettsia-endothelial cell interaction. Following rickettsia entry into host cells through induced phagocytosis, bacteria rapidly escape from the vacuole to gain the cytosolic compartment and possibly the eucaryotic nucleus where they replicate. For rickettsiae exhibiting a motile phenotype, cell-to-cell spreading is observed. T4SS translocate effectors that should contribute to the intracellular survival of the rickettsiae.

(i.e., *sca1, 2, 3*) together with *rOmpA* (*sca0*) and *rOmpB* (*sca5*), while *geneD* was renamed *sca4*. Using nine rickettsial genomic sequences, the "Sca protein family" was then extensively characterized and 17 subfamilies were established.[27] Their typical architecture (Fig. 2) comprises a N-terminal signal peptide and a C-terminal AT domain that promotes the export of the central passenger domain to the outside of the bacteria. With a few exceptions, including rOmpA and rOmpB (further detailed below), the function of these Sca proteins remains unknown. However, it was hypothesized that they should contribute to the specific recognition of different sets of host receptors.[27]

rickettsiae to host cells was further confirmed *ex vivo*.[33] Moreover, the recent comparative genomic analysis of *R. rickettsii* Sheila Smith (virulent) and Iowa (avirulent) strains highlighted a deletion resulting in defect of rOmpA expression in the latter.[14] Immunoblotting and immunofluorescence confirmed the absence of rOmpA from *R. rickettsii* Iowa. While this gene was initially present within *R. prowazekii* genome, its evolution led to its complete disappearance by degradation, leaving only traces of short homologous sequences.[34] Thus, and as confirmed from rickettsial genome sequencing, rOmpA is exclusive for the SFG rickettsiae.[12,27]

rOmpA

This 190 kDa immunodominant surface-exposed protein was thought to be involved in adhesion of rickettsiae to host cells, based on the protective effect against rickettsial infections in animal models immunized with the recombinant truncated rOmpA or DNA plasmid encoding this protein.[28–32] The critical role displayed by rOmpA in the attachment of

rOmpB

As rOmpA, rOmpB was long associated with both antigenicity and pathogenicity of these bacteria.[35] The gene *ompB* coding for this autotransporter belongs to the core genes of *Rickettsia*.[12] In fact, among the 17 members of rickettsial cell surface antigens (*sca* family) identified within available rickettsial genomes, *rompB* was the unique conserved one.[27] This

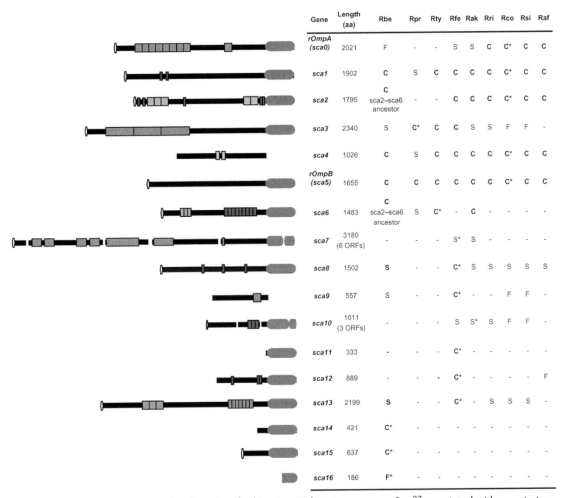

Gene	Length (aa)	Rbe	Rpr	Rty	Rfe	Rak	Rri	Rco	Rsi	Raf
rOmpA (sca0)	2021	F	-	-	S	S	C	C*	C	C
sca1	1902	C	S	C	C	C	C	C*	C	C
sca2	1795	C sca2–sca6 ancestor	-	-	C	C	C	C*	C	C
sca3	2340	S	C*	C	C	S	S	F	F	-
sca4	1026	C	S	C	C	C	C	C*	C	C
rOmpB (sca5)	1655	C	C	C	C	C	C	C*	C	C
sca6	1483	C sca2–sca6 ancestor	S	C*	-	C	-	-	-	-
sca7	3180 (6 ORFs)	-	-	-	S*	S	-	-	-	-
sca8	1502	S	-	-	C*	S	S	S	S	S
sca9	557	S	-	-	C*	-	-	F	F	-
sca10	1011 (3 ORFs)	-	-	-	S	S*	S	F	F	-
sca11	333	-	-	-	C*	-	-	-	-	-
sca12	889	-	-	-	C*	-	-	-	-	F
sca13	2199	S	-	-	C*	-	S	S	S	-
sca14	421	C*	-	-	-	-	-	-	-	-
sca15	637	C*	-	-	-	-	-	-	-	-
sca16	186	F*	-	-	-	-	-	-	-	-

Figure 2. The 17 *sca* gene families identified in nine *Rickettsia* genomes. See[27]; reprinted with permission, Oxford Journals, Oxford University Press licence number 1954711133562. The structural domains of the Sca proteins are schematized on the left. The yellow diamonds, thick black lines, and the blue ovals represent the predicted peptide signals, passenger domains, and AT domains, respectively. Interruptions in the thick black lines or the blue ovals indicate the occurrence of in-frame stop codons in the coding sequence. Colored boxes show the presence of repeated peptide motifs. Boxes of same color refer to similar peptide motifs. The table on the right summarizes the names, lengths of the peptide products, and the presence or absence of the *sca* genes in the *Rickettsia* genomes. The characters "C," "S," "F," and "-" indicate whether the gene is complete, split, fragment, or absent, respectively, in a given genome. Genes were defined as split if the entire protein is encoded by successive ORFs and as fragment if the gene size was less than 50% of that of the longest ortholog. Asterisks indicate the genes from which the length and the structural domains of the peptide products are shown. For Sca7 and Sca10, the protein lengths were obtained after concatenating the successive ORFs.

gene encodes a large precursor subsequently processed into the mature 120-kDa rOmpB and the 32 kDa β-peptide, respectively.[36,37] Recent experiments showed that expression of rOmpB in *Escherichia coli* allowed adherence and entry of transformed bacteria in epithelial cells.[38] The comparative analysis of virulent and avirulent strains of *R. prowazekii* suggested that rOmpB methylation could be associated with the virulent phenotype.[39] A relationship was further evidenced between the defect of methylation observed in the avirulent MadridE and the presence of a mutation within the gene encoding the lysine methyltransferase,[18] impairing expression of this enzyme.[19] Through overlay assays carried out with biotinylated endothelial cells, we recently evidenced that the β-peptide was a putative rickettsial ligand. This interaction was not observed with the avirulent *R. rickettsii* Iowa strain[40] that is defective in the processing of rOmpB.[14,37] While such interaction was somewhere in contradiction with the theoretical location of the β-peptide,[41] a positive immunofluorescence staining of rickettsiae outer membrane was observed with anti-β-peptide antibodies (unpublished data).

Adr1 and Adr2 Rickettsial Adhesins

Overlay assays coupled with high resolution 2D-PAGE and mass spectrometry analysis also permitted to point out two putative rickettsial adhesins of 30 kDa encoded by the paralogous genes RC1281 and RC1282 in *R. conorii* and, respectively, designed as Adr1 and Adr2.[40] As rOmpB, these proteins were found ubiquitously present within the *Rickettsia* genus.[12] While initially annotated of unknown function, BLAST analysis further evidenced homologies between these proteins and other bacterial adhesins including the adhesin/virulence factor Hek of *Escherichia coli* UTI89 (ZP_00726099), the putative invasin of *Lawsonia intracellularis* (YP_595216), and the possible outer membrane adhesin of *Salmonella enterica* subsp. (ZP_02675271). Moreover, we observed that polyclonal antibodies raised against the recombinant *R. conorii* Adr1 inhibited the bacterial entry into the host cells, estimated by plaque formation (unpublished data).

Eukaryotic Ligands

Only a few experiments were aimed at identifying the eukaryotic receptor of rickettsiae. It was demonstrated that the Ku70 subunit of DNA-dependent protein kinase, a protein present in the nucleus, cytoplasm, plasma membrane, and lipid raft microdomains might be involved in rickettsia entry within non-phagocytic mammalian cells.[42] While the cascade of signalling events leading to rickettsial phagocytosis remains to be characterized, the rOmpB protein was identified as the rickettsial ligand that interacted with Ku70.

Regulation of Rickettsial Ligand Expression

During their life cycle, bacteria from the *Rickettsia* genus *may* adapt to diverse environments in the ticks and mammals. Their adaptation strategy most probably results from a selective gene expression, as depicted for *Borrelia burgdorferi*.[43] Accordingly, we observed that rOmpA expression can undergo major changes, as being strongly detected when rickettsiae propagated within Vero cells while being poorly expressed in bacteria that was collected from tick hemolymph.[44] Variation in rOmpA, but not in rOmpB expression, was also evidenced in *R. massiliae* during the *Rhipicephalus turanicus* life cycle.[45] When inoculated from arthropod vectors to human beings, rickettsiae most probably exhibit a proteic profile different to that observed from bacteria grown in culture. *Ex-vivo* experiments aimed at characterizing this host-pathogen interaction should thus be analyzed with caution.

Phagosomal Escape

As several other pathogens of the genus *Listeria*, *Shigella*, and *Mycobacterium*, *Rickettsia* rapidly gain access to the cytosol of infected cells through phagosomal vacuole escape. The involvement for a phospholipase A_2 (PLA_2) in the entry vesicle lysis has for long been proposed for *R. rickettsii*[46,47] and then extended to both *R. conorii* and *R. prowazekii*.[48] Therefore, and despite the completion of corresponding genomes, any PLA_2-encoding gene was found. The first phospholipase identified within a rickettsial genome was the *R. conorii* phospholipase

D (PLD).[49] This dimeric protein belongs to a new clade of PLD superfamily and is characterized by the presence, on each monomer, of only one HKD motif that is critical for the biochemical activity.[50] Recent published data demonstrating that Salmonella isolates transformed with the *R. prowazekii* PLD genes were able to escape phagosomal vacuoles confirmed that PLD is likely to be the major effector of rickettsial phagosomal escape.[51] Of note is that this gene is conserved in all species of the *Rickettsia* yet sequenced.

Besides PLD ortholog, the analysis of *R. typhi* genome highlighted the presence of another putative phospholipase-like protein exhibiting significant similarity to the patatin family of proteins.[52] Patatin is the major storage glycoprotein found in potatoes and is endowed for phospholipase A_2 (PLA_2) activity.[53] While only one patatin-like protein gene (*pat1*) is present in rickettsial genomes including *R. conorii, R. rickettsii, R. prowazekii, R. bellii, R. akari, R. sibirica, R. africae,* and *R. akari,*[54] three copies 100% identical were found in *R. felis.*[55] The gene *pat1* is located on the chromosome, and the two others, designed *pat2A* and *pat2B*, are located on the two *R. felis* plasmids. Alignment of all the rickettsial patatin-like proteins with characterized patatins from plants evidenced that the amino acid residues accounting for phospholipase A_2 activity are highly conserved.[54] Accordingly, McLeod and colleagues[52] hypothesized that patatin-like proteins might be responsible for the PLA_2 activity and thus involved in escape of the organism from the phagolysosome. Therefore, in contrast to what was observed for *pld*, the *pat1* gene is not transcriptionally expressed in *R. prowazekii* during the peak time of escape.[51] Another candidate with potential membranolytic activities and susceptible to intervene in such a process is tlyC.[51]

Actin-Based Motility

Exploitation of the host-cell actin cytoskeleton is crucial for several microbial pathogens to enter and to disseminate within cells, thus avoiding the host immune response.[56,57] The capacity of rickettsiae to use the actin-based motility system for promoting cell-to-cell spreading was evidenced for several SFG rickettsiae including *R. conorii, R. rickettsii, R. montanensis, R. parkeri, R. australis,* and *R. monacensis.*[58–60] It was long considered that actin-based motility was confined to the SFG rickettsiae. Accordingly, the rickettsial factor susceptible to be responsible for actin polymerization was identified through the comparative analysis of *R. conorii* (SFG) and *R. prowazekii* (TG) genomes.[26] The so-called RickA protein contains a domain with homologies with Wiskott-Aldrich Syndrome Protein (WASP)-family proteins and was thought to function as a nucleation-promoting factor that directly activates the Arp2/3 complex.[61,62] In this respect, rickettsiae have evolved a strategy similar to that described for *Listeria monocytogenes.*[63] From *in vitro* actin branching assay performed with recombinant RickA, the involvement of additional bacterial or eukaryotic factors in reorganizing Arp2/3 complex generated Y-branched networks into parallel arrays was also suggested.[62]

Because genetic manipulations are still unfeasible, the role of RickA in the motility of rickettsiae has not been formerly demonstrated. Its function was in part supported by the absence of motility of *R. peacockii*, a strain for which *rickA* is disrupted by an insertion sequence of 1,095 nucleotides termed IRSpe1.[64] Therefore, some points remain unclear. Thus, and while RickA was found to be expressed on the bacterial surface,[65] both signal sequence and hydrophobic domain that are respectively required for secretion and membrane anchorage of this protein are lacking.[56,57] Thus, the putative involvement of the type IV secretion factor (T4SS) in the secretion of RickA to the rickettsial membrane was evoked.[61] Other bacterial components known to be responsible for intracellular motility as IcsA, ActA, or BimA, exhibited a polarized distribution.[66–68] Such polarization was not observed for RickA that was found to be expressed over the entire bacterial surface of

R. conorii,[61] a result consistent with the fact that stationary rickettsiae are usually surrounded by a uniform actin coat.[69] It can be speculated that a polarized distribution of RickA is sequentially achieved through the activity of a cofactor. For example, the unipolar distribution of IcsA that acts as the actin nucleation factor for the gram-negative bacterium *Shigella flexneri* relies on both a membrane protease and also onto the LPS structure.[70] Another key element came from *R. typhi* analysis. Short and occasional actin tails (<1%) were observed for these TG rickettsiae,[58,59] which were able to move approximately at the same rate as *R. rickettsii*, at least some of them, while others exhibited rather erratic movements.[71] However, *R. typhi* genome sequencing confirmed the absence of *rickA*,[52] thus reinforcing the role for another protein in actin-based motility. Whether rickettsial motility is facilitated by a bacterial or a host factor remains to be elucidated. Experiments achieved on *R. raoultii*, a newly isolated rickettsiae classified within the SFG,[72] evidenced that the motile phenotype could be dependent on the host cells and unrelated to the level of RickA expression.[73]

Specific Features of Motile Rickettsiae

The propulsive force generated by actin tail assembly could favor entry of SFG rickettsiae within the nucleus of eucaryotic cells. Accordingly, TG rickettsiae cannot penetrate in this cellular compartment.[4] Once inside the nucleus, the bacteria then become trapped, a phenomenon that should result from the lack of Arp2 and Arp3 proteins. In this respect, within the nucleus of Vero cells, *R. rickettsii* displayed irregular actin tails that was not accompanied with bacterial motility and tends to form high-density microcolonies.[69] The intranuclear growth of *R. bellii* was also observed, resulting in an intranuclear colony growth that should be favored by a nutrient enriched environment.[74]

As described for other microbial pathogens, including *Listeria monocytogenes* and *Shigella flexneri*, the intracellular actin-based motility *is also exploited by rickettsiae* to escape the host cell.[10,59,65] The filaments of actin push the rickettsiae to the surface of the host cell, where the host cell membrane is deformed outward and invaginates into the adjacent cell. Disruption of both cell membranes then enables the rickettsia to enter the adjoining cell without being exposed to the extracellular environment. The ability to spread from cell to cell without passing through the intercellular space enable bacteria to evade the immune response and thus contribute to the development of the infection. Through such long and thin cell projections, rickettsiae can exit via the luminal surface of blood vessels into the bloodstream without lysing the host cell. In contrast, TG rickettsiae devoid of motility escape the host cell by multiplying in such large numbers that they cause endothelial cell burst with subsequent release of bacteria into the blood.[10]

The reductive evolution of rickettsial genomes led to the lost of *rickA* from TG rickettsiae, namely *R. typhi* and *R. prowazekii*,[12] the latter being the most deadly of the rickettsiae infecting humans.[75–77] This observation somewhere contradicts the recent classification of RickA as a virulence factor.[78] We believe that this protein might rather play a critical role under specific situations, including long-term survival in arthropods, while not being a main actor of bacterial pathogenicity.

Type IV Secretion System

Several ORFs related to the T4SS[79] belong to the core gene set of rickettsiae.[12] T4SS are complex multiprotein structures spanning the bacterial envelope and composed of up to 12 individual protein building blocks classified into three groups,[80] each represented in this bacterial genus. Thus, proteins exposed to the cytoplasm of the cells and providing the energy for the biogenesis of the transporter (VirB4, VirB11, VirD4) are conserved in all *Rickettsia* sequenced genomes as those involved in the building of the translocation channel (VirB6, VirB8, VirB9, VirB10). Among the surface-exposed proteins, we noticed the presence of the genes encoding the major pilus component VirB2 and the pilus-associated protein VirB3. In contrast, VirB5 and VirB7 are lacking. The periplasmic VirB5$_{Ti}$ subunits contribute to the translocation of DNA substrates to the cell surface, and VirB7 are small lipoproteins only found in a subset of T4SS.[79]

The precise function of these transporters, which are ancestrally related to bacterial conjugation systems, have diverged during evolution. Three T4SS subfamilies are yet described.[80] Two of them, namely the conjugation system and the recently discovered "DNA uptake and release system" ensure genetic exchanges between bacteria, the latter functioning independently of contact with a target cell. The third T4SS subfamily corresponds to the "effector translocator systems" also called "injectisomes" and has been adopted by several bacterial pathogens for the delivery of virulence factors targeting eukaryotic host cells.[80,81] Since T4SS components are conserved in *Rickettsia* genomes that lack plasmids, their primary suspected role was the secretion of virulence factors rather than conjugation.[55] The T4SS were divided into two distinct subgroups, type IVA and type IVB, respectively.[82] Based on homologies with the *virB/virD4* secretion system of the plant pathogen *Agrobacterium tumefaciens* the T4SS conserved within the genus *Rickettsia* belongs to the type IVA.

What are the rickettsial substrates susceptible to, to be exported by such a secretion system? A high homology between *L. pneumophila* RalF and the Sec7 proteins of *R. prowazekii* (RP374) and *R. typhi* (RT0362) was reported.[52,83] The precise role of an effector known to contribute to the establishment of a replicative organelle by inhibiting the phagosome-lysosome fusion[84] is questionable in rickettsiae, since these bacteriae are growing into the cytoplasm of infected cells.[4] This protein is not conserved within all rickettsial genomes. Thus, besides *R. typhi* and *R. prowazekii*, *sec7* is also present in *R. felis* and

R. akari[85] (http://www.igs.cnrs-mrs.fr/mgdb/Rickettsia/rig/). Interestingly, two orthologous genes were found in *R. bellii*, a bacterium able to survive within ameba.[74] Miscroscopy examination of *Acanthameba polyphaga* coinfected by *R. bellii* and L. pneumophila revealed a co-localization of both bacteria within the amebal vacuole. In other SFG rickettsiae, Sec7 is either split or degraded.

We also noticed that other translocated effectors of the *L. pneumophila* Dot/Icm secretion system (Type IVB secretion system), namely LepA (RC0359) and LepB (RC0156), are present in all *Rickettsia* genome sequenced. These peptides are not required for *L. pneumophila* replication in mammalian cells, but rather promote the release of bacteria from protozoa through an exocytic pathway, thus favoring the pathogen dissemination via "faecal" or "respirable" infectious vesicles.[86] Again, this observation fits well with the probable ancestral location of rickettsiae within ameba.[74] As mentioned above, *R. bellii* can replicate within protozoan hosts, but this is not the case for other rickettsia species. Accordingly, whether these proteins are associated to the pathogenicity or parasitic lifestyle of rickettsiae during their interaction with eukaryotic host is not yet established.

VipD is patatin domain-containing protein that perturbs membrane trafficking and was recently identified as another effector of *L. pneumophila*.[87] This protein was found to modulate the intracellular bacterial growth.[88] As previously mentioned, *Rickettsia* also possesses patatin-like proteins with a conserved consensus phospholipase domain[54] and exhibits homologies with VipD including oxyanion hole (GGGXK/R), the active site serine (GXSXG), and the active site aspartate (DXG) regions. Similarly to what was observed in the L. pneumophila Philadelphia-1 genome,[88] three paralogs were found in *R. felis*.[55] The role of rickettsial patatin in the vacuole escape was discarded.[51] However, these proteins should be required in other steps of the infectious process.

While increasing number of T4SS effectors are described,[80] putative rickettsial effectors identified through the examination of available genomes are exclusively related to *Legionella* effectors. In contrast with other bacterial pathogens, including rickettsiae that possess a type IVA secretion system, *L. pneumophila* uses a type IVB secretion system, a specificity also observed for *Coxiella burnetii*.[98] Since relationships were evidenced between type IVA and IVB secretion systems,[89] it is conceivable that Dot/Icm-like substrates could be translocated through VirB/D4 system. The rationale for why effectors known to pervert the host cell endosomal pathways and promote growth of bacteria into intracellular compartments found in *Rickettsia* is not explained.

To date, the regulation of T4SS in intracellular pathogens has been poorly studied. It was shown that expression of *Brucella suis* and *Bartonella henselae* T4SS were specifically induced when the bacteria were located within their host cells.[90,91] Due to the obligate intracellular nature of rickettsiae, such a transcriptomic comparison cannot be achieved. However, from a global proteomic analysis conducted on whole *R. felis* extract, we identified 134 proteins among which 4 components were of the T4SS.[92] Detection of these proteins indicated that they were majoritary expressed, suggesting their role as main actors of the rickettsia life. Moreover, we recently evidenced the upregulation of the *virB* operon in *R. conorii* maintained in Vero cells and exposed to a nutrient stress.[93] This result is consistent with what was reported for *Brucella suis* when incubated in minimal medium.[90] Accordingly, it could be hypothesized that factors secreted by the T4SS should promote rickettsia survival by triggering synthesis of nutrients from the host cell or used for another purpose allowing adaptation of rickettsiae to intracellular or extracellular environments. A detailed understanding of the regulation of Rickettsia transcriptome would facilitate the identification of the effector functions, which enable this pathogen to parasitize eukaryotic cells.

Conclusions

The post-genomic analysis of bacteria from the *Rickettsia* genus achieved the last few years allowed to identify several proteins susceptible to be involved in their interaction with host cells. Functional studies of these factors would provide a better knowledge about the strategies devised by such obligate intracellular pathogens in colonizing their hosts.

Conflicts of Interest

The authors declare no conflicts of interest.

References

1. Ricketts, H.T. 1906. The transmission of Rocky Mountain spotted fever by the bite of the wood-tick (*Dermacentor occidentalis*). *J. Am. Med. Assoc.* **47:** 358.
2. Walker, D.H. 2004. Ricketts creates rickettsiology, the study of vector-borne obligately intracellular bacteria. *J. Infect. Dis.* **189:** 938–955.
3. Harden, V.A. 1987. Koch's postulates and the etiology of rickettsial diseases. *J. Hist. Med. Allied Sci.* **42:** 277–295.
4. Raoult, D. & V. Roux. 1997. Rickettsioses as paradigms of new or emerging infectious diseases. *Clin. Microbiol. Rev.* **10:** 694–719.
5. La Scola, B. & D. Raoult. 1997. Laboratory diagnosis of rickettsioses: current approaches to diagnosis of old and new rickettsial diseases. *J. Clin. Microbiol.* **35:** 2715–2727.
6. Parola, P., C.D. Paddock & D. Raoult. 2005. Tick-borne rickettsioses around the world: emerging diseases challenging old concepts. *Clin. Microbiol. Rev.* **18:** 719–756.
7. Fournier, P.E., Y. Zhu, H. Ogata & D. Raoult. 2004. Use of highly variable intergenic spacer sequences for multispacer typing of *Rickettsia conorii* strains 264. *J. Clin. Microbiol.* **42:** 5757–5766.
8. Walker, T.S. & H.H. Winkler. 1978. Penetration of cultured mouse fibroblasts (L cells) by *Rickettsia prowazekii*. *Infect. Immun.* **22:** 200–208.
9. Teysseire, N., J.A. Boudier & D. Raoult. 1995. *Rickettsia conorii* entry into Vero cells. *Infect. Immun.* **63:** 366–374.
10. Valbuena, G., H.M. Feng & D.H. Walker. 2002. Mechanisms of immunity against rickettsiae. New perspectives and opportunities offered by unusual intracellular parasites. *Microbes. Infect.* **4:** 625–633.

11. Wood, D.O. & A.F. Azad. 2000. Genetic Manipulation of *Rickettsiae*: a Preview. *Infect. Immun.* **68:** 6091–6093.

12. Blanc, G. *et al.* 2007. Reductive genome evolution from the mother of *Rickettsia*. *PloS Genet.* **3:** e14.

13. Andersson, S.G. *et al.* 1998. The genome sequence of *Rickettsia prowazekii* and the origin of mitochondria. *Nature* **396:** 133–140.

14. Ellison, D.W. *et al.* 2008. Genomic comparison of virulent *Rickettsia rickettsii* Sheila Smith and avirulent *Rickettsia rickettsii* Iowa. *Infect. Immun.* **76:** 542–550.

15. Winkler H.H. & R.M. Daugherty. 1983. Cytoplasmic distinction of avirulent and virulent *Rickettsia prowazekii*: fusion of infected fibroblasts with macrophage-like cells. *Infect. Immun.* **40:** 1245–1247.

16. Balayeva, N.M., M. Eremeeva & D. Raoult. 1994. Genomic identification of *Rickettsia slovaca* among spotted fever group rickettsia isolates from *Dermacentor marginatus* in Armenia. *Acta. Virol.* **38:** 321–325.

17. Ge, H. *et al.* 2004. Comparative genomics of *Rickettsia prowazekii* Madrid E and Breinl Strains. *J. Bacteriol.* **186:** 556–565.

18. Zhang, J.Z., J.F. Hao, D.H. Walker & X.J. Yu. 2006. A mutation inactivating the methyltransferase gene in avirulent Madrid E strain of *Rickettsia prowazekii* reverted to wild type in the virulent revertant strain. *Evir. Vaccine* **24:** 2317–2323.

19. Chao, C.C., *et al.* 2007. Insight into the virulence of Rickettsia prowazekii by proteomic analysis and comparison with an avirulent strain. *Biochim. Biophys. Acta.* **1774:** 373–381.

20. Jacques, M. 1996. Role of lipo-oligosaccharides and lipopolysaccharides in bacterial adherence. *Trends Microbiol.* **4:** 408–409.

21. Feng, H.-M., T. Whitworth, V.L. Popov & D.H. Walker. 2004. Fc-dependent polyclonal antibodies and antibodies to outer membrane proteins A and B, but not to lipopolysaccharide, protect SCID mice against fatal *Rickettsia conorii* infection. *Infect. Immun.* **72:** 2222–2228.

22. Li, H. & D.H. Walker. 1992. Characterization of rickettsial attachment to host cells by flow cytometry. *Infect. Immun.* **60:** 2030–2035.

23. Palmer, E.L., M.L. Martin & L. Mallavia. 1974. Ultrastucture of the surface of *Rickettsia prowazeki* and *Rickettsia akari*. *Appl. Microbiol.* **28:** 713–716.

24. Ching, W.-M., M. Carl & G.A. Dasch. 1992. Mapping of monoclonal antibody binding sites on CNBr fragments of the S-layer protein antigens of *Rickettsia typhi* and *Rickettsia prowazekii*. *Mol. Immunol.* **29:** 95–105.

25. Teyssiere, N. & D. Raoult. 1992. Comparison of Western immunoblotting and microimmunofluorescence for diagnosis of Mediterranean spotted fever. *J. Clin. Microbiol.* **30:** 455–460.

26. Ogata, H. *et al.* 2001. Mechanisms of evolution in *Rickettsia conorii* and *R. prowazekii*. *Science* **293:** 2093–2098.

27. Blanc, G., M. *et al.* 2005. Molecular evolution of Rickettsia surface antigens: Evidence of positive selection. *Mol. Biol. Evol.* **22:**2073–2083.

28. McDonald, G.A., R.L. Anacker & K. Garjian. 1987. Cloned gene of *Rickettsia rickettsii* surface antigen: candidate vaccine for Rocky Mountain spotted fever. *Science* **235:** 83–85.

29. Li, H., B. Lenz & D.H. Walker. 1988. Protective monoclonal antibodies recognize heat-labile epitopes on surface proteins of spotted fever group rickettsiae. *Infect. Immun.* **56:** 2587–2593.

30. Vishwanath, S., G.A. McDonald & N.G. Watkins. 1990. A recombinant *Rickettsia conorii* vaccine protects guinea pigs from experimental boutonneuse fever and Rocky Mountain spotted fever. *Infect. Immun.* **58:** 646–653.

31. Sumner, J.W., K.G. Sims, D.C. Jones & B.E. Anderson. 1995. Protection of guinea-pigs from experimental Rocky Mountain spotted fever by immunization with baculovirus-expressed *Rickettsia rickettsii* rOmpA protein. *Vaccine* **13:** 29–35.

32. Crocquet-Valdes, P.A. *et al.* 2001. Immunization with a portion of rickettsial outer membrane protein A stimulates protective immunity against spotted fever rickettsiosis. *Vaccine* **20:** 979–988.

33. Li, H. & D.H. Walker. 1998. rOmpA is a critical protein for the adhesion of Rickettsia rickettsiito host cells. *Microbial. Pathogenesis* **24:** 289–298.

34. Renesto, P. *et al.* 2005. Some lessons from Rickettsia genomics. *FEMS Microbiol. Rev.* **29:** 99–117.

35. Bourgeois, A.L. & G.A. Dasch. 1981. The species-specific surface protein antigen in *Rickettsia typhi*: immunogenicity and protecting efficacy in guinea-pigs. In *Rickettsiae and Rickettsial Diseases*. W. Burgdorfer & R.L. Anacker, Eds.: 71–80. New York.

36. Gilmore, R.D., Jr., W.J. Cieplak, P.F. Policastro & T. Hackstadt. 1991. The 120 kilodalton outer membrane protein (rOmp B) of *Rickettsia rickettsii* is encoded by an unusually long open reading frame: evidence for protein processing from a large precursor. *Mol. Microbiol.* **5:** 2361–2370.

37. Hackstadt, T., R. Messer, W. Cieplak & M.G. Peacock. 1992. Evidence for proteolytic cleavage of the 120-kilodalton outer membrane protein of rickettsiae: identification of an avirulent mutant deficient in processing. *Infect. Immun.* **60:** 159–165.

38. Uchiyama, T., H. Kawano & Y. Kusuhara. 2006. The major outer membrane protein rOmpB of spotted fever group rickettsiae functions in the rickettsial adherence to and invasion of Vero cells. *Microbes. Infect.* **8:** 801–809.

39. Ching, W.M., H. Wang, J. Davis & G.A. Dasch. 1993. Amino acid analysis and multiple methylation of lysine rsidues in the surface protein antigen of *Rickettsia prowazekii*. In *Techniques in Protein Chemistry*. R.H. Angeletti, Ed.: 307–314.

40. Renesto, P. *et al*. 2006. Identification of two putative rickettsial adhesins by proteomic analysis. *Res. Microbiol*. **158**: 605–612.

41. Wells, T.J., J.J. Tree, G.C. Ulett & M.A. Schembri. 2007. Autotransporter proteins: novel targets at the bacterial cell surface. *FEMS Microbiol. Lett.* **274**: 163–172.

42. Martinez, J.J. *et al*. 2005. Ku70, a component of DNA-dependent protein kinase, is a mammalian receptor for *Rickettsia conorii*. *Cell* **123**: 1016–1023.

43. Fikrig, E. & S. Narasimhan. 2006. *Borrelia burgdorferi* – Traveling incognito? *Microbes Infection* **8**: 1390–1399.

44. Rovery, C. *et al*. 2005. Preliminary transcriptional analysis of *spoT* gene family and of membrane proteins in *Rickettsia conorii* and *Rickettsia felis*. *Ann. N.Y. Acad. Sci.* **1063**: 79–82.

45. Ogawa, M., K. Matsumoto, P. Parola & P. Brouqui. 2006. Expression of rOmpA and rOmpB protein in *Rickettsia massiliae* during the *Rhipicephalus turanicus* life cycle. *Ann. N.Y. Acad. Sci.* **1078**: 352–356.

46. Winkler, H.H. & E.T. Miller. 1982. Phospholipase A and the interaction of *Rickettsia prowazekii* and mouse fibroblasts (L-929 cells). *Infect. Immun.* **38**: 109–113.

47. Silverman, D.J., L.A. Santucci, N. Meyers & Z. Sekeyova. 1992. Penetration of host cells by *Rickettsia rickettsii* appears to be mediated by a phospholipase of rickettsial origin. *Infect. Immun.* **60**: 2733–2740.

48. Walker, D.H., H.M. Feng & V.L. Popov. 2001. Rickettsial phospholipase A2 as a pathogenic mechanism in a model of cell injury by typhus and spotted fever group rickettsiae. *Am. J. Trop. Med. Hyg.* **65**: 936–942.

49. Renesto, P. *et al*. 2003. Identification and characterization of a phospholipase D-superfamily gene in rickettsiae. *J. Infect. Dis.* **188**: 1276–1283.

50. Ponting, C.P. & I.D. Kerr. 1996. A novel family of phospholipase D homologues that includes phospholipid synthases and putative endonucleases: identification of duplicated repeats and potential active site residues. *Protein Sci.* **5**: 914–922.

51. Whitworth, T. *et al*. 2005. Expression of the *Rickettsia prowazekii* pld or tlyC gene in *Salmonella enterica* serovar Typhimurium mediates phagosomal escape. *Infect. Immun.* **73**: 6668–6673.

52. McLeod, M.P. *et al*. 2004. Complete genome sequence of *Rickettsia typhi* and comparison with sequences of other rickettsiae 282. *J. Bacteriol.* **186**: 5842–5855.

53. Hirschberg, H.J., J.W. Simons, N. Dekker & M.R. Egmond. 2001. Cloning, expression, purification and characterization of patatin, a novel phospholipase A. *Eur. J. Biochem.* **268**: 5037–5044.

54. Blanc, G., P. Renesto & D. Raoult. 2005. Phylogenic analysis of rickettsial patatin-like protein with conserved phospholipase A2 active sites. *Ann. N.Y. Acad. Sci.* **1063**: 83–86.

55. Ogata, H. *et al*. 2005. The genome sequence of *Rickettsia felis* identifies the first putative conjugative plasmid in an obligate intracellular parasite. *PLoS Biology* **3**: e248.

56. Stevens, J.M., E.E. Galyov & M.P. Stevens. 2006. Actin-dependent movement of bacterial pathogens. *Nat. Rev. Microbiol.* **4**: 91–101.

57. Carlsson, F. & E.J. Brown. 2006. Actin-based motility of intracellular bacteria, and polarized surface distribution of the bacterial effector molecules. *J. Cell Physiol.* **209**: 288–296.

58. Teysseire, N. & D. Raoult. 1992. Comparison of Western immunoblotting and microimmunofluorescence for diagnosis of Mediterranean spotted fever. *Infect. Immun.* **30**: 455–460.

59. Heinzen, R.A., S.F. Hayes, M.G. Peacock & T. Hackstadt. 1993. Directional actin polymerization associated with spotted fever group Rickettsia infection of Vero cells. *Infect. Immun.* **61**: 1926–1935.

60. Baldridge, G.D. *et al*. 2005. Analysis of fluorescent protein expression in transformants of *Rickettsia monacensis*, an obligate intracellular tick symbiont. *Appl. Environ. Microbiol.* **71**: 2095–2105.

61. Gouin, E. *et al*. 2004. The RickA protein of *Rickettsia conorii* activates the Arp2/3 complex. *Nature* **427**: 457–461.

62. Jeng, R.L. *et al*. 2004. A Rickettsia WASP-like protein activates the Arp2/3 complex and mediates actin-based motility. *Cell Microbiol.* **6**: 761–769.

63. Gouin, E., M.D. Welch & P. Cossart. 2005. Actin-based motility of intracellular pathogens. *Curr. Opin. Microbiol.* **8**: 35–45.

64. Simser, J.A., M.S. Rahman, S.M. Dreher-Lesnick & A.F. Azad. 2005. A novel and naturally occurring transposon, ISRpe1 in the *Rickettsia peacockii* genome disrupting the *rickA* gene involved in actin-based motility. *Mol. Microbiol.* **58**: 71–79.

65. Gouin, E., H. Gantelet, C. Egile, *et al*. 1999. A comparative study of the actin-based motilities of the pathogenic bacteria *Listeria monocytogenes*, *Shigella flexneri* and *Rickettsia conorii*. *J. Cell Sci.* **112**: 1697–1708.

66. Goldberg, M.B., O. Barzu, C. Parsot & P.J. Sansonetti. 1993. Unipolar localization and ATPase activity of IcsA, a *Shigella flexneri* protein involved in intracellular movement. *J. Bacteriol.* **175**: 2189–2196.

67. Kocks, C. *et al*. 1993. Polarized distribution of *Listeria monocytogenes* surface protein ActA at the site of directional actin assembly. *J. Cell Sci.* **105**: 699–710.

68. Stevens, M.P. *et al*. 2005. Identification of a bacterial factor required for actin-based motility of *Burkholderia pseudomallei*. *Mol. Microbiol*. **56:** 40–53.

69. Heinzen, R.A., S.S. Grieshaber, L.S. Van Kirk & C.J. Devin. 1999. Dynamics of actin-based movement by *Rickettsia rickettsii* in vero cells. *Infect. Immun*. **67:** 4201–4207.

70. Monack, D.M. & J.A. Theriot. 2001. Actin-based motility is sufficient for bacterial membrane protrusion formation and host cell uptake. *Cell Microbiol*. **3:** 633–647.

71. Heinzen, R.A. 2003. Rickettsial Actin-Based Motility: Behavior and Involvement of Cytoskeletal Regulators. *Ann. N. Y. Acad. Sci*. **990:** 535–547.

72. Mediannikov, O. *et al*. 2008. *Rickettsia raoultii* sp. nov., a new spotted fever group rickettsia associated with *Dermacentor* ticks in Europe and Russia. *Int. J. Syst. Evol. Microbiol*.

73. Balraj, P. *et al*. 2008. RickA expression is not sufficient to promote actin-based motility of *Rickettsia raoultii*. *PLoS ONE* **3:** e2582.

74. Ogata, H. *et al*. 2006. Genome sequence of *Rickettsia bellii* illuminates the role of amoebae in gene exchanges between intracellular pathogens. *PLoS Genet*. **2:** e76.

75. Duma, R.J. *et al*. 1981. Epidemic typhus in the United States associated with flying squirrels. *JAMA* **245:** 2318–2323.

76. Raoult, D. *et al*. 1998. Outbreak of epidemic typhus associated with trench fever in Burundi. *Lancet* **352:** 353–358.

77. Netesov, S.V. & J.L. Conrad. 2001. Emerging infectious diseases in Russia, 1990–1999. *Emerg. Infect. Dis*. **7:** 1–5.

78. Hybiske, K. & R.S. Stephens. 2008. Exit strategies of intracellular pathogens. *Nat. Rev. Microbiol*. **6:** 99–110.

79. Christie, P.J. *et al*. 2005. Biogenesis, architecture, and function of bacterial type IV secretion systems. *Annu. Rev. Microbiol*. **59:** 451–85.

80. Cascales, E. & P.J. Christie. 2003. The versatile bacterial type IV secretion systems. *Nat. Rev. Microbiol*. **1:** 137–149.

81. Burns, D.L. 2003. Type IV transporters of pathogenic bacteria. *Curr. Opin. Microbiol*. **6:** 29–34.

82. Christie, P.J. & J.P. Vogel. 2000. Bacterial type IV secretion: conjugation systems adapted to deliver effector molecules to host cells. *Trends Microbiol*. **8:** 354–360.

83. Sexton, J.A. & J.P. Vogel. 2002. Type IVB secretion by intracellular pathogens. *Traffic* **3:** 178–185.

84. Nagai, H., J.C. Kagan, R.A. Kahn & C.R. Roy. 2002. A bacterial guanine nucleotide exchange factor activates ARF on Legionella phagosomes. *Science* **295:** 679–682.

85. http://www.igs.cnrs-mrs.fr/mgdb/Rickettsia/rig/

86. Chen, J. *et al*. 2004. *Legionella* effectors that promote nonlytic release from protozoa. *Science* **303:** 1358–1361.

87. Shohdy, N., J.A. Efe, S.D. Emr & H.A. Shuman. 2005. Pathogen effector protein screening in yeast identifies Legionella factors that interfere with membrane trafficking. *Proc Natl Acad Sci USA* **102:** 4866–4871.

88. Vanrheenen, S.M., Z.Q. Luo, T. O'Connor & R.R. Isberg. 2006. Members of a *Legionella pneumophila* family of proteins with ExoU (phospholipase A) active sites are translocated to target cells. *Infect. Immun*. **74:** 3597–3606.

89. Segal, G., M. Feldman & T. Zusman. 2005. The Icm/Dot type-IV secretion systems of *Legionella pneumophila* and *Coxiella burnetii*. *FEMS Microbiol. Rev*. **29:** 65–81.

90. Boschiroli, M.L. *et al*. 2002. The *Brucella suis virB* operon is induced intracellularly in macrophages. *Proc. Natl. Acad. Sci. USA* **99:** 1544–1549.

91. Schmiederer, M. *et al*. 2001. Intracellular induction of the *Bartonella henselae virB* operon by human endothelial cells. *Infect. Immun*. **69:** 6495–6502.

92. Ogawa, M. *et al*. 2007. Proteome analysis of *Rickettsia felis* highlights the expression profile of intracellular bacteria. *Proteomics* **8:** 1232–1248.

93. La, M.V. *et al*. 2007. Development of a method for recovering rickettsial RNA from infected cells to analyze gene expression profiling of obligate intracellular bacteria. *J. Microbiol. Methods* **71:** 292–297.

Type IV Secretion System of *Anaplasma phagocytophilum* and *Ehrlichia chaffeensis*

Yasuko Rikihisa, Mingqun Lin, Hua Niu, and Zhihui Cheng

Department of Veterinary Biosciences, College of Veterinary Medicine, The Ohio State University, Columbus, Ohio 43210, USA

The intracellular bacterial pathogens *Ehrlichia chaffeensis* and *Anaplasma phagocytophilum* have evolved to infect leukocytes and hijack biological compounds and processes of these host defensive cells. Bacterial type IV secretion (T4S) system transports macromolecules across the membrane in an ATP-dependent manner and is increasingly recognized as a virulence factor delivery mechanism that allows pathogens to modulate eukaryotic cell functions for their own benefit. Genes encoding T4S system homologous to those of a plant pathogen *Agrobacterium tumefaciens* have been identified in *E. chaffeensis* and *A. phagocytophilum*. Upon interaction with new host cells, *E. chaffeensis* and *A. phagocytophilum* genes encoding the T4S apparatus are upregulated. The delivered macromolecules are referred to as T4S substrates, or effectors, because they affect and alter basic host cellular processes, resulting in disease development. Recently, *A. phagocytophilum* 160-kDa AnkA protein was to be delivered by T4S system into the host cytoplasm. Thus, dynamic signal transduction events are likely induced by T4S substrates in the host cells for successful establishment of intracellular infection. Further studies on *Ehrlichia* and *Anaplasma* T4S effectors cognate host cell molecules will undoubtedly advance our understanding of the complex interplay between obligatory intracellular pathogens and their hosts. Such data can be applied toward treatment, diagnosis, and control of ehrlichiosis and anaplasmosis.

Key words: A. phagocytophilum; E. chaffeensis; type IV secretion

Introduction

Ehrlichia chaffeensis and *Anaplasma phagocytophilum* are gram-negative bacteria belonging to the family *Anaplasmataceae*. *E. chaffeensis* is the agent of human monocytic ehrlichiosis (HME)[1,2] and *A. phagocytophilum* is the agent of human granulocytic anaplasmosis (HGA).[3,4] HME and HGA are systemic diseases characterized by fever, headache, myalgia, anorexia, and chills, and frequently are accompanied by leukopenia with a leftward shift, thrombocytopenia, anemia, and elevations in serum hepatic aminotransferases. The severity of the disease varies from asymptomatic seroconversion to frequently documented severe morbidity to death.[5,6] HME and HGA are prevalent, life-threatening tick-borne zoonoses in North America and were designated as a nationally notifiable diseases in 1998.[7] The disease continues to be a public health problem, since wild animals such as white-tailed deer and white-footed mice are reservoirs of these bacteria.[8,9] *E. chaffeensis* has been identified most commonly in the Lone Star tick (*Amblyomma americanum*).[8,10] *A. phagocytophilum* has been found in the deer tick (*Ixodes scapularis*) and other *Ixodes* spp.[9,11]

Signaling Events in the Infected Host Cells

A. phagocytophilum and *E. chaffeensis* are obligatory intracellular bacteria that replicate inside

Address for correspondence: Yasuko Rikihisa, Department of Veterinary Biosciences, College of Veterinary Medicine, The Ohio State University, 1925 Coffey Road, Columbus, Ohio 43210. Voice: +614-292-9677; fax: +614-292-6473. rikihisa.1@osu.edu

Rickettsiology and Rickettsial Diseases-Fifth International Conference: Ann. N.Y. Acad. Sci. 1166: 106–111 (2009).
doi: 10.1111/j.1749-6632.2009.04527.x © 2009 New York Academy of Sciences.

mammalian granulocytes and monocytes-macrophages, respectively; primary immune defensive cells that normally are responsible for powerful innate antimicrobial defenses. Recently, unique strategies employed by these intravacuolar bacteria for successful parasitism have begun to be unraveled.[12,13] A common mechanism shared by these bacteria is the ability to subvert multiple innate immune responses of host cells.[13] Furthermore, this group of bacteria inhibits host cell apoptosis to maximize intracellular bacterial reproduction.[14–17] *A. phagocytophilum* and *E. chaffeensis* induce their internalization into host cells without eliciting signals that induce microbicidal activities. For internalization, these bacteria usurp caveolae-mediated endocytosis, which directs pathogens to an intracellular compartment secluded from late endosome or lysosome markers and NADPH oxidase components.[18–22] Both early and replicative *E. chaffeensis* and *A. phagocytophilum* inclusions are co-localized with tyrosine-phosphorylated proteins and PLC-γ2, which are required for infection of host cells.[18,23] Despite sharing several common features as described above, *E. chaffeensis* and *A. phagocytophilum* inclusions are distinct from each other, and thus, the 2 species never co-localize in the same inclusions even after co-infection of the same HL-60 cell.[21] *E. chaffeensis* inclusions retain the early endosome characteristics including rab5 and early endosome antigen 1 (EEA1), and fuse with transferrin receptor (TfR) endosomes.[20,21] Exogenous iron-loaded transferrin (Tf) actually enters into the *E. chaffeensis* replicative inclusion through the TfR-Tf endosome recycling pathway.[20] In contrast, the inclusions of *A. phagocytophilum* are negative for these endosomal markers.[21] Recently, several hallmarks of early autophagosomes were detected in *A. phagocytophilum* replicative inclusions, including a double lipid bilayer membrane, and co-localization with GFP-tagged LC3 and Beclin 1, the human homologs of *Saccharomyces cerevisiae* autophagy-related proteins Atg8 and Atg6, respectively.[24] Stimulation of autophagy by ra-

pamycin favors *A. phagocytophilum* infection. Inhibition of the autophagosomal pathway by 3-methyladenine does not inhibit *A. phagocytophilum* internalization, but reversibly arrests its growth.[24] Although autophagy is considered part of the innate immune response that clears a variety of intracellular pathogens, *A. phagocytophilum* subverts this system to establish itself in an early autophagosome-like compartment, segregated from lysosomes, to facilitate its proliferation.

How do these bacteria down-regulate a number of critical innate immune responses and modify vesicular traffic to create a sheltered niche in host cells? Our central hypothesis is that the bacterial type IV secretion (T4S) system has an important role in these processes. For analysis of *A. phagocytophilum* and *E. chaffeensis* factors, we now have much better tools than ever before, since several members of genus *Rickettsia* and family *Anaplasmataceae* have been sequenced. Complete genome sequences of *A. phagocytophilum* (1.47 Mbp) and *E. chaffeensis* (1.18 Mbp) were obtained and compared to each other and to the published Rickettsiales genome sequences. *E. chaffeensis* and *A. phagocytophilum* genomes are syntenic. The 2 species share approximately 640 genes[25] with approximately 470–580 genes that are unique to each species. These latter genes are mostly of unknown function and presumably are responsible for the important phenotypic differences between these 2 organisms.

T4S System

T4S system transports macromolecules across the membrane in an ATP-dependent manner and is ancestrally related to the conjugation system of gram-negative bacteria. The T4S system is increasingly recognized as a virulence factor delivery mechanism that allows pathogens to modulate eukaryotic cell functions for their own benefit.[26] There are at least 2 ancestral lineages for the T4S system: the *virB/virD* system of *Agrobacterium tumefaciens*

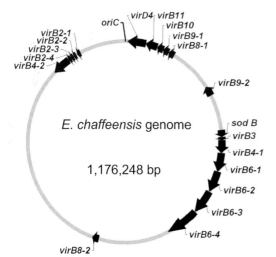

Figure 1. *virB/D* gene loci on the *E. chaffeensis* genome. The genome map of *E. chaffeensis* is shown as a circle. The putative origin of replication is shown as oriC. The *virB/D* gene loci are shown as black arrows. The length of each arrow is enlarged to approximately 10 times of the size in the genome.

and the *dot/icm* system of *Legionella pneumophila*, sometimes referred as T4aS and T4bS systems, respectively. For facultative intracellular bacteria, including *Legionella, Bartonella,* and *Brucella* species, the T4S system is essential for their intracellular survival.[27–29] In the most extensively studied T4aS system from *Ag. tumefaciens*, the single *virB* operon, along with *virD4*, encodes 12 membrane-associated proteins that form a transmembrane channel complex.[30] Genes encoding T4aS system: *vir* orthologs (*virB2, B3, B4, B6, B8, B9, B10, B11,* and *D4*), have been identified in *E. chaffeensis* and *A. phagocytophilum*.[25,31,32] These *virB/D* genes are split into 2 major operons: *sodB-virB3–virB4-virB6–1-virB6–2-virB6–3-virB6–4* and *virB8–1-virB9–1-virB10-virB11–virD4*. Between these 2 operons, there are *virB4–2, multiple virB2, virB8–2,* and *virB9–2* (A genomic map of *E. chaffeensis virB/D* is shown in Fig. 1). Analysis of recent whole-genome sequence databases indicates conservation of this split operon structure in other members of the order *Rickettsiales*.[33–37] The *A. phagocytophilum* T4aS system is expected to function during mammalian leukocyte infection *in vitro* and *in vivo*, since 1) both *virB8–*

virD4 and *sodB–virB6* operons are polycistronically transcribed in *A. phagocytophilum* replicating in HL-60 promyelocytic leukemia cells,[32] 2) *A. phagocytophilum virB9* gene is transcribed in peripheral blood leukocytes from HGA patients and from experimentally infected animals,[32] 3) in the closely related monocyte-tropic *Ehrlichia canis, virB9* is expressed in the blood from infected dogs and infected canine monocyte DH82 cell cultures,[38] and 4) *A. phagocytophilum* AnkA protein can be delivered into the host cell cytoplasm in a VirB/D-dependent manner.[39]

The expression of T4S system is not constitutive, but is regulated during the *A. phagocytophilum* and *E. chaffeensis* intracellular life cycle.[31,40] Both *virB9* and *virB6* of *A. phagocytophilum* are up-regulated at the mRNA level and VirB9 at the protein level during infection of human neutrophils *in vitro*[31] and 5 *virB/D* loci (except VirB2s) were up-regulated during the exponential growth stage of *E. chaffeensis* synchronously cultured in THP-1 human monocytic leukemia cells.[40] In contrast, the majority of *A. phagocytophilum* spontaneously released from infected host cells poorly expresses the VirB9 protein.[31] Transcription of 5 *virB/D* loci is down-regulated prior to the release of *E. chaffeensis* from host THP-1 cells.[40] In fact, proteomic analysis identified a unique DNA binding protein, EcxR, which coordinately regulates 5 *virB/D* loci of *E. chaffeensis*.[40] Thus, this modulation of bacterial *virB/D* gene expression during the establishment of bacterial infection may promote intracellular survival and rapid replication in a safe haven and resistance when exposed to the extracellular environment, and/or the next round of infection of host cells. In addition, the T4aS system is expected to function during tick infection as well, since *virB9* is expressed by *E. canis* in tick tissues.[38] Some of duplicated *virB* paralogs of these bacteria may be reserved to function specifically during tick stages. Recently, differential transcription of several *A. phagocytophilum* VirB2 paralogs in mammalian and ISE6 tick cells were reported.[41]

The delivered macromolecules are referred to as T4S substrates or effectors because they affect and alter basic host cellular processes, resulting in disease development. Two T4aS effector molecules, CagA of *Helicobacter pyroli*[42] and pertussis toxin,[43] have been shown to play a major role in mammalian disease pathogenesis. The T4S system has been demonstrated as being essential for the creation of cytoplasmic replicative compartments unique to each of several facultative intracellular bacteria such as *Brucella, Bartonella,* and *Legionella.*[44,45] There is direct evidence that over 30 effector molecules are translocated into the host cell during *Legionella* infection.[45] Particularly, a large and diverse family of proteins containing ankyrin-repeat homology domains of *L. pneumophila* and *Coxiella burnetii* are translocated into eukaryotic cells by pathogen-associated T4bS system. The *L. pneumophila* AnkX protein prevented microtubule-dependent vesicular transport to interfere with fusion of the *L. pneumophila*-containing vacuole with late endosomes after infection of macrophages.[46] Recently, we demonstrated that *A. phagocytophilum* 160-kDa ankyrin repeat protein, AnkA is delivered by a VirB/D-dependent manner into the host leukocyte cytoplasm and subsequently is tyrosine phosphorylated.[39] AnkA binds to Abl-interactor 1 that interacts with Abl-1 tyrosine kinase, thus mediating AnkA phosphorylation. AnkA and Abl-1 are critical for *A. phagocytophilum* infection, as infection was inhibited upon host cytoplasmic delivery of anti-AnkA antibody, Abl-1 knockdown with targeted siRNA, or treatment with a specific pharmacological inhibitor of Abl-1.[39] Studies showed that *A. phagocytophilum* specifically induces tyrosine phosphorylation of a 190-kDa AnkA (AnkA molecular size is bacterial strain-dependent), which then interact with the host cell tyrosine phosphatase SHP-1.[47] AnkA also was reported to localize within nuclei of infected HL-60 cells and bind to the internucleosomal region of HL-60 cell DNA and DNA fragments containing genes encoding ATPase, tyrosine phosphatase and NADH dehydrogenase-like functions, and nuclear proteins in a cell-free system.[48,49] *Ag. tumefaciens* VirD4, a membrane-associated ATPase, is involved in the recognition of substrates of *Ag. tumefaciens* T4aSV system.[50,51] Our recent study identified several additional T4S effector candidates in *A. phagocytophilum* and *E. chaffeensis* via bacterial 2-hybrid system using *A. phagocytophilum* and *E. chaffeensis* VirD4 as bait. One of them is an *A. phagocytophilum* hypothetical protein, named <u>A</u>naplasma <u>T</u>ranslocation <u>S</u>ubstrate 1 (Ats-1). Ats-1 is expressed by *A. phagocytophilum* in the inclusion, translocated across the inclusion membrane, and localized in the mitochondria of infected human neutrophils and HL-60 cells. Ats-1 in mitochondria inhibits etoposide-induced apoptosis and cytochrome *c* release from mitochondria.[24,52] Further research dissecting the functional role of these candidates will lead to a better understanding of the host processes that facilitate obligatory intracellular bacterial survival and infection.

Acknowledgments

Some of studies in the authors' laboratory reported in this review were supported by grants R01 AI054476 from the National Institutes of Health.

Conflicts of Interest

The authors declare no conflicts of interest.

References

1. Dawson, J.E. *et al.* 1991. Isolation and characterization of an *Ehrlichia* sp. from a patient diagnosed with human ehrlichiosis. *J. Clin. Microbiol.* **29:** 2741–2745.

2. Maeda, K. *et al.* 1987. Human infection with *Ehrlichia canis*, a leukocytic rickettsia. *N. Engl. J. Med.* **316:** 853–856.

3. Chen, S.M. *et al.* 1994. Identification of a granulocytotropic *Ehrlichia* species as the etiologic agent of human disease. *J. Clin. Microbiol.* **32:** 589–595.

4. Goodman, J.L. *et al.* 1996. Direct cultivation of the causative agent of human granulocytic ehrlichiosis. *N. Engl. J. Med.* **334:** 209–215.

5. Paddock, C.D. & J.E. Childs. 2003. *Ehrlichia chaffeensis*: a prototypical emerging pathogen. *Clin. Microbiol. Rev.* **16:** 37–64.

6. Bakken, J.S. *et al.* 1996. Clinical and laboratory characteristics of human granulocytic ehrlichiosis. *JAMA* **275:** 199–205.

7. Gardner, S.L. *et al.* 2003. National Surveillance for the human ehrlichioses in the United States, 1997–2001, and proposed methods for evaluation of data quality. In *Ann. N. Y. Acad. Sci.*, Vol. 990. K.E. Hechemy *et al.*, Eds.: 80–89. N.Y. Acad. Sci. New York, NY.

8. Ewing, S.A. *et al.* 1995. Experimental transmission of *Ehrlichia chaffeensis* (*Rickettsiales: Ehrlichieae*) among white-tailed deer by *Amblyomma americanum* (Acari: Ixodidae). *J. Med. Entomol.* **32:** 368–374.

9. Telford, S.R., 3rd *et al.* 1996. Perpetuation of the agent of human granulocytic ehrlichiosis in a deer tick-rodent cycle. *Proc. Natl. Acad. Sci. USA* **93:** 6209–6214.

10. Anderson, B.E. *et al.* 1993. *Amblyomma americanum*: a potential vector of human ehrlichiosis. *Am. J. Trop. Med. Hyg.* **49:** 239–244.

11. Pancholi, P. *et al.* 1995. *Ixodes dammini* as a potential vector of human granulocytic ehrlichiosis. *J. Infect Dis.* **172:** 1007–1012.

12. Rikihisa, Y. 2003. Mechanisms to create a safe haven by members of the family *Anaplasmataceae*. *Ann. N. Y. Acad. Sci.*, Vol. 990. K.E. Hechemy *et al.*, Eds.: 548–555. N.Y. Acad. Sci. New York, NY.

13. Rikihisa, Y. 2006. Ehrlichia subversion of host innate responses. *Curr. Opin. Microbiol.* **9:** 95–101.

14. Ge, Y. & Y. Rikihisa. 2006. *Anaplasma phagocytophilum* delays spontaneous human neutrophil apoptosis by modulation of multiple apoptotic pathways. *Cell Microbiol.* **8:** 1406–1416.

15. Ge, Y. *et al.* 2005. *Anaplasma phagocytophilum* inhibits human neutrophil apoptosis via upregulation of *bfl-1*, maintenance of mitochondrial membrane potential and prevention of caspase 3 activation. *Cell Microbiol.* **7:** 29–38.

16. Yoshiie, K. *et al.* 2000. Intracellular infection by the human granulocytic ehrlichiosis agent inhibits human neutrophil apoptosis. *Infect Immun.* **68:** 1125–1133.

17. Xiong, Q., X. Wang & Y. Rikihisa. 2007. High-cholesterol diet facilitates *Anaplasma phagocytophilum* infection and up-regulates macrophage inflammatory protein-2 and CXCR2 expression in apolipoprotein E-deficient mice. *J. Infect Dis.* **195:** 1497–1503.

18. Lin, M. & Y. Rikihisa. 2003. Obligatory intracellular parasitism by *Ehrlichia chaffeensis* and *Anaplasma phagocytophilum* involves caveolae and glycosylphosphatidylinositol-anchored proteins. *Cell Microbiol.* **5:** 809–820.

19. Lin, M. & Y. Rikihisa. 2007. Degradation of p22phox and inhibition of superoxide generation by *Ehrlichia chaffeensis* in human monocytes. *Cell Microbiol.* **9:** 861–874.

20. Barnewall, R.E., Y. Rikihisa & E.H. Lee. 1997. *Ehrlichia chaffeensis* inclusions are early endosomes which selectively accumulate transferrin receptor. *Infect Immun.* **65:** 1455–1461.

21. Mott, J., R.E. Barnewall & Y. Rikihisa. 1999. Human granulocytic ehrlichiosis agent and *Ehrlichia chaffeensis* reside in different cytoplasmic compartments in HL-60 cells. *Infect Immun.* **67:** 1368–1378.

22. Mott, J., Y. Rikihisa & S. Tsunawaki. 2002. Effects of *Anaplasma phagocytophila* on NADPH oxidase components in human neutrophils and HL-60 cells. *Infect Immun.* **70:** 1359–1366.

23. Lin, M., M.X. Zhu & Y. Rikihisa. 2002. Rapid activation of protein tyrosine kinase and phospholipase C-γ2 and increase in cytosolic free calcium are required by *Ehrlichia chaffeensis* for internalization and growth in THP-1 cells. *Infect Immun.* **70:** 889–898.

24. Niu, H., M. Yamaguchi, and Y. Rikihisa. 2008. Subversion of cellular autophagy by *Anaplasma phagocytophilum*. *Cell Microbiol.* 10: 593–605.

25. Dunning Hotopp, J.C. *et al.* 2006. Comparative genomics of emerging human ehrlichiosis agents. *PLoS Genetics* **2:** e21.

26. Cascales, E. & P.J. Christie. 2003. The versatile bacterial type IV secretion systems. *Nat. Rev. Microbiol.* **1:** 137–149.

27. Roy, C.R., K.H. Berger & R.R. Isberg. 1998. *Legionella pneumophila* DotA protein is required for early phagosome trafficking decisions that occur within minutes of bacterial uptake. *Mol. Microbiol.* **28:** 663–674.

28. Schulein, R. & C. Dehio. 2002. The VirB/VirD4 type IV secretion system of *Bartonella* is essential for establishing intraerythrocytic infection. *Mol. Microbiol.* **46:** 1053–1067.

29. Celli, J. *et al.* 2003. *Brucella* evades macrophage killing via VirB-dependent sustained interactions with the endoplasmic reticulum. *J. Exp. Med.* **198:** 545–556.

30. Christie, P.J. 1997. *Agrobacterium tumefaciens* T-complex transport apparatus: a paradigm for a new family of multifunctional transporters in eubacteria. *J. Bacteriol.* **179:** 3085–3094.

31. Niu, H. *et al.* 2006. Differential expression of VirB9 and VirB6 during the life cycle of *Anaplasma phagocytophilum* in human leucocytes is associated with differential binding and avoidance of lysosome pathway. *Cell Microbiol.* **8:** 523–534.

32. Ohashi, N. *et al.* 2002. Characterization and transcriptional analysis of gene clusters for a type IV secretion machinery in human granulocytic and monocytic ehrlichiosis agents. *Infect Immun.* **70:** 2128–2138.

33. Andersson, S.G. *et al.* 1998. The genome sequence of *Rickettsia prowazekii* and the origin of mitochondria. *Nature* **396:** 133–140.

34. Collins, N.E. *et al.* 2005. The genome of the heartwater agent *Ehrlichia ruminantium* contains multiple tandem repeats of actively variable copy number. *Proc. Natl. Acad. Sci. USA* **102:** 838–843.

35. Brayton, K.A. *et al.* 2005. Complete genome sequencing of *Anaplasma marginale* reveals that the surface is skewed to two superfamilies of outer membrane proteins. *Proc. Natl. Acad. Sci. USA* **102:** 844–849.

36. Foster, J. *et al.* 2005. The *Wolbachia* genome of *Brugia malayi*: endosymbiont evolution within a human pathogenic nematode. *PLoS Biol.* **3:** e121.

37. Ogata, H. *et al.* 2001. Mechanisms of evolution in *Rickettsia conorii* and *R. prowazekii*. *Science* **293:** 2093–2098.

38. Felek, S., H. Huang & Y. Rikihisa. 2003. Sequence and expression analysis of *virB9* of the type IV secretion system of *Ehrlichia canis* strains in ticks, dogs, and cultured cells. *Infect Immun.* **71:** 6063–6067.

39. Lin, M. *et al.* 2007. *Anaplasma phagocytophilum* AnkA secreted by type IV secretion system is tyrosine phosphorylated by Abl-1 to facilitate infection. *Cell Microbiol.* **9:** 2644–2657.

40. Cheng, Z., X. Wang & Y. Rikihisa. 2008. Regulation of type IV secretion apparatus genes during *Ehrlichia chaffeensis* intracellular development by a previously unidentified protein. *J. Bacteriol.* **190:** 2096–2105.

41. Nelson, C.M. *et al.* 2008. Whole genome transcription profiling of *Anaplasma phagocytophilum* in human and tick host cells by tiling array analysis. *BMC Genomics* **9:** 364.

42. Odenbreit, S. *et al.* 2000. Translocation of *Helicobacter pylori* CagA into gastric epithelial cells by type IV secretion. *Science* **287:** 1497–1500.

43. Kotob, S.I., S.Z. Hausman & D.L. Burns. 1995. Localization of the promoter for the ptl genes of *Bordetella pertussis*, which encode proteins essential for secretion of pertussis toxin. *Infect Immun.* **63:** 3227–3230.

44. Backert, S. & T.F. Meyer. 2006. Type IV secretion systems and their effectors in bacterial pathogenesis. *Curr. Opin. Microbiol.* **9:** 207–217.

45. Ninio, S. & C.R. Roy. 2007. Effector proteins translocated by *Legionella pneumophila*: strength in numbers. *Trends Microbiol.* **15:** 372–380.

46. Pan, X. *et al.* 2008. Ankyrin repeat proteins comprise a diverse family of bacterial type IV effectors. *Science* **320:** 1651–1654.

47. IJdo, J., A.C. Carlson & E.L. Kennedy. 2007. *Anaplasma phagocytophilum* AnkA is tyrosine-phosphorylated at EPIYA motifs and recruits SHP-1 during early infection. *Cell Microbiol.* **9:** 1284–1296.

48. Caturegli, P. *et al.* 2000. *ankA*: an *Ehrlichia phagocytophila* group gene encoding a cytoplasmic protein antigen with ankyrin repeats. *Infect Immun.* **68:** 5277–5283.

49. Park, J. *et al.* 2004. *Anaplasma phagocytophilum* AnkA binds to granulocyte DNA and nuclear proteins. *Cell Microbiol.* **6:** 743–751.

50. Christie, P.J. 2001. Type IV secretion: intercellular transfer of macromolecules by systems ancestrally related to conjugation machines. *Mol. Microbiol.* **40:** 294–305.

51. Llosa, M. *et al.* 2002. Bacterial conjugation: a two-step mechanism for DNA transport. *Mol. Microbiol.* **45:** 1–8.

52. Niu, H. & Y. Rikihisa. Amer. Soc. Microbiology. 2009. Ats-1, a substrate of type IV secretion system of *Anaplasma phagocytophilum*, targets host cell mitochondria. Presented at the *108th General Meeting*. Boston, MA, June 4. Abstract No. D-146.

Ixodes ovatus Ehrlichia Exhibits Unique Ultrastructural Characteristics in Mammalian Endothelial and Tick-derived Cells

Ulrike G. Munderloh,[a] **David J. Silverman,**[b]
Katherine C. MacNamara,[d] **Gilbert G. Ahlstrand,**[c]
Madhumouli Chatterjee,[d] **and Gary M. Winslow**[d]

[a] *Department of Entomology, University of Minnesota, St. Paul, Minnesota 55108, USA*

[b] *Department of Microbiology and Immunology, University of Maryland School of Medicine, Baltimore, Maryland 21201, USA*

[c] *Imaging Center, University of Minnesota, St. Paul, Minnesota 55108, USA*

[d] *Wadsworth Center, New York State Department of Health, Albany, New York 12208, USA*

Tick-borne pathogens in the genus *Ehrlichia* cause emerging zoonoses. Although laboratory mice are susceptible to *Ehrlichia* infections, many isolates do not cause clinical illness. In contrast, the *Ixodes ovatus Ehrlichia*-like agent (IOE) causes disease and immune responses in mice comparable to the human illness caused by *Ehrlichia chaffeensis*. No culture system had been developed for IOE, however, which limited studies of this pathogen. We reasoned that endothelial and tick cell lines could potentially serve as host cells, since the IOE is found in ticks and in endothelial cells in mice. Infected spleen cells from RAG-deficient mice were overlaid onto ISE6 and RF/6A cultures, and colonies typical of *Ehrlichia* were noted in RF/6A cells within 2 weeks. Infection of ISE6 cells was established after transfer of IOE from RF/6A cells. Electron microscopy revealed densely packed inclusions in infected RF/6A and ISE6 cells; these inclusions contained copious amounts of filamentous structures, apparently originating from *Ehrlichial* cells. In particular, within RF/6A cells the structures assumed an ordered morphology of finely combed hair. IOE from RF/6A cells, when inoculated into C57BL/6 and RAG-deficient mice, induced fatal disease. These data reveal unique structural features of IOE that may contribute to the pathogen's high virulence.

Key words: *Ehrlichia*; tick cell; endothelial cell; bacterial infection; ultrastructure

Introduction

The ehrlichiae comprise a genus of obligate intracellular bacteria within the family *Anaplasmataceae*.[1] Propagation of these agents requires that the bacteria infect and multiply within eukaryotic cells. Since the ehrlichiae are well-known to reside in macrophages and other phagocytic blood cells (e.g., *E. ewingii* infects neutrophils and eosinophils), propagation is commonly performed in human myleomonocytic cell lines such as HL-60,[2] or in macrophage cell lines such as DH82[3] and THP-1 cells.[4] Although many of the ehrlichiae have been cultured from clinical isolates or laboratory-infected mice, establishment of these organisms in cell lines has often been difficult, and some isolates have resisted culturing.

Address for correspondence: Gary Winslow, Wadsworth Center, 120 New Scotland Avenue, Albany, NY 12208. Voice: +518-473-2795; fax: +518-486-9858. gary.winslow@wadsworth.org.

This work was supported by US Public Health Service grant R01AI47963-01 to GMW and R01 AI042792-09 to UGM.

Rickettsiology and Rickettsial Diseases-Fifth International Conference: Ann. N.Y. Acad. Sci. 1166: 112–119 (2009).
doi: 10.1111/j.1749-6632.2009.04520.x © 2009 New York Academy of Sciences.

Among these is the *Ixodes ovatus Ehrlichia*-like agent, IOE, a bacterium identical or closely related to "*Candidatus Neoehrlichia mikurensis*."[5] IOE was originally identified in *Ixodes ovatus* ticks in Japan and was shown to fatally infect mice.[6] IOE is a particularly pathogenic ehrlichia that can induce a fatal disease in mice that resembles human monocytotropic ehrlichiosis.[7,8] Thus, the bacterial isolate has provided a very useful model for examination of aspects of immunity and immunopathology.[9–14] Until now, however, it had not been possible to culture IOE, and passage of the bacteria in mice has been necessary; this limitation has precluded detailed genetic and ultrastructural analyses. Since IOE has been shown to infect not only monocytic cells, but also endothelial cells and macrophages, we reasoned that non-myelomonocytic cell lines would be good candidates for *in vitro* culture. In this study, we demonstrate the culture of IOE in the rhesus monkey (*Macaca mulatta*) endothelial cell line RF/6A,[15] and in the tick cell line ISE6.[16] Furthermore, our data reveal unique ultrastructural features of IOE that may be associated with the organism's high virulence in laboratory mice.

Materials and Methods

Cell Culture

RF/6A cells were obtained from the American Tissue Type Culture Association (ATCC, Manassas, VA, USA; ATCC CRL-1780) and were cultured in L15B300[16] supplemented with 5% FBS (heat-inactivated; Harlan, Indianapolis, IN, USA), 5% TPB (Difco, Detroit, MI, USA), 0.1% lipoprotein concentrate (MP Biomedical, Irvine, CA, USA), 25 mM HEPES, 0.25% NaHCO$_3$, adjusted to pH ~7.5, in the absence of antibiotics at 37°C in a 5% CO$_2$-atmosphere. The tick cell line ISE6 was routinely propagated in the same medium, but without HEPES and NaHCO$_3$, in tightly capped flasks at 34°C. For IOE culture, however, 25 mM HEPES and 0.25% NaHCO$_3$

were included in tick cell culture medium as well, as described.[16] Subsequent passage of RF/6A was performed in Complete Tumor Medium, as described previously.[17]

IOE and *Ehrlichia muris* Isolation

IOE and *Ehrlichia muris* were obtained from spleens of infected C57BL/6 RAG-deficient mice on day 9 post-infection. Spleen tissue was mechanically disrupted, erythrocytes were lysed, and mononuclear cells were suspended in Complete Tumor Medium.[17] Splenocytes were collected by centrifugation at 1000 × *g* for 15 min., and resuspended in L15B300 supplemented as stated above; spleen cells infected with either *Ehrlichia* species were then overlaid separately on RF/6A and ISE6 cell cultures. Antibiotics and antifungals were not used. Quantitative PCR analyses indicated that the spleen cell suspension contained 8.2 × 10^4 IOE copies per 10 ng total DNA (equivalent to approximately 2000 host cells).

Ultrastructural Analyses

Cells in culture were prepared for electron microscopy when the cultures were approximately 70–90% infected. After removal of the growth medium, cell layers were flooded with modified Ito's fixative,[18] and fixed for 15 min. on ice. Cells were carefully scraped off the substrate, collected by centrifugation at 100 × *g* for 10 min, and resuspended in fresh fixative. After washing 3 times by centrifugation in phosphate buffer, pH 7.2, the cells were post-fixed in 1% osmium tetroxide in sodium phosphate buffer, pH 7.2 for 1 hr at room temperature, dehydrated in an ascending ethanol series and embedded in Epon 812. Ultrathin sections were cut on a Sorvall MT-1 ultramicrotome, stained with uranyl acetate and lead citrate, and examined and photographed in a JEOL 1200 EX or FEI CM12 electron microscope operating at 60 kV.

Light Microscopy

To confirm infection, we centrifuged infected cells onto microscope slides (Cytospin, Shandon Southern Instruments, Sewickley, PA), fixed them in methanol, and stained them with Giemsa's solution. Preparations were examined with an Olympus BH2 microscope, and images were captured with a Scion Greyscale digital camera (model CFW-1310M) and Scion Visicapture software (Scion Corporation, Frederick, MD, USA) running on an Apple iMac (Apple Computer, Inc., Cupertino, CA, USA).

Immunofluorescence Detection

The IOE cultured in the RF/6A were detected using a biotinylated anti-OMP-19 antibody (Ec18.1[19]) followed by streptavidin-Alexa-fluor 488 (Molecular Probes, Invitrogen, Carlsbad, CA, USA). The cells were permeabilized with 0.1% saponin and nonspecific binding was inhibited with a streptavidin-biotin blocking kit (Vector Laboratories, Burlingame, CA, USA).

Mice and Infections

C57BL/6 and C57BL/6-Rag1^{tm1Mom}/J mice were obtained from Jackson Laboratories (Bar Harbor, ME, USA) and were maintained in the Animal Care Facility at the Wadsworth Center under microisolator conditions in accordance with institutional guidelines for animal welfare. Mice were gender-matched for each experiment and were 6 to 12 weeks in age. For infections, RF/6A cells were harvested from infected cultures using a cell scraper and disrupted using a Braun-Sonic 2000 sonicator (40 W for 2 mins on ice). The cell lysate was clarified by low-speed centrifugation (600 × g), and the bacteria were harvested by high-speed centrifugation (10,000 × g). The pelleted bacteria were resuspended in sucrose-phosphate-glutamate (SPG) buffer (0.0038 M KH_2PO_4/0.0072 M K_2HPO_4/0.0049 M L-glutamate-0.218M sucrose, pH 7.2) and injected intraperitonally into

mice. Moribund mice judged to be incapable of surviving infection; indicated by ruffled coat, immobility, and hunched posture, and were humanely sacrificed.

Results

Infection of RF/6A and ISE6 Cells with IOE and *E. muris*

Of the primary cultures initially seeded with IOE or *E. muris*-infected splenocytes, one RF/6A and one ISE6 culture of IOE, as well as one ISE6 culture of *E. muris*, appeared to be productively infected and were chosen for expansion. Productive infection with IOE was first noted in RF/6A cells by phase contrast microscopy of intact cell layers 2 weeks after addition of IOE obtained from spleen cells from a RAG-deficient C57BL/6 mouse. Initially, inclusions suggestive of ehrlichial morulae were small, and there usually were several in each infected cell. These subsequently grew until the entire cytoplasm was filled with numerous bacteria. Giemsa-stained cell spreads confirmed the presence of multiple small IOE-morulae in RF/6A rhesus endothelial cells (Fig. 1A) and ISE6 tick cells (Fig. 1B). Notably, IOE within tick cells clustered inside their inclusion, leaving an apparently empty "halo" around the bacteria; the halo could also be seen in live cultures (data not shown). In contrast, *E. muris* produced one or two large inclusions in each tick cell (Fig. 1C). No IOE were recovered from the primary culture of ISE6 tick cells, but subsequent passage of IOE from RF/6A to ISE6 cells was successful. Although IOE were originally isolated in RF/6A cells with L15B300, they were later propagated successfully in RPMI1640 with 25 mM HEPES buffer and 10% heat-inactivated FBS, and in Complete Tumor Medium composed of Eagle's MEM supplemented with 10 μM 2-mercaptoethanol, 10% Mishell-Dutton Nutrient cocktail,[20] and 10% FBS.

Electron microscopic analyses revealed an accumulation of copious amounts of fibrillar

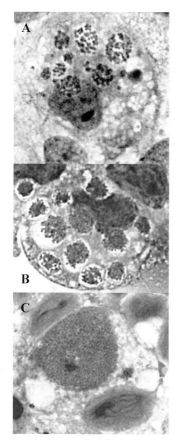

Figure 1. Detection of IOE and *E. muris* in RF/6A and tick-derived ISE6 cells. Light microscopic appearance of the *Ixodes ovatus* ehrlichia in rhesus monkey endothelial cells (**A**) and ISE6 tick cells (**B**), and of *Ehrlichia muris* in ISE6 cells (**C**). Bar in C = 15 μm. Arrow heads in **A** and **B** point to several of multiple morulae in each cell. Note the "empty" space surrounding the morulae of the *I. ovatus* ehrlichia-like agent in **B**; such an appearance is also visible by phase contrast microscopy of living cultures (not shown). For comparison, panel **C** depicts *Ehrlichia muris* in ISE6 tick cell culture, typically presenting a single, large morula in one cell. N = host cell nucleus; M = morula.

material in IOE morulae. This appearance was most striking in RF/6A cells, where the material displayed an orderly appearance of fine, combed hair (Fig. 2A, B). The structures seemed to be streaming from the bacteria, obscuring details of their cell wall in most cases, and individual bacteria were extremely pleomorphic and condensed to varying degrees. In tick cells also (Fig. 2C), fibrillar material was

evident inside the inclusions, but, here, it was arranged in a disorganized, random fashion. The inset in Figure 2, panel C, shows a cross section of an individual bacterium, revealing the typical structure of the ehrlichial cell wall.[5] For comparison, sections of *E. muris*-infected ISE6 tick cells are shown in panels D and E. The *E. muris* morulae lacked fibrillar material, and ehrlichiae were only moderately pleomorphic compared to IOE. The *E. muris* bacteria had an ultrastructural organization typical of organisms in the genus *Ehrlichia*. The inclusions in panel D contain a mixture of reticulated and dense core forms, while the inclusions in panel E are entirely composed of reticulated organisms bounded by flaccid membranes.

IOE Cultured in RF/6A Cells Retained Antigenicity

To confirm that the cultured IOE retain antigenicity, immunohistochemical analyses of the IOE in RF/6A cells, was performed with the anti-OMP-19 antibody Ec18.1.[19] Although the antibody was raised against OMP-19 from *E. chaffeensis*, the antibody epitope is conserved in IOE.[21] Infected cells containing many morulae were detected, indicating that OMP-19 expression was maintained in the endothelial cell line (Fig. 3).

IOE Cultured in RF/6A Cells Is Fully Competent to Infect Immunocompromised and Immunocompetent Mice

IOE grown in RF/6A cells readily infected C57BL/6 and RAG-deficient mice and caused mortality within 9–14 days post-infection, as observed in previous studies that used mouse-passaged bacteria.[9,14] For confirmation that the IOE grown in RF/6A cells were infectious, cell-free ehrlichiae obtained after ultrasonic disruption were used to infect C57BL/6 RAG-deficient mice via the peritoneum. Retrospective quantitative PCR analyses revealed that mice were infected with a range of 4–6 $\log_{10}$

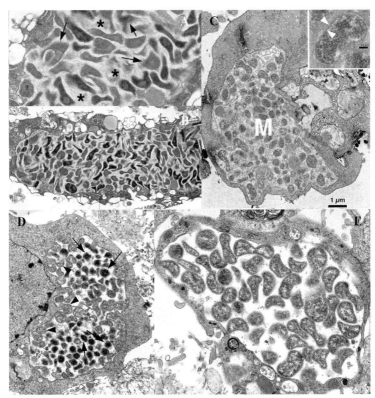

Figure 2. Ultrastructural analysis of IOE and *E. muris*. Panels **A** and **B**: *Ixodes ovatus* ehrlichia in rhesus monkey endothelial cells, line RF/6A. Arrows in **A** indicate dense, fur-like material streaming from the ehrlichiae. Asterisks mark a more lightly packed fibrous substance between the bacteria. Panel **B**: Overview of *I. ovatus* ehrlichiae in cell line RF/6A. Panel **C**: Large morula (M) of the *I. ovatus Ehrlichia*-like agent in tick cell line ISE6 from *Ixodes scapularis*. **Inset**: Cross section of a single bacterium demonstrating the typical bilayer membrane structure, arrow heads. Bar = 0.1 μm. For comparison, panels **D** and **E** depict *Ehrlichia muris* in tick cells, line ISE6. Note absence of "fur" and fibrous material in the morulae. Arrows in **D** indicate condensed bacterial cells among reticulated forms (arrow heads).

bacterial copies. All RAG-deficient infected mice were judged to be moribund and incapable of surviving infection within 9 days postinfection, indicating that the RF/6A-grown bacteria were fully infectious (Fig. 4). Similar inoculations performed with C57BL/6 mice also induced fatal disease (data not shown). Bacteria isolated from the spleens of infected RAG-deficient mice were successfully recultured *in vitro* in RF/6A cells (data not shown).

Discussion

The present report details the successful culture of the IOE agent *in vitro*. This accomplishment will facilitate research that entails the use of large numbers of purified bacteria, such as genetic transformation and analysis, and biochemical studies. Even though methods are becoming more widely used that permit analysis of the behavior of pathogens *in vivo* (e.g., tissue-specific gene expression assays using quantitative reverse transcription PCR), studies that utilize large numbers of pure microbes typically require a source of bacteria from *in vitro* cultures. In addition, cell culture provides an opportunity to observe the organisms in a living state or with minimal manipulation. Although myelomonocytic cells are often considered to be the chief targets of IOE and related

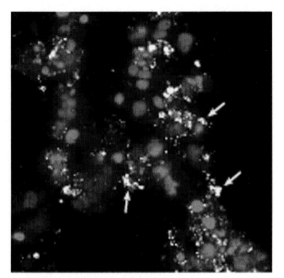

Figure 3. Immunofluoresence microscopy of IOE. RF/6A cells containing IOE were stained with the monoclonal antibody Ec18.1, which recognizes OMP-19. Numerous morulae can be detected in the cells (arrows).

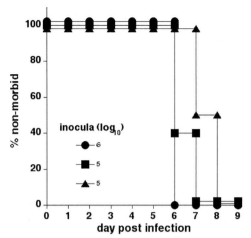

Figure 4. IOE cultured in RF/6A endothelial cells is fully competent to infect mice. C57BL/6 RAG-deficient mice were infected with 4–6 $\log_{10}$ copies of IOE, via the peritoneum. Moribund mice were those judged to be incapable of surviving the infection. Three mice were used per group.

ehrlichiae *in vivo*, IOE are known to infect cell types, including endothelial cells and hepatocytes.[22] This likely explains the ability of IOE to establish infection in the rhesus monkey endothelial cell line RF/6A and suggests that other endothelial cell lines could be susceptible to infection. RF/6A also supported the growth of related tick-borne pathogens (i.e., *Anaplasma phagocytophilum* and *A. marginale*),[23] and, thus, it may be broadly suitable for other Anaplasma. Since endothelial cells can present major histocompatibility complex (MHC) processed peptide antigens, infecting bacteria could potentially interfere with this pathway, thereby altering the immune response in the pathogen's favor.[24] We conclude that endothelial cell cultures provide a relevant and useful *in vitro* model whose utilization will facilitate investigation of the biology, pathogenesis, and immunological aspects of infection with the IOE and related bacteria.

Culture was also successful in the tick-derived cell line ISE6, a line that has been used to propagate other *Ehrlichia* and *Anaplasma* species.[16,25] In those cases, however, IOE were not recovered in tick cells from the primary inoculum of infected blood, but only after transfer from RF/6A cells. Whether that result was due to the prior mouse-to-mouse passage history of the isolate and concomitant adaptation to the mammalian host, or whether it reflected a lower degree of susceptibility of the tick cells relative to the RF/6A cells, will require additional investigation. Regardless, the availability of two culture systems representing both the mammalian host and the arthropod vector will benefit studies that seek to examine the entire life cycle of the IOE *in vitro*, and those that focus on IOE in either the mammal or the tick. It is likely that the IOE differentially expresses specific subsets of genes or gene variants necessary for survival in cells from these very different hosts, as has been shown to be the case for related pathogens.[25,26] This assumption is supported by the different appearances of the IOE between tick cells and mammalian cells (see Figs. 1A, B and 2A, B, and C). Notably, in RF/6A cells, the bacteria filled the entire inclusion, whereas in ISE6 tick cells, some of the inclusions showed a clear zone next to or surrounding a group of IOE. The most striking feature, visible upon electron microscopic examination of sectioned material, was a matrix of regularly arrayed fibrils embedding the IOE. In places, these converged into dense bundles (see Fig. 2A, arrows). Although IOE morulae within tick cells also contained an undefined material admixed in with the bacteria, such material was irregular and stringy and flocculent in appearance, quite unlike the highly structured fibrils seen in RF/6A cells. *Ehrlichia muris*, grown in ISE6 cells under identical conditions and processed at the same time and in the same manner, did not contain such material in their morulae, suggesting that it was unique to the IOE. The function of these structures, especially in the RF/6A cells, remains unknown. Other investigators have demonstrated the presence of amorphous material among *E. chaffeensis* inside morulae,[27–29] but none of those studies documented the highly regularly structured fibrils described here. We propose that they are a unique feature of the biology of IOE and are possibly linked to the organism's high pathogenicity in mice.

Acknowledgments

The authors wish to thank Kathryn Hogle and Shelia Le of the Wadsworth Center for excellent technical assistance, and the Wadsworth Center Animal Care Facility.

The authors have no competing financial interests.

Conflicts of Interest

The authors declare no conflicts of interest.

References

1. Dumler, J.S. *et al*. 2001. Reorganization of genera in the families Rickettsiaceae and Anaplasmataceae in the order Rickettsiales: Unification of some species of Ehrlichia with Anaplasma, Cowdria with Ehrlichia and Ehrlichia with Neorickettsia, descriptions of six new species combinations and designation of *Ehrlichia equi* and 'HGE agent' as subjective synonyms of *Ehrlichia phagocytophila*. *Int. J. Syst. Evol. Microbiol.* **51:** 2145–2165.

2. Goodman, J.L. *et al*. 1996. Direct cultivation of the causative agent of human granulocytic ehrlichiosis. *N. Engl. J. Med.* **334:** 209–215.

3. Heimer, R., D. Tisdale & J.E. Dawson. 1998. A single tissue culture system for the propagation of the agents of the human ehrlichioses. *Am. J. Trop. Med. Hyg.* **58:** 812–815.

4. Barnewall, R.E. & Y. Rikihisa. 1994. Abrogation of gamma interferon-induced inhibition of *Ehrlichia chaffeensis* infection in human monocytes with iron transferrin. *Infect. Immun.* **62:** 4804–4810.

5. Kawahara, M. *et al*. 2004. Ultrastructure and phylogenetic analysis of '*Candidatus Neoehrlichia mikurensis*' in the family Anaplasmataceae, isolated from wild rats and found in *Ixodes ovatus* ticks. *Int. J. Syst. Evol. Microbiol.* **54:** 1837–1843.

6. Shibata, S. *et al*. 2000. New Ehrlichia species closely related to *Ehrlichia chaffeensis* isolated from *Ixodes ovatus* ticks in Japan. *J. Clin. Microbiol.* **38:** 1331–1338.

7. Okada, H. *et al*. 2003. Distribution of Ehrlichiae in tissues as determined by in-situ hybridization. *J. Comp. Pathol.* **128:** 182–187.

8. Okada, H. *et al*. 2001. Ehrlichial proliferation and acute hepatocellular necrosis in immunocompetent mice experimentally infected with the HF strain of Ehrlichia, closely related to *Ehrlichia chaffeensis*. *J. Comp. Pathol.* **124:** 165–171.

9. Ismail, N. *et al*. 2004. Overproduction of TNF-alpha by CD8+ type 1 cells and down-regulation of IFN-gamma production by CD4+ Th1 cells contribute to toxic shock-like syndrome in an animal model of fatal monocytotropic ehrlichiosis. *J. Immunol.* **172:** 1786–1800.

10. Ismail, N., H.L. Stevenson & D.H. Walker. 2006. Role of tumor necrosis factor alpha (TNF-{alpha}) and interleukin-10 in the pathogenesis of severe murine monocytotropic ehrlichiosis: Increased resistance of TNF Receptor p55- and p75-deficient mice to fatal ehrlichial infection. *Infect. Immun.* **74:** 1846–1856.

11. Stevenson, H.L. *et al*. 2006. An intradermal environment promotes a protective type-1 response against lethal systemic monocytotropic ehrlichial infection. *Infect. Immun.* **74:** 4856–4864.

12. Bitsaktsis, B., B. Nandi & G. Winslow. 2007. T Cell-independent humoral immunity is sufficient for protection against fatal intracellular ehrlichia infection. *Infect. Immun.* **75:** 4933–4941.

13. Bitsaktsis, C. & G. Winslow. 2006. Fatal recall responses mediated by CD8 T cells during intracellular bacteria infection. *J. Immunol.* **177:** 4644–4651.

14. Bitsaktsis, C., J. Huntington & G.M. Winslow. 2004. Production of Interferon-g by CD4 T cells is essential for resolving ehrlichia infection. *J. Immunol.* **172:** 6894–6901.

15. Lou, D.A. & F.N. Hu. 1987. Specific antigen and organelle expression of a long-term rhesus endothelial cell line. *In Vitro Cell. Dev. Biol.* **23:** 75–85.

16. Munderloh, U.G. *et al.* 1999. Invasion and intracellular development of the human granulocytic ehrlichiosis agent in tick cell culture. *J. Clin. Microbiol.* **37:** 2518–2524.

17. Mix, D. & G.M. Winslow. 1996. Proteolytic processing activates a viral superantigen. *J. Exp. Med.* **184:** 1549–1554.

18. Kurtti, T.J. *et al.* 1994. Ultrastructural analysis of the invasion of tick cells by Lyme disease spirochetes (*Borrelia burgdorferi*) in vitro. *Can. J. Zool.* **72:** 977–994.

19. Li, J.S. *et al.* 2001. Outer membrane protein specific monoclonal antibodies protect SCID Mice from fatal infection by the obligate intracellular bacterial pathogen *Ehrlichia chaffeensis*. *J. Immunol.* **166:** 1855–1862.

20. Mishell, R.I. & R.W. Dutton. 1967. Immunization of dissociated spleen cell cultures from normal mice. *J. Exp. Med.* **126:** 423–442.

21. Nandi, B. *et al.* 2007. CD4 T cell epitopes associated with protective immunity induced following vaccination of mice with an ehrlichia variable outer membrane protein. *Infect. Immun.* **75:** 5453–5459.

22. Sotomayor, E.A. *et al.* 2001. Animal model of fatal human monocytotropic ehrlichiosis. *Am. J. Pathol.* **158:** 757–769.

23. Munderloh, U.G. *et al.* 2004. Infection of endothelial cells with *Anaplasma marginale* and *A. phagocytophilum*. *Vet. Microbiol.* **101:** 53–64.

24. Vachiery, N. *et al.* 1998. Inhibition of MHC class I and class II cell surface expression on bovine endothelial cells upon infection with *Cowdria ruminantium*. *Vet. Immunol. Immunopathol.* **61:** 37–48.

25. Singu, V., H. Liu, C. Cheng & R. Ganta. 2005. *Ehrlichia chaffeensis* expressed macrophage- and tick cell-specific 28-kilodalton outer membrane proteins. *Infect. Immun.* **73:** 79–87.

26. Lohr, C.V. *et al.* 2002. Expression of *Anaplasma marginale* Major Surface Protein 2 operon-associated proteins during mammalian and arthropod infection. *Infect. Immun.* **70:** 6005–6012.

27. Popov, V.L. *et al.* 1995. Ultrastructural variation of cultured *Ehrlichia chaffeensis*. *J. Med. Microbiol.* **43:** 411–421.

28. Popov, V.L. *et al.* 1998. Ultrastructural differentiation of the genogroups in the genus Ehrlichia. *J. Med. Microbiol.* **47:** 235–251.

29. Zhang, J.Z. *et al.* 2007. The developmental cycle of *Ehrlichia chaffeensis* in vertebrate cells. *Cell Microbiol.* **9:** 610–618.

Bartonella Endocarditis

A Pathology Shared by Animal Reservoirs and Patients

Bruno B. Chomel,[a] R.W. Kasten,[a] C. Williams,[b] A.C. Wey,[c] J.B. Henn,[d] R. Maggi,[e] S. Carrasco,[f] J. Mazet,[f] H.J. Boulouis,[g] R. Maillard,[g] and E.B. Breitschwerdt[e]

[a]*Department of Population Health and Reproduction, School of Veterinary Medicine, University of California, Davis, California 95616, USA*

[b]*Animal Surgical and Emergency Center, 1535 S. Sepulveda Blvd, Los Angeles, California 90025, USA*

[c]*Upstate Veterinary Specialties, PLLC, 222 Troy-Schenectady Road, Latham, New York 12110, USA*

[d]*Napa County Public Health, 2344 Old Sonoma Road, Building F, Napa, California 94559, USA*

[e]*College of Veterinary Medicine, North Carolina State University, Raleigh, North Carolina 27606, USA*

[f]*Department of Medicine and Epidemiology, School of Veterinary Medicine, University of California, Davis, California 95616, USA*

[g]*Ecole Nationale Vétérinaire d'Alfort, Maisons-Alfort, 94704, France*

Bartonellae were first recognized to cause endocarditis in humans in 1993 when cases caused by *Bartonella quintana, B. elizabethae,* and *B. henselae* were reported. Since the first isolation of *Bartonella vinsonii* subspecies *berkhoffii* from a dog with endocarditis, this organism has emerged as an important pathogen in dogs and an emerging pathogen in people. Subsequently, four types of *B. vinsonii* subsp. *berkhoffii* have been described, all of which have been associated with endocarditis in dogs. A limited number of dog endocarditis cases have also been associated with *B. clarridgeiae, B. washoensis, B. quintana,* and *B. rochalimae.* The second canine *B. clarridgeiae* endocarditis case is presented. The clinical and pathological characteristics of *Bartonella* endocarditis in dogs are similar to disease observed in humans, more often affecting the aortic valve, presenting with highly vegetative lesions with accompanying calcification, and in most instances high antibody titers. Pathological features in dogs include a combination of fibrosis, mineralization, endothelial proliferation, and neovascularization with variable inflammation. Endocarditis has also been described in animal species, which are the natural reservoir of specific *Bartonella* species, once thought to be solely healthy carriers of these pathogens. A few *Bartonella* endocarditis cases, including *B. henselae,* have been reported in cats in the USA and Australia. The second case of *B. henselae* type Houston I identified in the USA is presented. Furthermore, two cases of *B. bovis* endocarditis were recently described in adult cows from France. Finally, on-going investigation of valvular endocarditis in free-ranging Alaskan sea otters suggests the involvement of *Bartonella* species.

Key words: Bartonella; endocarditis; dogs; cats; cattle; reservoir

Address for correspondence: Bruno B. Chomel, D.V.M., Ph.D., Department of Population Health and Reproduction, School of Veterinary Medicine, University of California, Davis, Davis, CA 95616. Voice: +530-752-8112; fax: +530-752-2377. bbchomel@ucdavis.edu

Rickettsiology and Rickettsial Diseases-Fifth International Conference: Ann. N.Y. Acad. Sci. 1166: 120–126 (2009).
doi: 10.1111/j.1749-6632.2009.04523.x © 2009 New York Academy of Sciences.

Introduction

Bartonella spp. are fastidious hemotropic gram-negative bacteria which are mainly transmitted by arthropod vectors. Among the 13 species or subspecies known or suspected to be pathogenic for humans, 8 have been associated with endocarditis or cardiopathy, including *Bartonella henselae*,[1] *B. quintana*,[2] *B.(Rochalimaea) elizabethae*,[3] *B. vinsonii* subsp. *berkhoffii*,[4] *B. vinsonii* subsp. *arupensis*,[5] *B. koehlerae*,[6] *B. alsatica*,[7] and *B. washoensis*.[8] However, most of human cases of endocarditis are caused by *Bartonella henselae* or *B. quintana*.[9–11] Only a few published human cases of endocarditis or myocarditis have been associated with *B. elizabethae* (1 case), *B. vinsonii* subsp. *berkhoffii* (1 case), *B. vinsonii* subsp. *arupensis* (1 case), *B. koehlerae* (1 case), *B. washoensis* (1 case), and *B. alsatica* (1 case). A second human case of endocarditis caused by *B. alsatica* was recently presented.[12] Overall, *Bartonella* endocarditis prevalence follows a northern to southern gradient, with a very low prevalence at most northern latitudes (0% in Sweden, 1.1% in the United Kingdom, 3% in France and in Germany) and the highest prevalence in more southern latitudes (≥10% in Northern Africa).[13] Most human cases of *Bartonella* endocarditis are associated with high antibody titers.[14] It has been suggested that human *B. henselae* endocarditis occurs in cat scratch disease patients with preexisting abnormalities of the heart valves.[15]

Bartonella Endocarditis in Dogs

In animals, most cases of endocarditis have been reported in dogs (Table 1). Since the isolation of *Bartonella vinsonii* subspecies *berkhoffii* from a dog with endocarditis in 1993,[16,17] this organism has emerged as an important pathogen in dogs[18] and as an emerging pathogen in people.[18,19] Several cases of endocarditis caused by *B. vinsonii* subsp. *berkhoffii* have been reported from dogs both on the eastern and western parts of the USA,[20–23] as well as a case from Canada.[24] Similarly, a limited

TABLE 1. *Bartonella* Species Associated with Endocarditis in Animals

Bartonella sp.	Animal species (location)	Isolation/ PCR/serology
B. quintana	Dogs (USA, NC; New Zealand)	PCR
B. clarridgeiae	Dogs (USA)	Isolation/PCR
B. rochalimae	Dog (USA)	PCR
B. vinsonii berkhoffii		
type 1	Dogs (USA)	Isolation/PCR
type 2	Dogs (USA)	Isolation/PCR
type 3	Dogs (USA)	PCR
type 4	Dogs (Canada) USA (Colorado)	PCR
B. washoensis	Dog (USA, CA)	Isolation
B. henselae	Cats (USA; Australia)	Isolation, PCR serol.
	Dogs (Belgium)	PCR
	Dogs (USA, CO)	
B. bovis	Cows (France)	PCR
B. volans-like	Sea otters (USA, AK)	PCR

number of endocarditis cases have also been associated with *B. clarridgeiae*,[25] *B. washoensis*,[26] *B. rochalimae*,[27] and *B. quintana*[28] in the USA and New Zealand. Furthermore, four distinct types of *B. vinsonii* subsp. *berkhoffii* have been described, all of which have been associated with endocarditis in dogs.[24,29,30] The first cases of *B. henselae* endocarditis in dogs were recently detected in a dog from Belgium and in dogs from Colorado (Breitschwerdt, personal communication) and seropositivity for *B. henselae* was detected in three of four dogs with endocarditis in the USA.[31] So far, no dog endocarditis cases have been published yet from other parts of the world, more likely by lack of detection rather than absence of such infection in dogs. In northern California, two studies indicated that *Bartonella* infection accounted for 18% to 28% of all cases of endocarditis in dogs,[22,23] a prevalence rate much higher than has been reported for humans.[13]

The clinical and pathological characteristics of endocarditis in dogs are very similar to abnormalities observed in human patients, including the aortic valve being more frequently affected, highly vegetative lesions with accompanying calcification, and in most instances infection associated with high *Bartonella* antibody titers.[11,14,18] The clinical abnormalities reported in dogs with endocarditis due to *Bartonella* spp. are commonly a murmur (89%), fever (72%), leukocytosis (78%), hypoalbuminemia (67%), thrombocytopenia (56%), elevated liver enzymes (56%), lameness (43%), azotemia (33%), respiratory abnormalities (28%), and weakness and collapse (17%).[22] Dogs with endocarditis secondary to infection with *Bartonella* spp. are often afebrile, more likely to develop congestive heart failure, rarely having mitral valve involvement, and having shorter survival times.[23] Features of *Bartonella* endocarditis in dogs include a combination of fibrosis, mineralization, endothelial proliferation, and neovascularisation with variable inflammation.[32]

Dogs appear to be excellent sentinels of *Bartonella* infections, as they are mainly infected with the same *Bartonella* species causing endocarditis in humans.[18]

New Case Reports

We report the second case of endocarditis caused by *B. clarridgeiae* in a dog and a case of *B. vinsonii* subsp. *berkhoffii* endocarditis characterized by a perforation of the mitral valve in another dog.

Case Reports

Case 1

A 5 year-old-spayed female German shepherd living in Southern California was diagnosed with aortic valve endocarditis (calcified, thickened, proliferative aortic valve cups) and biventricular heart failure in November 2005. *Bartonella* serology was performed at that time using an immunofluorescence test, as previously described,[22] and titers were 1:512 for *B. clarridgieae* and 1:64 for *B. henselae*, respectively. The dog died in February 2006 of acute respiratory distress syndrome. A necropsy was performed and heart (aortic valve and ventricular

wall) and lung tissues were collected. Conventional PCR testing was performed after DNA extraction from fragments of the aortic valve using primers targeting the citrate synthase gene (*glt*A), as previously described.[23,25,26] *Bartonella* DNA was amplified from the aortic valve tissues, producing a very intense characteristic 400 bp band. Amplified DNA was sequenced, and the partial sequence was identical to *B. clarridgeiae* (sequence BCU84386 in GenBank).

Case 2

A 3.5-year-old spayed female Newfoundland from Southern California was diagnosed with endocarditis of the mitral valve, and *Bartonella* infection was suspected. On May 7, 2007 a blood sample was submitted to the University of California, Davis for blood culture and serological testing for *Bartonella* antibodies. The blood culture did not yield a *Bartonella* isolate, but the dog had very high antibody titers (*B. clarridgeiae*: 1:2048; *B. vinsonii* subsp. *berkhoffii* and *B. henselae*: 1:1024), and a *Corynebacterium* sp. was isolated from the blood. Almost a month later (June 3, 2007), the dog died of acute respiratory distress syndrome and pulmonary thromboembolism. At necropsy, a massive hole in the supravalvular region of the mitral valve was observed immediately upon opening of the left heart (Figs. 1 and 2). *Bartonella* DNA was amplified from the mitral valve tissues, producing a very intense characteristic 400-bp band, while amplification from the aortic and pulmonic valve tissues did not yield *Bartonella* DNA. Amplified DNA was sequenced, and partial sequence was identical to *B. vinsonii* subsp. *berkhoffii*.

Bartonella Endocarditis in Cats

Domestic cats are the natural reservoir of *B. henselae* and are usually considered as healthy carriers of this bacterium, as are humans for *B. quintana*.[18] However, clinical signs have been associated with *Bartonella* infection, mainly based on serological studies involving naturally infected cats or experimentally infected cats.[19]

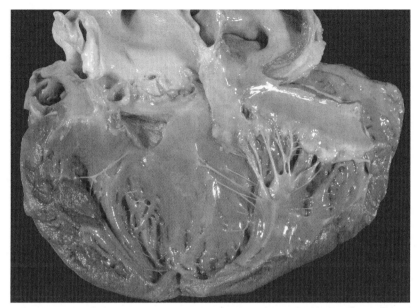

Figure 1. Heart of dog with *Bartonella vinsonii* subspecies *berkhoffii* endocarditis on mitral valve (see perforation in mitral valve) Photo: Bill Thomas, UCD Case referred by Dr. Cathy Williams.

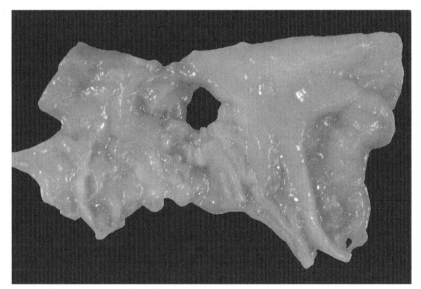

Figure 2. Mitral valve with major perforation in the supravalvular region of the mitral valve.

Endocarditis is rarely diagnosed in cats; however, in a case series study conducted in Australia, *Bartonella* sp. were isolated from two cats with endocarditis of the aortic valve; however, direct causality was not proven.[33] A few years later, the first confirmed case of *B. henselae* endocarditis was reported from California.[34] We report here the second confirmed case of endocarditis in a cat, caused by *B. henselae* in North America.

Case Report

A 10-year-old castrated male "indoor/ outdoor" cat from New York State was clinically diagnosed with a large hyperechoic vegetative lesion on the aortic valve detected by electrocardiography. The aortic valve cups were thickened, and severe aortic insufficiency was detected. A small hyperechoic thickening was also apparent on the anterior leaflet of the mitral valve, and mild mitral regurgitation was observed directed toward the caudal lateral left atrial wall. These findings were consistent with vegetative endocarditis of the aortic and possibly mitral valves with secondary valvular insufficiencies, left ventricular volume overload, and congestive heart failure. Conventional PCR testing was performed after DNA extraction on fragments of the aortic, mitral, and pulmonic valves using primers targeting the citrate synthase gene, as previously described.[34] *Bartonella* DNA was amplified from the aortic and mitral valve tissues, producing a very intense, characteristic 400 bp band, while amplification from the pulmonic valve tissue did not yield any *Bartonella* DNA. Amplified DNA was sequenced, and partial sequence was identical to *B. henselae* genotype I. It is of interest to note that this second case of *B. henselae* endocarditis in a cat in North America is also caused by genotype I, a genotype suspected to be more likely to induce visceral lesions in humans.[35] As for other cases of endocarditis in dogs and humans, the *Bartonella* antibody titer was very high (Western blot 4+, on a scale of 0 to 4+, as performed by Dr. Hardy, National Veterinary Laboratory, Inc., New Jersey, USA).

In addition, *B. henselae* was isolated from a young cat with aortic valve endocarditis in North Carolina (Breitschwerdt *et al.*, unpublished data). Following antibiotic treatment, there was total resolution of the heart murmur and the valvular lesion, as assessed by echocardiography.

Bartonella Endocarditis in Cattle

Cattle have also been found to be the natural reservoir of *Bartonella* species, mainly *B. bovis* and *B. chomelii*.[36,37] Bacteria-induced vegetative valvular endocarditis is one of the main cardiac disorders in adult cattle, and the prevalence of endocarditis may reach 5.2 cases per 10,000 cows, but the disease is often misdiagnosed and only discovered during the slaughtering process or at necropsy.[38] The first two cases of endocarditis caused by *B. bovis* were diagnosed recently in two French cows aged 13 and 15 years old, respectively.[38] Both cows had high antibody titers and were PCR positive for *B. bovis*. This study demonstrated that *B. bovis* is a potential bovine pathogen and that *B. bovis* can induce endocarditis in the animal reservoir host, as previously shown for *B. henselae* and *B. vinsonii* subsp. *berkhoffii* in cats and dogs, respectively.[18]

Emergence of *Bartonella* as a Possible Agent of Endocarditis in Wildlife

Bartonella species have been isolated or detected from a wide range of wild mammals,[19] including sea mammals.[39] However, no reports of endocarditis associated with *Bartonella* infection have been published yet in wildlife. Since 2002, an unusual mortality event of more than 300 northern sea otter (*Enhydra lutris kenyoni*) has been under investigation in Alaska. Postmortem examinations indicate that vegetative valvular endocarditis was a main factor for mortality.[40] In addition to other organisms isolated from the lesions, a *Bartonella* species close to *B. volans* by partial sequencing of amplified DNA has been detected.[41] An evaluation of the *Bartonella* frequency in sea otter lesions is underway, which will include further molecular characterization of the *Bartonella* species involved.

Conclusion

Bartonella species have a specific tropism for erythrocytes and endothelial cells and have been shown to cause vasculoproliferative lesions. These organisms also appear to have a specific tropism for cardiovascular valves in humans and several domestic animals, including species that are the natural reservoir for these bacteria. The spectrum of animal species for which endocarditis lesions are associated to *Bartonella* is expending, including for the first time the identification for *Bartonella* spp. infection of heart valves in free-ranging wildlife.

Acknowledgments

The authors thank V. A. Gill, A. M. Doroff and K. A. Burek from the US Fish and Wildlife Service, Marine Mammals Management, Anchorage, AK, and Alaska Veterinary Pathology Services, Eagle River, AK, for their collaboration on the Alaskan sea otters.

Conflicts of Interest

The authors declare no conflicts of interest.

References

1. Hadfield, T.L. *et al*. 1993. Endocarditis caused by *Rochalimaea henselae*. *Hum. Pathol*. **24:** 1140–1141.
2. Spach, D.H. *et al*. 1993. Endocarditis caused by *Rochalimaea quintana* in a patient infected with human immunodeficiency virus. *J. Clin. Microbiol*. **31:** 692–694.
3. Daly, J.S. *et al*. 1993. *Rochalimaea elizabethae* sp. nov. isolated from a patient with endocarditis. *J. Clin. Microbiol*. **31:** 872–881.
4. Roux, V., S.J. Eykyn, S. Wyllie & D. Raoult. 2000. *Bartonella vinsonii* subsp. *berkhoffii* as an agent of afebrile blood culture-negative endocarditis in a human. *J. Clin. Microbiol*. **38:** 1698–1700.
5. Fenollar, F., S. Sire & D. Raoult. 2005. *Bartonella vinsonii* subsp. *arupensis* as an agent of blood culture-negative endocarditis in a human. *J. Clin. Microbiol*. **43:** 945–947. Erratum in: J. Clin. Microbiol. 43: 4923.
6. Avidor, B. *et al*. 2004. *Bartonella koehlerae*, a new cat-associated agent of culture-negative human endocarditis. *J. Clin. Microbiol*. **42:** 3462–3468.
7. Raoult, D. *et al*. 2006. First isolation of *Bartonella alsatica* from a valve of a patient with endocarditis. *J. Clin. Microbiol*. **44:** 278–279.
8. Kosoy, M. *et al*. 2003. *Bartonella* strains from ground squirrels are identical to *Bartonella washoensis* isolated from a human patient. *J. Clin. Microbiol*. **41:** 645–650.
9. Raoult, D. *et al*. 1996. Diagnosis of 22 new cases of *Bartonella* endocarditis. *Ann. Intern. Med*. **125:** 646–652. Erratum in: Ann. Intern. Med. 1997;127:249.
10. La Scola, B. & D. Raoult. 1999. Culture of *Bartonella quintana* and *Bartonella henselae* from human samples: a 5-year experience (1993 to 1998). *J. Clin. Microbiol*. **37:** 1899–1905.
11. Fournier, P.E. *et al*. 2001. Epidemiologic and clinical characteristics of *Bartonella quintana* and *Bartonella henselae* endocarditis: a study of 48 patients. *Medicine (Baltimore)* 80: 245–251.
12. JeanClaude, D. *et al*. 2008. *Bartonella alsatica* endocarditis in a French patient in close contact with rabbits. *Poster #267, 5ᵗʰ International Meeting on Rickettsiae and Rickettsial Diseases*, Marseille, France, May 18–20, 2008.
13. Brouqui, P. & D. Raoult. 2006. New insight into the diagnosis of fastidious bacterial endocarditis. *FEMS Immunol. Med. Microbiol*. **47:** 1–13.
14. Fournier, P.E., J.L. Mainardi & D. Raoult. 2002. Value of microimmunofluorescence for diagnosis and follow-up of *Bartonella* endocarditis. *Clin. Diagn. Lab. Immunol*. **9:** 795–801.
15. Gouriet, F. *et al*. 2007. From cat scratch disease to endocarditis, the possible natural history of *Bartonella henselae* infection. *BMC Infect. Dis*. **7:** 30.
16. Breitschwerdt, E.B. *et al*. 1995. Endocarditis in a dog due to infection with a novel *Bartonella* subspecies. *J. Clin. Microbiol*. **33:** 154–160.
17. Kordick, D.L. *et al*. 1996. *Bartonella vinsonii* subsp. *berkhoffii* subsp. nov., isolated from dogs; *Bartonella vinsonii* subsp. *vinsonii*; and emended description of *Bartonella vinsonii*. *Int. J. Syst. Bacteriol*. **46:** 704–709.
18. Chomel, B.B., H.J. Boulouis, S. Maruyama & E.B. Breitschwerdt. 2006. *Bartonella* spp. in pets and effect on human health. *Emerg. Infect. Dis*. 12: 389–394.
19. Boulouis, H.J. *et al*. 2005. Factors associated with the rapid emergence of zoonotic *Bartonella* infections. *Vet. Res*. **36:** 383–410.
20. Breitschwerdt, E.B. *et al*. 1999. *Bartonella vinsonii* subsp. *berkhoffii* and related members of the alpha subdivision of the Proteobacteria in dogs with cardiac arrhythmias, endocarditis, or myocarditis. *J. Clin. Microbiol*. **37:** 3618–3626.
21. Chomel, B.B. *et al*. 2003. Clinical impact of persistent *Bartonella* bacteremia in humans and animals. *Ann. N. Y. Acad. Sci*. **990:** 267–278.
22. MacDonald, K.A. *et al*. 2004. A prospective study of canine infective endocarditis in northern California (1999–2001): emergence of *Bartonella* as a prevalent etiologic agent. *J. Vet. Intern. Med*. **18:** 56–64.

23. Sykes, J.E. *et al*. 2006. Evaluation of the relationship between causative organisms and clinical characteristics of infective endocarditis in dogs: 71 cases (1992–2005). *J. Am. Vet. Med. Assoc.* **228:** 1723–1734.

24. Cockwill, K.R. *et al*. 2007. *Bartonella vinsonii* subsp. *berkhoffii* endocarditis in a dog from Saskatchewan. *Can. Vet. J.* **48:** 839–844.

25. Chomel, B.B. *et al*. 2001. Aortic valve endocarditis in a dog due to *Bartonella clarridgeiae*. *J. Clin. Microbiol.* **39:** 3548–3554.

26. Chomel, B.B., A.C. Wey & R.W. Kasten. 2003. Isolation of *Bartonella washoensis* from a dog with mitral valve endocarditis. *J. Clin. Microbiol.* **41:** 5327–5332.

27. Henn, J.B. *et al*. 2009. Infective endocarditis in a dog and the phylogenetic relationship of the associated "Bartonella rochalimae" strain with isolates from dogs, gray foxes, and a human. *J. Clin. Microbiol.* **47:** 787–790.

28. Kelly, P. *et al*. 2006. *Bartonella quintana* endocarditis in dogs. *Emerg. Infect. Dis.* **12:** 1869–1872.

29. Maggi, R.G. *et al*. 2006. A *Bartonella vinsonii berkhoffii* typing scheme based upon 16S-23S ITS and Pap31 sequences from dog, coyote, gray fox, and human isolates. *Mol. Cell. Probes.* **20:** 128–134.

30. Cadenas, M.B. *et al*. 2008. Molecular characterization of *Bartonella vinsonii* subsp. *berkhoffii* genotype III. *J. Clin. Microbiol.* **46:** 1858–1860.

31. Goodman, R.A. & E.B. Breitschwerdt. 2005. Clinicopathologic findings in dogs seroreactive to *Bartonella henselae* antigens. *Am. J. Vet. Res.* **66:** 2060–2064.

32. Pesavento, P.A. *et al*. 2005. Pathology of *Bartonella* endocarditis in six dogs. *Vet. Pathol.* **42:** 370–373.

33. Malik, R. *et al*. 1999. Vegetative endocarditis in six cats. *J. Feline Med. Surg.* **1:** 171–180.

34. Chomel, B.B. *et al*. 2003. Fatal case of endocarditis associated with *Bartonella henselae* type I infection in a domestic cat. *J. Clin. Microbiol.* **41:** 5337–5339.

35. Chang, C.C. *et al*. 2002. Molecular epidemiology of *Bartonella henselae* infection in human immunodeficiency virus-infected patients and their cat contacts, using pulsed-field gel electrophoresis and genotyping. *J. Infect. Dis.* **186:** 1733–1739.

36. Chang, C.C. *et al*. 2000. *Bartonella* spp. isolated from wild and domestic ruminants in North America. *Emerg. Infect. Dis.* **6:** 306–311.

37. Maillard, R. *et al*. 2004. *Bartonella chomelii* sp. nov., isolated from French domestic cattle (*Bos taurus*). *Int. J. Syst. Evol. Microbiol.* **54:** 215–220.

38. Maillard, R. *et al*. 2007. Endocarditis in cattle caused by *Bartonella bovis*. *Emerg. Infect. Dis.* **13:** 1383–1385.

39. Maggi, R.G. *et al*. 2005. *Bartonella henselae* in porpoise blood. *Emerg. Infect. Dis.* **11:** 1894–1898.

40. Gill, V.A. 2006. *Marine Mammal Unusual Mortality Event Initiation Protocol in Northern Sea Otters.* Marine Mammals Management Office. Anchorage, Alaska, p. 11.

41. Carrasco, S.E. *et al*. 2008. Investigation of *Bartonella* spp. in northern sea otters (*Enhydra lutris kenyoni*) with vegetative valvular endocarditis in Alaska. *Poster #280, 5th International Meeting on Rickettsiae and Rickettsial Diseases*, Marseille, France, May 18–20, 2008.

Insights in *Bartonella* Host Specificity

Muriel Vayssier-Taussat, Danielle Le Rhun, Sarah Bonnet, and Violaine Cotté

UMR Bipar, Afssa 23 rue du Général de Gaulle 94 700 Maisons-Alfort. France

The genus *Bartonella* comprises a unique group of emerging gram-negative, intracellular bacteria that can cause a long-lasting intraerythrocytic bacteremia in their reservoir hosts. In recent years, the widespread occurrence and diversity of these bacteria has been increasingly recognized. This has resulted in a dramatic expansion of the genus *Bartonella* to 24 currently described species or subspecies, among which at least half have been associated with human disease. *Bartonella* infections have been observed in virtually all species examined, extending from humans to carnivores, ungulates, rodents, lagomorphs, insectivores, and bats. Adaptation by *Bartonellae* to such a diverse range of mammals has resulted in host specificity, and all validated *Bartonella* species described to date are capable of parasitizing only a limited number of animal species. In this review, the possible mechanisms explaining the specificity of each *Bartonella* species for its reservoir host are discussed.

Key words: *Bartonella*; arthropod host; mammalian host; specificity

The Natural History of *Bartonella* Infection

Bartonellae are small gram-negative bacilli belonging to the alpha-2 subdivision of *Proteobacteria*. *Bartonella bacilliformis* has been known as a human pathogen for a century (Barton, 1909) and was the only recognized species of the genus until the beginning of the 1990s. Since then, reclassification of species previously classified in other genera (*Rochalimae, Gahamella*)[1,2] and the description of novel species isolated from various vertebrate reservoirs have resulted in a major expansion of the genus to the current 24 species or subspecies among which 13 have been associated with human disease[3] (Table 1). *Bartonella* sp. are mainly transmitted through the bite of an arthropod; human body lice for *B. quintana* (the agent of trench fever), sand flies for *B. bacilliformis* (the agent of Oroya fever), fleas and ticks for *B. henselae* (the agent of cat scratch disease), and fleas for *B. taylorii*

and *B. grahamii* (mouse adapted species).[4][8] For other species, transmission via vectors is suspected, but not yet demonstrated.

A wide range of mammalian hosts serves as reservoirs for *Bartonella* species. However, humans are the only reservoir for *B. bacilliformis* and *B. quintana*. The hallmark of *Bartonella* infection in their reservoir hosts is the induction of a long-lasting intraerythrocytic bacteremia that does not cause immediate detriment to the host. When infecting incidental hosts, *Bartonella* sp. infection results in acute clinical manifestations, with no evidence of intraerythrocytic localization, as typically observed in reservoir hosts. The severity of the clinical manifestation correlates well with the status of the host's immune system.

All 22 validated *Bartonella* sp. described to date are only capable of infecting a limited number of mammalian species (Table 1). However some hosts are able to be infected by several *Bartonella* species, that is, cats can be infected by *B. henselae*, *B. clarridgeiae* and *B. khoelerae*, and rodents such as wood mice and bank voles can carry at least 4 different *Bartonella* species. The molecular basis for host specificity

Address for correspondence: Dr. Muriel Vayssier-Taussat, UMR Bipar, Afssa 23 rue du Général de Gaulle 94 700 Maisons-Alfort, France. mvayssier@vet-alfort.fr

Rickettsiology and Rickettsial Diseases-Fifth International Conference: Ann. N.Y. Acad. Sci. 1166: 127–132 (2009).
doi: 10.1111/j.1749-6632.2009.04531.x © 2009 New York Academy of Sciences.

is not known; however, different mechanisms are suspected: (i) the host range of the arthropod vector of any given *Bartonella* species can influence the host range of this species (ii) the resistance/sensitivity pattern of *Bartonella* species to innate immune defenses of potential mammalian hosts, and (iii) *Bartonella*-specific factors determining the host specificity.

The Different Mechanisms Suspected to Be Responsible for *Bartonella* sp. Mammalian Reservoir Specificity

Is Mammalian Host Specificity of *Bartonella* Due to Its Vector Specificity?

Arthropods play an essential role in the natural cycle of *Bartonella* sp. by serving as vectors and possibly as reservoirs. Their natural host range might be responsible for the host specificity of *Bartonella*. It has long been reported that each *Bartonella* sp. is transmitted to its mammalian host via the bite of a specific species of arthropod. *B. bacilliformis*, associated with Carrion disease in the inhabitants of Andean Cordillera of South America, is transmitted by one sand fly species, *Lutzomyia verrucarum*. *L. verrucarum* is highly anthropophylic and is found in a limited geographical area. No animal reservoir has yet been described for *B. bacilliformis*.[7] *B. quintana*, the agent of Trench fever, is also known to be transmitted to humans by a single vector species, the human-specific body louse *Pediculus humanus corporis*.[4] Recently, *B. quintana* infection was described in cats;[9–11] which implies that a vector other than the human body louse exists for *B. quintana*. This means that the specificity of *B. quintana* for its vector is not as strict as previously thought, changing our understanding of the epidemiology of this infection.

Similarly, the specificity of *B. henselae* does not seem to be restricted to the cat flea, *Ctenocephalides felis*.[5,6] Epidemiological evidence has implicated ticks belonging to *Ixodes* genus, which bite a very wide variety of hosts, as a putative vector for *B. henselae*.[7,12–14] *B. henselae* DNA was recently detected in a tick removed from a dog,[15] and two cases of "cat" scratch disease arising from domestic dogs have been reported.[16,17] Finally, we have recently shown that European *Ixodes ricinus* ticks can transmit *B. henselae* via salivary glands under experimental conditions, demonstrating for the first time that arthropods other than fleas could be competent for transmission of *B. henselae*.[18] Considering transmission by ticks is complex, requiring (i) conservation of intact bacteria through molting (transstadial transmission), (ii) bacterial migration in the salivary glands, and (iii) transmission of infective bacteria during the feeding steps; demonstration of *I. ricinus* competence for *B. henselae* leads us to speculate whether *B. henselae* transmission by ticks is not more widespread than thought.

Although specificity of any one *Bartonella* species for any one arthropod species may exist in nature, other vectors of *Bartonella*, not yet experimentally proven due to a lack of suitable experimental models, must be considered.

In conclusion, the specificity of *Bartonella* for its mammalian host could be partly explained by the capacity of the bacteria to be transmitted by an arthropod, which has its own specific host range. However, under laboratory conditions without the use of vectors, the mammalian host specificity observed in nature seems to be reproduced, at least for the few models studied (*B. henselae* in mice, mainly).[19] Other mechanisms involved in *Bartonella* host specificity separate from the vector-vertebrate host specificity might thus exist.

Is Mammalian Host Specificity of *Bartonella* Due to Resistance to Complement?

To explain the host specificity of *Bartonella* species, we can speculate that an innate protective response of the host exists that is specific to the *Bartonella* species. Complement activation is one of the innate immune defenses of the host, resulting in pathogen killing. Pathogenic

TABLE 1. List of the *Bartonella* Species (Subspecies and *Candidatus*), Their Natural Hosts (Reservoirs), Vectors, and Diseases in Human

Species	Natural Hosts	Vectors *: suspected	Disease in human
B. alsatica	Rabbit	Unknown	Endocarditis
B. australis	Kangaroo	Unknown	Not described
B. bacilliformis	Human	Phlebotome, *Lutzomyia verrucarum*	Oroya fever
B. birtlesii	Mice (*Apodemus*)	Flea*	Not described
B. bovis	Ruminants	Unknown	Not described
B. capreoli	Ruminants	Unknown	Not described
B. chomelii	Ruminants	Unknown	Not described
B. clarridgeiae	Cats	Fleas (*Ctenocephalides felis*)	Cat scratch disease
B. doshiae	Mice (microtus)	Unknown	Not described
B. elizabethae	Rat	Flea* (*Xenopsylla cheopis*)	Endocarditis
B grahamii	Bank vole	Flea (*Ctenophthalmus nobilis*)	Ocular manifestations
B. henselae	Cat	Fleas (*Ctenocephalides felis*)	Cat scratch disease and complications
		Ticks (*Ixodes ricinus*)	
B. koehlerae	Cat	Unknown	Cat scratch disease Endocartitis
B. phoceensiis	Rat	Unknown	Not described
B. peromysci	Small mammals	Unknown	Not described
B. quintana	Human	Body lice	Trench fever, endocarditis
B. rattimasiliensis	Rat	Unknown	Not described
B. schoenbuchensis	Ruminant	Fly* (*Lipoptena cervi*)	Not described
B. talpae	Shrew mole	unknown	Note described
B. taylorii	Mice (*Apodemus*)	Flea (*Ctenophthalmus nobilis*)	Not described
B. tribocorum	Rat	Unknown	Not described
B. vinsonii subsp arupensis	Mice	Unknown	Fever+bacteremia Endocarditis
B. vinsonii subsp berkhoffii	Dog	Ticks*	Endocarditis
B. vinsonii subsp vinsonii	Mice	Flea (*Trombicula microti*)	Fever + bacteremai
Candidatus species			
B. melophagii	Sheep	*Melophagus ovinus**	Not described
B. rochalimae	Unknown	Unknown	Fever

bacteria have developed protective mechanisms against serum complement-mediated lysis. Therefore, resistance to host complement appears to be a strategy for pathogens to persist in their hosts, as described for *Yersinia enterolitica*[20] and *Porphyromonas gengivalis*.[21] Resistance to host complement also appears to play a key role in the specific association of bacteria to hosts.[22] This is the case for strains of *Borrelia burgdorferi* sensu lato (*B. burgdorferi* s.l.) that differ in their resistance or sensitivity patterns to complement from different vertebrate species. Indeed, a clear pattern of resistance or sensitivity to complement within *B. burgdorferi* s.l. has emerged that is consistent with pattern of transmissibility.[23–26] The molecular mechanism of this protection has been dissected, and bacterial membrane proteins have been shown to bind to complement control proteins preventing the formation of the membrane-attack complex. The deflection of the complement system is now considered to be 1 of the key determinant of the niche of *B. burgdorferi* s.l. Little is known about *Bartonella* sp. resistance or sensitivity to complement. It will be of great interest to investigate the putative role of complement in the susceptibility of the mammalian host to *Bartonella* sp. infection and the consequences on the global epidemiology of bartonellosis.

Does *Bartonella* sp. Derive Its Host Specificity through Expression of Specific Factors?

For many bacterial species, comparative whole-genomic analyses have revealed differences in the contents of genes and genomic islands in closely related strains or species with different host ranges and/or virulence characteristics.[27–32] In order to define putative genes or genomic islands involved in host specificity, Lindroos and colleagues[33] compared, using whole-genomic microarrays, the genetic composition of *Bartonella* species that share the same host-vector (cat-flea) combination: *B. koehlerae* and *B. henselae*, with the human pathogen *B. quintana* transmitted by human body lice. No obvious relationship was found between the gene content and the host adaptation pattern, and only 1 gene, *parA1* encoding a plasmid partitioning protein, is absent in *B. quintana* and shared by *B. henselae* and *B. koehlerae*. Upstream of the *parA1* gene, 2 noncoding regions are present solely in the feline-associated species.[34] The role of these coding and noncoding regions in the specific association of these species to felines remains to be investigated.

An alternative is that the host specificity could be conferred with genes belonging to all species, with sequence variations. Putative candidates are surface proteins that could mediate host cell interactions. Several surface proteins encoded by multicopy genes with intragenic repeats are present in *Bartonella* genus. These could easily be modified to fit any given host cell receptor. This is the case for BadA, the highly repetitive nonfimbrial adhesin, in *B. henselae*[35,36] and Vomp in *B. quintana*.[37] Variation of Vomp expression is achieved by deletion across the repeated sequences.[37] The essential role of BadA in interactions with endothelial cell cultures was demonstrated using mutants where BadA was disrupted,[35] and both proteins are required for bloodstream infection.[38,34,39] This adhesin family could have evolved to provide diversity that can direct host tropism and specificity.

Another potential suspect for host specificity that also harbors sequence changes is the Trw system of *Bartonella*. This type IV secretion system (T4SS) is unique in that several genes in the cluster are duplicated: *trwL* is present in a variable number of copies according to species, and a segment belonging *trwJ, H, I* is present in variable copy numbers in the different species. By homology with other T4SS, TrwJ of *Bartonella* is thought to mediate host cell attachment, whereas TrwH and TrwI are thought to be associated with anchoring the pilus to the membrane.[40,41] Interestingly, in *B. tribocorum*, the *trwE* gene has been shown to be required for establishing bacteremia and for erythrocyte invasion. Currently, it appears that all structural variants are exposed simultaneously on the cell surface of the bacteria, suggesting an increased binding potential to the erythrocytes. Mammalian erythrocytes are known to have highly variable glycoprotein surface proteins within and between individual host species. Due to the extreme variation of the *trwJ* gene copies within and between isolates,[34] the Trw pilus is a prime suspect as a factor required for a *Bartonella* species to recognize and to infect erythrocytes according to their animal origin.

Conclusion

Host specificity of *Bartonella* species is likely due to a combination of different mechanisms resulting from the interrelationships between the 3 partners: the vector, the bacterium, and the host. Due to *in vivo* and *in vitro* infection models, effective molecular tools, and the availability of complete genome sequence data for increasing numbers of *Bartonella* sp., we can certainly predict a huge increase in our understanding of the mechanisms of *Bartonella* specificity for its reservoir hosts. This will be facilitated by the expansion of a community of enthusiastic scientists exploring new insights in *Bartonella* biology.

Conflicts of Interest

The authors declare no conflicts of interest.

References

1. Birtles, R.J. *et al.* 1995. Proposals to unify the genera *Grahamella* and *Bartonella*, with descriptions of *Bartonella talpae* comb. nov., *Bartonella peromysci* comb. nov., and three new species, *Bartonella grahamii* sp. nov., *Bartonella taylorii* sp. nov., and *Bartonella doshiae* sp. nov. *Int. J. Syst. Bacteriol.* **45:** 1–8.

2. Brenner, D.J. *et al.* 1993. Proposals to unify the genera *Bartonella* and *Rochalimaea*, with descriptions of *Bartonella quintana* comb. nov., *Bartonella* vinsonii comb. nov., *Bartonella henselae* comb. nov., and *Bartonella elizabethae* comb. nov., and to remove the family Bartonellaceae from the order Rickettsiales. *Int. J. Syst. Bacteriol.* **43:** 777–786.

3. Boulouis, H.J. *et al.* 2007. Persistent *Bartonella* infection: epidemiological and clinical implications. *Bull. Acad. Natl. Med.* **191:** 1037–1044; discussion 1047–9.

4. Fournier, P.E. *et al.* 2001. Experimental model of human body louse infection using green fluorescent protein-expressing *Bartonella quintana*. *Infect Immun.* **69:** 1876–1879.

5. Finkelstein, J.L. *et al.* 2002. Studies on the growth of *Bartonella henselae* in the cat flea (Siphonaptera: Pulicidae). *J. Med. Entomol.* **39:** 915–919.

6. Foil, L. *et al.* 1998. Experimental infection of domestic cats with Bartonella henselae by inoculation of Ctenocephalides felis (Siphonaptera: Pulicidae) feces. *J. Med. Entomol.* **35:** 625–628.

7. Ihler, G.M. 1996. *Bartonella bacilliformis*: dangerous pathogen slowly emerging from deep background. *FEMS Microbiol. Lett.* **144:** 1–11.

8. Bown, K.J., M. Bennet & M. Begon. 2004. Flea-borne *Bartonella grahamii* and *Bartonella taylorii* in bank voles. *Emerg. Infect Dis.* **10:** 684–687.

9. La, V.D. *et al.* 2005. *Bartonella quintana* in domestic cat. *Emerg. Infect Dis.* **11:** 1287–1289.

10. Chomel, B.B. *et al.* 2006. *Bartonella* infection in domestic cats and wild felids. *Ann. N. Y. Acad. Sci.* **1078:** 410–415.

11. Breitschwerdt, E.B. *et al.* 2007. Isolation of *Bartonella quintana* from a woman and a cat following putative bite transmission. *J. Clin. Microbiol.* **45:** 270–272.

12. Eskow, E., R.V. Rao & E. Mordechai. 2001. Concurrent infection of the central nervous system by *Borrelia burgdorferi* and *Bartonella henselae*: evidence for a novel tick-borne disease complex. *Arch. Neurol.* **58:** 1357–1363.

13. Holden, K. *et al.* 2006. Co-detection of *Bartonella henselae*, *Borrelia burgdorferi*, and *Anaplasma phagocy-tophilum* in *Ixodes pacificus* ticks from California, USA. *Vector Borne Zoonotic Dis.* **6:** 99–102.

14. Lucey, D. *et al.* 1992. Relapsing illness due to *Rochalimaea henselae* in immunocompetent hosts: implication for therapy and new epidemiological associations. *Clin. Infect Dis.* **14:** 683–688.

15. Podsiadly, E. *et al.* 2007. *Bartonella henselae* in *Ixodes ricinus* ticks removed from dogs. *Vector Borne Zoonotic Dis.* **7:** 189–192.

16. Chen, T.C. *et al.* 2007. Cat scratch disease from a domestic dog. *J. Formos Med. Assoc.* **106:** S65–S68.

17. Yamanouchi, H. *et al.* 2004. A case of *Bartonella henselae* infection from a dog. *Kansenshogaku Zasshi* **78:** 270–273.

18. Cotté, V., S. Bonnet, D. Le Rhun, *et al.* 2008. Transmission of *Bartonella henselae* by *Ixodes ricinus*. *Emerg. Infect Dis.* **14**.

19. Velho, P.S. *et al.* 1998. Baccilary Angiomatosis: Negative results using normal Balb/c and Balb/c nude mice. *Braz J. Infect Dis.* **2:** 300–303.

20. Roggenkamp, A. *et al.* 2003. Molecular analysis of transport and oligomerization of the *Yersinia enterocolitica* adhesin YadA. *J. Bacteriol.* **185:** 3735–3744.

21. Slaney, J.M. & M.A. Curtis. 2008. Mechanisms of evasion of complement by *Porphyromonas gingivalis*. *Front Biosci.* **13:** 188–196.

22. Kurtenbach, K. *et al.* 2002. Host association of *Borrelia burgdorferi* sensu lato–the key role of host complement. *Trends Microbiol.* **10:** 74–79.

23. Kurtenbach, K. *et al.* 1998. Serum complement sensitivity as a key factor in Lyme disease ecology. *Infect Immun.* **66:** 1248–1251.

24. Lane, R.S. & G.B. Quistad. 1998. Borreliacidal factor in the blood of the western fence lizard (*Sceloporus occidentalis*). *J. Parasitol.* **84:** 29–34.

25. Kuo, M.M., R.S. Lane & P.C. Giclas. 2000. A comparative study of mammalian and reptilian alternative pathway of complement-mediated killing of the Lyme disease spirochete (*Borrelia burgdorferi*). *J. Parasitol.* **86:** 1223–1228.

26. Nelson, D.R. *et al.* 2000. Complement-mediated killing of *Borrelia burgdorferi* by nonimmune sera from sika deer. *J. Parasitol.* **86:** 1232–1238.

27. Dziejman, M. *et al.* 2002. Comparative genomic analysis of *Vibrio cholerae*: genes that correlate with cholera endemic and pandemic disease. *Proc. Natl. Acad. Sci. USA* **99:** 1556–1561.

28. Hinchliffe, S.J. *et al.* 2003. Application of DNA microarrays to study the evolutionary genomics of *Yersinia pestis* and *Yersinia pseudotuberculosis*. *Genome Res.* **13:** 2018–2029.

29. Porwollik, S., R.M. Wong & M. McClelland. 2002. Evolutionary genomics of *Salmonella*: gene acquisitions revealed by microarray analysis. *Proc. Natl. Acad. Sci. USA* **99:** 8956–8961.

30. Salama, N. *et al.* 2000. A whole-genome microarray reveals genetic diversity among *Helicobacter pylori* strains. *Proc. Natl. Acad. Sci. USA* **97:** 14668–14673.

31. Wolfgang, M.C. *et al.* 2003. Conservation of genome content and virulence determinants among clinical and environmental isolates of *Pseudomonas aeruginosa*. *Proc. Natl. Acad. Sci. USA* **100:** 8484–8489.

32. Zhang, C. *et al.* 2003. Genome diversification in phylogenetic lineages I and II of *Listeria monocytogenes*: identification of segments unique to lineage II populations. *J. Bacteriol.* **185:** 5573–5584.

33. Lindroos, H.L. *et al.* 2005. Characterization of the genome composition of *Bartonella koehlerae* by microarray comparative genomic hybridization profiling. *J. Bacteriol.* **187:** 6155–6165.

34. Nystedt, B. *et al.* 2008. Diversifying selection and concerted evolution of a type IV secretion system in *Bartonella*. *Mol. Biol. Evol.* **25:** 287–300.

35. Riess, T. *et al.* 2004. *Bartonella* adhesin mediates a proangiogenic host cell response. *J. Exp. Med.* **200:** 1267–1278.

36. Riess, T. *et al.* 2007. Analysis of *Bartonella* adhesin A expression reveals differences between various *B. henselae* strains. *Infect Immun.* **75:** 35–43.

37. Zhang, P. *et al.* 2004. A family of variably expressed outer-membrane proteins (Vomp) mediates adhesion and autoaggregation in *Bartonella quintana*. *Proc. Natl. Acad. Sci. USA* **101:** 13630–13635.

38. MacKichan, J.K. *et al.* 2008. A SacB mutagenesis strategy reveals that the *Bartonella quintana* variably expressed outer membrane proteins are required for bloodstream infection of the host. *Infect Immun.* **76:** 788–795.

39. Saenz, H.L. *et al.* 2007. Genomic analysis of *Bartonella* identifies type IV secretion systems as host adaptability factors. *Nat. Genet.* **39:** 1469–1476.

40. Krall, L. *et al.* 2002. Detergent extraction identifies different VirB protein subassemblies of the type IV secretion machinery in the membranes of *Agrobacterium tumefaciens*. *Proc. Natl. Acad. Sci. USA* **99:** 11405–11410.

41. Cascales, E. & P.J. Christie. 2004. Definition of a bacterial type IV secretion pathway for a DNA substrate. *Science* **304:** 1170–1173.

The Science and Fiction of Emerging Rickettsioses

Christopher D. Paddock

Infectious Disease Pathology Branch, Division of Viral and Rickettsial Diseases, Centers for Disease Control and Prevention, Atlanta, Georgia 30333, USA

As newly recognized rickettsial diseases and rickettsial pathogens increase in scope and magnitude, several elements related to the concept of emerging rickettsioses deserve consideration. Newly identified rickettsiae may be mildly pathogenic, or perhaps even nonpathogenic, and have little direct impact on human or animal health, yet nonetheless wield considerable influence on the epidemiology and ecology of historically recognized diseases. In this context "new" rickettsioses provide a lens through which "old" rickettsioses are more accurately represented. Predicting pathogen from nonpathogen is not an exact science, particularly as so few rickettsiae have been broadly accepted as nonpathogenic by contemporary rickettsiologists. However, various factors relating to specific physiologic requirements and molecular machinery of the particular rickettsia, as well as characteristics of its invertebrate host that either position or exclude the rickettsia from infecting a human host, must be considered. Close inspection of mild or atypical forms of historically recognized rickettsioses and a greater emphasis on culture- and molecular-based diagnostic techniques are the keys to identifying future rickettsial agents of disease.

Key words: rickettsiosis; *Rickettsia*; emerging infections

The term "emerging infection" has been interpreted broadly and somewhat subjectively since its inception in the 1990s. Rickettsiology encompasses many inarguable examples of newly recognized pathogens that were unknown to science or medicine as recently as 25 years ago, exemplified by *Ehrlichia chaffeensis*, *Rickettsia felis*, *Rickettsia aeschlimannii*, *Rickettsia massiliae*, and *Rickettsia monacencis*.[1-6] This discipline also includes other agents like *Rickettsia slovaca* and *Rickettsia parkeri*, recognized for several decades, yet only recently associated with disease in humans.[7,8] Finally, rickettsiologists continue to uncover novel aspects of "old" rickettsioses that influence the incidence, distribution, and ecology of historically recognized diseases. Recent examples of these discoveries include an epidemic of Rocky Mountain spotted fever (RMSF)—in a high desert community of eastern Arizona caused by a newly recognized North American vector of *Rickettsia rickettsii*—[9,10] and the isolation of *Rickettsia prowazekii* from an *Amblyomma* sp. tick in Mexico.[11]

Considering these examples, the criteria for an emerging rickettsiosis are relatively fluid, constrained only by the parameters defined by the particular investigator. The following discussion will focus on a few general topics relating to the expanding spectrum of newly recognized rickettsioses, including the direct and indirect importance of these infections, an appraisal of various factors that determine emergence of these bacteria as pathogens in human hosts, and strategies for future discovery of novel rickettsioses.

Address for correspondence: Christopher D. Paddock, M.D., Infectious Diseases Pathology Branch, Mailstop G-32, Centers for Disease Control and Prevention, 1600 Clifton Road Atlanta, GA 30333. Voice: +404-639-1309; fax: +404-639-3043. CPaddock@cdc.gov

Rickettsiology and Rickettsial Diseases-Fifth International Conference: Ann. N.Y. Acad. Sci. 1166: 133–143 (2009).
doi: 10.1111/j.1749-6632.2009.04529.x © 2009 New York Academy of Sciences.

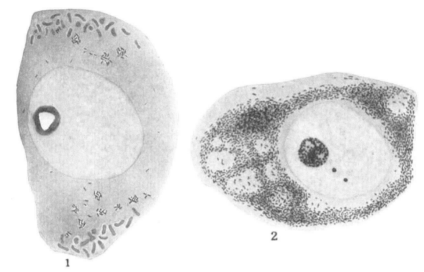

Figure 1. *Rickettsia*-like bacteria in the cytoplasm of oocytes of *Amblyomma americanum*, stained with Giemsa stain (1) and iron hematoxylin (2), described by E.V. Cowdry in 1923.[13]

The Importance of Emerging Rickettsioses

The discovery of a new rickettsial pathogen may generate considerable scientific excitement but have little direct impact on human health. Nonetheless, these agents have considerable indirect importance by: providing a lens through which "old" rickettsioses are more accurately represented; competing with more virulent rickettsiae for limited niches within arthropods, and; potentially immunizing vertebrate hosts involved in the circulation of highly pathogenic rickettsiae in nature.

Some, and perhaps many, of the novel rickettsial species identified by contemporary investigators were seen or documented by scientists many decades before the particular bacterium was formally described or characterized. Willy Burgdorfer and colleagues are credited with the discovery of *Rickettsia amblyommii*, a spotted fever group (SFG) rickettsia broadly and commonly distributed among lone star ticks (*Amblyomma americanum*) in the United States, and in other *Amblyomma* spp. in the Western Hemisphere;[12] however, this microbe may have been first recognized in the early 1920s by E.V. Cowdry during a bacteriological survey of multiple arthropod species (Fig. 1).[13] In a similar fashion, it is likely that rickettsiologists in the 1920s discovered *Rickettsia montanensis*, *Rickettsia bellii*, or *Rickettsia peacockii* in Rocky Mountain wood ticks (*Dermacentor andersoni*) long before formal recognition of these species[14–17]

Most emerging rickettsioses circulate in human populations long before these are discovered as unique infections, and these are often misidentified as a clinically similar and historically recognizable disease. Because the most virulent pathogens are typically the first to be identified and characterized, subsequently discovered agents can be erroneously associated with the initially described disease until an astute investigator recognizes subtle differences or performs confirmatory tests that provide an agent-specific diagnosis. In this context, cases of murine typhus were frequently misidentified as louse-borne typhus until the recognition of *Rickettsia typhi*,[18] just as some cases of *R. felis* infection are now misidentified as infections caused by *R. typhi*.[3,19] In a similar manner, infections caused by *Rickettsia africae*, *R. massiliae*, *R. aeschlimannii*, and *R. monacensis* were for many decades classified incorrectly as Mediterranean spotted fever (MSF) by clinicians, rickettsiologists, and epidemiologists.[20]

TABLE 1. Frequency of *Rickettsia rickettsii* Infection in Selected Tick Species, Determined by Culture, Mouse Serotyping, or PCR

Tick species	Location, year	Detection technique	No. evaluated (% infected)	Reference
Dermacentor andersoni	Western Montana, 1977	Culture and serotyping	3705 (0.3)	21
	Western Montana, 1992	PCR	226 (0.6)	22
Dermacentor variabilis	Maryland, 1951–53	Culture	17,649 (0.25)	23
	Maryland, 2002	PCR	392 (0)	24
	Ohio, 1981	Culture and serotyping	155 (1.9)	25
	North Carolina, not specified	Culture and serotyping	2123 (0.05)	26
Dermacentor occidentalis	Northern California, 1980	Culture and serotyping	327 (0)	27
	Southern California, 2006–07	PCR	366 (0.3)	28
Amblyomma cajennense	São Paulo, Brazil, 2000–01	PCR	1468 (0)	29
Amblyomma aureolatum	São Paulo, Brazil, 2000–02	PCR	669 (0.6)	30

TABLE 2. Frequency of Infection with Selected Spotted Fever Rickettsiae in Certain Human-Biting Ticks in the Western Hemisphere

Agent	Tick species	Location, Year(s)	Detection technique	No. evaluated (% infected)	References
Rickettsia parkeri	*Amblyomma maculatum*	Bulloch County, Georgia (1999–2005)	PCR	60 (16.7)	34
		Franklin County, Florida (2004–07)	PCR	95 (10.5)	34; CDC, unpublished
	Amlyomma triste	Delta Paranense, Argentina (2007)	PCR	223 (7.6)	35
Rickettsia amblyommii	*Amblyomma americanum*	New York (1998–2003)	PCR	475 (41.7)	36
		Georgia (2002–05)	PCR	704 (37.1)	
		North Carolina (2002–03)	PCR	391 (56.1)	
Strain 364D	*Dermacentor occidentalis*	Northern California (1980)	Culture and serotyping	327 (2.8)	27
		Southern California (2006–07)	PCR	365 (7.7)	28

It is conceivable that the most severe SFG rickettsioses are rarely encountered when compared with the occurrence of milder rickettsial infections. The relative frequencies of SFG rickettsiae in nature support this concept. Contemporary surveys detect *R. rickettsii* in less than 1% of human biting ticks evaluated for this infection (Table 1)[21–30] while levels of tick infection >1% are considered exceptional.[31–33] In contrast, other SFG rickettsiae in the Western Hemisphere of proven or suspected pathogenicity, including *R. parkeri*, *R. amblyommii*, and strain 364D, are found in human-biting ticks at levels 10 to 100 greater than those observed for *R. rickettsii* (Table 2).[27,28,34–36]

With these ecologic data in mind, how does one reconcile the rapidly increasing numbers of RMSF cases in the USA reported during the past decade? The answer may be that many and possibly most of these cases represent infections with other agents. During 2002–2007, >1000 cases of RMSF were reported annually to the Centers for Disease Control and Prevention, including 2221 in 2007,[37] the largest yearly total since national surveillance for RMSF began in 1920. Only about 5% of confirmed cases of RMSF are actually identified by assays that accurately differentiate the various SFG rickettsiae indigenous to the USA.[38] The full impact of this level of nonspecific testing on the epidemiologic accuracy of RMSF is unknown;

however, antibodies to SFG rickettsiae are detected in the general US population at relatively high frequencies—approximately 5% to 10% in some studies—[39,40] suggesting that confirmatory methods more rigorous than existing serologic techniques should be considered when diagnosing patients with a presumed spotted fever rickettsiosis.

Because a serum sample that shows significant reactivity with *R. rickettsii* antigens is also likely to react significantly with *R. parkeri, R. amblyommii*, or other SFG antigens,[38] cases of infection caused by agents other than *R. rickettsii* could be attributed to *R. rickettsii* simply because most serologic tests provided commercially or by state health departments use only *R. rickettsii* as the reacting antigen. Indeed, when investigators have assessed serologic responses of patients with presumed RMSF to *R. amblyommii* antigen, higher titers and more seroconversions are identified than with *R. rickettsii* antigen.[41] When molecular- or culture-based diagnostic methods are used, as seen recently in a series of patients with *R. parkeri* rickettsiosis,[38] the number of true RMSF cases could be diminished even further.

The impact of incorrect diagnoses extends beyond simple case counts. During 1997–2002 the reported US RMSF case fatality rate was 1.4%;[42] however, it is likely that this estimate is far from valid, considering the historically identifiable severity of RMSF, and the unfortunate reality that most US physicians have considerable difficulty making a correct diagnosis of this life-threatening infection during the early stage of the illness. Using a hypothetical situation, consider that the estimated case-fatality rate of RMSF for a given year is 2%, based on 20 reported annual deaths and 1000 reported cases of RMSF, recognizing that approximately 95% or more of these cases will be confirmed by SFG-specific serologic assays. The assumption that each fatality is attributable to *R. rickettsii* is reasonable, considering that this is the only SFG rickettsia ever to be detected from a patient with fatal spotted fever acquired in the Western Hemisphere.[43] However, if the true composition of the 1000 "RMSF" reports comprising the denominator were 200 cases of *R. parkeri* rickettsiosis, 100 cases of 364D infection, and 500 cases of *R. amblyommii* infection, then the actual number of RMSF cases drops to 200, and the case-fatality rate during this hypothetical year increases to 10%, a statistic far more consistent with the recognized lethality of this disease. In this context, the effect of inaccurate case counts, created by nonspecific confirmatory assays, can compromise the validity of many of the assumed epidemiologic and clinical features of RMSF, including its incidence, distribution, and frequencies of death, hospitalization, or atypical disease manifestations.

Similar situations are likely to exist with historically recognized rickettsioses in other parts of the world. In a recent study from Portugal, the Malish strain of *R. conorii* was isolated in culture or detected by PCR from 71 patents diagnosed with MSF during 1994–2006.[44] The case-fatality rate among these Portuguese patients was 13%, more than 5 times higher than the conventionally recognized lethality of MSF.[20] Because *R. conorii* Malish is the strain most commonly detected in MSF patients from the Mediterranean basin,[20] the case-fatality rate determined from the Portuguese study is perhaps a more accurate and broadly applicable statistic than previously recognized. Two recent surveys of SPG rickettsiae in Spanish ticks suggest that the numbers of MSF cases reported in that country may be inaccurate. During a 7-year study in northwestern Spain, SPG rickettsiae were detected in ∼8% of 4049 ticks removed from 3685 persons. Sequencing revealed *R. slovaca, R. massiliae*, and *R. aeschlimannii* in most, but *R. conorii* in only 1 tick, despite 353 serologically-confirmed cases of MSF reported in this region during this same period.[45] In the second study, 2229 adult *Rhipicephalus sanguineus* were ticks collected off dogs in an area of western Andalusia, Spain, which was considered endemic for MSF; 18% of tick pools positive for SPG rickettsiae by PCR, and these were exclusively *R. massiliae*.[46]

TABLE 3. Characteristics of Selected North American Rickettsiae of Suspected or Undetermined Pathogenicity in Humans

Rickettsia species or strain	Tick(s) infected with rickettsia in nature	Frequency with which tick(s) will bite humans	Demonstrated pathogenicity of rickettsia in animals (route of infection)	Reference
Rickettsia bellii	Multiple genera, including *Dermacentor* and *Amblyomma*	Frequent	Eschars in rabbits and guinea pigs (ID)	57
Rickettsia canadensis	Multiple genera, including *Haemaphysalis* and *Dermacentor*	Infrequent to Frequent	Fever in guinea pigs (IP)	58
Strain 364D	*Dermacentor occidentalis*	Frequent	Scrotal erythema in guinea pigs (IP)	59
Strain Parumapertus	*Dermacentor parumapertus*	Infrequent	Fever and scotal erythema in guinea pigs (IP)	60
Strain Tillamook	*Ixodes pacificus*	Frequent	Death in mice (IP)	61
Rickettsia rhipicephali	Multiple genera, including *Dermacentor* and *Rhipicephalus*	Frequent	Fever, scrotal swelling, and death in meadow voles (IP)	54

ID = intradermal; IP = intraperitoneal

Nonpathogenic or mildly pathogenic rickettsiae may exert considerable influence on the natural history of more virulent rickettsiae by competition within the tick host for limited microhabitats in a process termed rickettsial interference[47,48] These interactions can profoundly affect the ecology, distribution, and incidence of rickettsioses, as exemplified by the relationship between *R. peacockii* and *R. rickettsii* in Rocky Mountain wood ticks, and the effect of this interaction on the distribution of RMSF in the Bitterroot Valley.[17,47] Correlates of rickettsial interference undoubtedly exist in other tick species. Early investigators determined that the lone star tick is a competent vector of *R. rickettsii* in the laboratory,[49,50] yet no contemporary studies have verified an infection with *R. rickettsii* in this broadly distributed and aggressive human-biting tick.[51,52] In contrast, *R. amblyommii* is identified on average in >40% of lone star ticks across its range, with infection prevalence in some areas of the USA that exceed 80%.[36] From these data, it is reasonable to assume that the frequent occurrence of *R. amblyommii* in *A. americanum* has effectively excluded *R. rickettsii* from commonly establishing residence in this tick, and it has muted considerably the role of *A. americanum* as a vector of RMSF.

Animals that are repeatedly exposed to rickettsiae of lesser virulence but greater ubiquity in nature theoretically could develop partial or complete protection against subsequent infection with uncommon but highly pathogenic rickettsiae. Guinea pigs and meadow voles experimentally infected with *R. montanensis*, *R. rhipicephali*, or *R. parkeri* develop immune responses that protect these animals against severe illness or death when later challenged with *R. rickettsii*;[53–56] however, the biological consequences of natural immunization of vertebrate hosts in the transmission cycles of virulent rickettsioses remain unknown.

Predicting Pathogen from Nonpathogen

Many historically recognized rickettsiae have not been definitively associated with infections in human hosts despite data that show pathogenic effects in animals infected experimentally with these bacteria (Table 3).[54,57–61] What are some of the factors that determine emergence of these bacteria as pathogens in human populations? Fundamentally, there must be reasonable opportunity for a human host to become infected with the microbe. *Neorickettsia risticii*, the etiologic agent of Potomac horse fever, cycles in nature within several trematode species that parasitize bats. The natural history of this agent, recently elucidated in a series of elegant ecological studies,[62,63] also involves freshwater snails and aquatic insects that serve as intermediate hosts for the immature flukes that are infected with *N. risticii*. In this context, the likelihood of human infection with *N. risticii* is extremely remote, unless a human host ingests a *N. risticii* –infected snail, caddisfly, mayfly, or bat liver. In a similar manner, even virulent rickettsiae that reside in hematophagous arthropods are unlikely to cause an emerging rickettsiosis if the arthropod does not take a blood meal from a human host. Newly identified rickettsiae and rickettsia-like bacteria continue to be discovered in a diverse and extremely broad range of invertebrate species, including, beetles, wasps, leeches, and amoebae.[64] It remains to be determined if some or any of these newly recognized bacteria cause diseases in vertebrate species under natural circumstances; however, without direct access to a vertebrate host, a discussion of pathogenicity becomes moot.

Physiologic requirements of particular rickettsiae may also influence the pathogenicity of these microbes in human or animal hosts. Some of the most virulent rickettsial agents, including *R. rickettsii*, *R. conorii*, and *Orientia tsutsugamushi* will grow at a wide range of temperatures, including the core human body temperature of $37°C$.[65–67] In contrast, some rickettsiae of undetermined pathogenicity, or presumed nonpathogenicty, including *R. bellii*, *Rickettsia helvetica*, and *R. peacockii*, grow poorly or not at all in mammalian cells cultured at $37°C$.[68–70] Restricted bacterial growth, imposed by normal core body temperatures, could potentially limit the ability of some temperature-sensitive rickettsiae to cause disease in a human host. Nonetheless, *R. felis* is one example of a rickettsia that grows in cultured cells optimally at temperatures $<32°C$ and does not proliferate at $37°C$, but causes disease and bacteremia in humans.[3,71–73] In this context, temperature endpoints for rickettsial growth, as predictors of pathogenicity, must be interpreted cautiously.

The ability of some rickettsiae to cause fever, scrotal swelling and erythema, or death in rodents experimentally infected with these agents has long been regarded as predictor of pathogenicity in human hosts. Indeed, the clinical response of guinea pigs following inoculation with *R. parkeri* led R.R. Parker to suggest that *R. parkeri* might be a cause of spotted fever-like disease in humans, more than 60 years before the first infection in a human patient was recognized.[53] In the USA, there are several distinct species and various as yet unnamed SFG rickettsiae that elicit disease in experimentally infected animals and represent candidate emerging pathogens (Table 3).[54,57–61] Two tick-borne rickettsiae in the western USA, believed initially to represent strains of *R. rickettsii*, deserve particular attention.

Strain 364D was first isolated from Pacific Coast ticks (*Dermacentor occidentalis*) collected in southern California in 1966 and subsequent surveys detected this rickettsia in approximately 3% to 8% of *D. occidentalis* collected from coastal and inland valley regions of California.[27,28,59] Recent molecular characterization of strain 364D reveals genetic differences that distinguish it from *R. rickettsii* and suggest that it is a unique rickettsial species.[74] Guinea pigs develop a mild-to-moderate, spotted fever-like disease when inoculated with strain 364D,[59] and its tick host *D. occidentalis* is a broadly distributed human-biting tick in California.[75] In 1981 investigators postulated that 364D may be a cause of a spotted fever-like disease in California, based on identification of 364D-infected *D. occidentalis* from a focus of spotted fever infections in Lake County in northern California and subsequent antibody cross-adsorption data using the patient serum that implicated 364D as the infecting agent.[30] In 2001, a patient from this same area was diagnosed with an eschar-associated spotted fever rickettsiosis, lending additional support to the hypothesis that 364D may be another cause of spotted fever in the western USA.[76] Strain Tillamook, isolated from *Ixodes pacificus* ticks collected from western Oregon and northern California, causes mild fever and scrotal swelling in guinea pigs, and it can be lethal to mice.[30,59,61] Because *I. pacificus* frequently bites humans, the role of strain Tillamook as a candidate emerging pathogen in the western USA deserves further study.[76]

Using similar criteria, are there rickettsiae that can be considered nonpathogenic? *R. peacockii*, a SFG rickettsia found in *D. andersoni* ticks from Montana and Colorado, shows a very close phylogenetic relationship to *R. rickettsii*, but it lacks many of the characteristics commonly associated with tick-borne rickettsial pathogens. Its distribution in its arthropod host is limited to the ovaries, posterior diverticulae of the midgut, and Malpighian tubules, restricting any obvious route of egress during blood feeding. Guinea pigs, mice, and voles inoculated with *R. peacockii* show no signs of illness or infection, and this rickettsia does not grow in embryonated eggs or mammalian cell lines.[17,47,70,77] On a molecular level, the *ompA* gene of *R. peacockii* multiple premature stop codons and a weakened ribosome binding site consensus sequence that prevent expression of functional ompA, a protein believed to play a key role in rickettsial adhesion to mammalian cells.[17,77,78] Recently, a naturally occurring insertion element (ISRpe1) that disrupts genes involved in actin-based motility (*rickA*) and cell adhesion (*sca1*) has been identified in the genome of *R. peacockii*.[79] Collectively, these findings support the concept that *R. peacockii* is a nonpathogen and suggest that other *Rickettsia* species may represent true endosymbionts of arthropods.

Prospectus

Investigators will undoubtedly continue to discover novel rickettsiae and distinguish new rickettsioses. Three important and closely linked considerations combine to stimulate these discoveries: (1) a multidisciplinary approach that includes analysis of the natural history of the specific rickettsia, (2) closer inspection of "mild" or "atypical" forms of historically recognized rickettsioses, and; (3) a greater emphasis on culture- and molecular-based diagnostic techniques.

To guide the search for emerging pathogens, investigators need to intensify efforts that more completely characterize the life histories of rickettsiae in the natural world. Fundamental studies regarding distribution of the microbe in the arthropod, host preferences of the suspected vector, or peculiar physiologic requirements of the rickettsial agent are early priorities in these evaluations. From a clinical perspective, it is important to convey to physicians that multiple forms of a rickettsial syndrome may exist in the same geographical region. Most rickettsioses demonstrate a collection of clinical features, including include fever, rash, and headache, that are shared manifestations of infections caused by multiple, but distinct, rickettsial species. However, when discrepant or unexpected manifestations are uncovered, such as the occurrence of an eschar in a rickettsiosis not often identified with eschars, or relatively mild, self-limiting cases of an illness that is historically associated with high rates of death or hospitalization, these warrant the use of assays that more specifically determine the causative agent. Indeed, historically recognized rickettsioses were included in the working diagnoses of many of the index patients of emerging rickettsioses (Table 4).[3–8,53,80–89]

Mice infected with a particular rickettsial species generate highly specific antibodies that typically react most intensely with the homologous rickettsial species, a characteristic that allows for microimmunofluorescence serotyping of rickettsiae.[90] However, and anti-rickettsial antibodies generated by most humans typically produce substantial titers to multiple closely related, but heterologous rickettsial antigens.[38] Current serologic assays do not generally

TABLE 4. Interval between Discovery of Selected Rickettsiae and Confirmation of These Agents as Pathogens of Humans

Agent	Year of discovery (initial designation)	Year reported as a confirmed pathogen (interval from discovery)	Initial diagnosis of index patient(s)	References
Rickettsia parkeri	1937 (maculatum agent)	2004 (67)	Rickettsialpox	8, 53
Rickettsia honei	1962 (TT-118)	1992 (30)	Queensland tick typhus	80–82
Rickettsia slovaca	1968 (strains B, D)	1997 (29)	Lyme borreliosis	7, 83
Rickettsia felis	1990 (ELB agent)	1994 (4)	Murine typhus	3, 84
Rickettsia massiliae	1992 (strains Mtu1, Mtu5)	2006 (14)	Mediterranean spotted fever	5, 85
Rickettsia aeschlimannii	1995 (strain PoTiR8)	2002 (7)	Mediterranean spotted fever	4, 86
Rickettsia raoultii	1999 (genotypes RpA4, DnS14, DnS28)	2006 (7)	Tick-borne lymphadenopathy	87, 88
Rickettsia monacensis	2002 *(R. monacensis)*	2007 (5)	Mediterranean spotted fever	6, 89

provide the granularity required to specifically identify a causative agent, and rickettsiology is replete with examples where dependence on serology has resulted in mistaken identity of the infecting agent.[1,38,82] Western blot assays and cross-adsorption methods provide more discriminative data, but most studies lack the appropriate controls needed to validate these techniques. Furthermore, as additional rickettsiae are discovered, the panel of antigens needed for an accurate determination becomes prohibitively large.

Cell culture and PCR are the best available tools to effectively unveil the true identity of an infecting microbe, particularly for patients with illnesses that clinically or epidemiologically resemble a locally acquired rickettsiosis, but for whom some aspect of the disease seems inconsistent in terms of temporal or spatial occurrence, or a manifestation that is unusual for the presumed infection.[91] The combination of classical and contemporary microbiologic tools will provide enormous rewards for investigators in rickettsiology, in terms of pathogen discovery, reappraising historically recognized rickettsioses and providing a better understanding of the complexity of these diseases in nature.

Conflicts of Interest

The author declares no conflicts of interest.

References

1. Maeda, K. *et al.* 1987. Human infection with *Ehrlichia canis*, a leukocytic rickettsia. *N. Engl. J. Med.* **316:** 853–856.
2. Bakken, J.S. *et al.* 1994. Human granulocytic ehrlichiosis in the upper Midwest United States: a new species emerging? *J. Am. Med. Assoc.* **272:** 212–218.
3. Schriefer, M.E. *et al.* 1994. Identification of a novel rickettsial infection in a patient diagnosed with murine typhus. *J. Clin. Microbiol.* **32:** 949–954.
4. Raoult, D., P.E. Fournier, P. Abboud & F. Caron. 2002. First documented human *Rickettsia aeschlimannii* infection. *Emerg. Infect. Dis.* **8:** 748–749.
5. Vitale, G., S. Mansueto, J.M. Rolain & D. Raoult. 2006. *Rickettsia massiliae* human isolation. *Emerg. Infect. Dis.* **12:** 174–175.
6. Jado, I. *et al.* 2007. *Rickettsia monacensis* and human disease, Spain. *Emerg. Infect. Dis.* **13:** 1405–1407.
7. Raoult, D. *et al.* 1997. A new tick transmitted disease due to *Rickettsia slovaca*. *Lancet* **350:** 112–113.
8. Paddock, C.D. *et al.* 2004. *Rickettsia parkeri*: a newly recognized cause of spotted fever rickettsiosis in the United States. *Clin. Infect. Dis.* **38:** 805–811.
9. Demma, L.J. *et al.* 2005. Rocky Mountain spotted fever from an unexpected vector in Arizona. *N. Engl. J. Med.* **353:** 587–594.
10. Demma, L.J. *et al.* 2006. Serologic evidence for exposure to *Rickettsia rickettsii* in eastern Arizona and recent emergence of Rocky Mountain spotted fever in this region. *Vector-Borne Zoonotic Dis.* **6:** 423–429.
11. Medina-Sanchez, A. *et al.* 2005. Detection of a typhus group *Rickettsia* in *Amblyomma* ticks in the state of Nuevo Leon, Mexico. *Ann. N.Y. Acad. Sci.* **1063:** 327–332.
12. Burgdorfer, W., S.F. Hayes & L.A. Thomas. 1981. A new spotted fever group rickettsia from the lone star

tick, *Amblyomma americanum*. *Rickettsiae and Rickettsial Diseases*. W. Burgdorfer & R.L. Anacker, Eds.: 595–602. Academic Press. New York, NY.

13. Cowdry, E.V. 1923. The distribution of *Rickettsia* in the tissues of insects and arachnids. *J. Exp. Med.* **37:** 431–56.

14. Parker, R.R. & Spencer R.R. 1926. Rocky Mountain spotted fever. A study of the relationship between the presence of *Rickettsia*-like organisms in tick smears and the infectiveness of the same ticks. *Public Health Rep.* **41:** 461–469.

15. Bell, E.J., G.M. Kohls, H.G. Stoenner & D.B. Lackman. 1963. Nonpathogenic rickettsias related to the spotted fever group isolated from ticks, *Dermacentor variabilis* and *Dermacentor andersoni* from eastern Montana. *J. Immunol.* **90:** 770–781.

16. Philip, R.N. *et al.* 1983. *Rickettsia bellii* sp. nov.: a tick-borne *Rickettsia* widely distributed in the United States, that is distinct from the spotted fever and typhus biogroups. *Int. J. Syst. Bacteriol.* **33:** 94–106.

17. Nieblyski, M.L. *et al.* 1997. *Rickettsia peacockii* sp. nov., a new species infecting wood ticks, *Dermacentor andersoni*, in Western Montana. *Int. J. Sys. Bacteriol.* **47:** 446–452.

18. Maxcy, K.F. 1929. Typhus fever in the United States. *Public Health Rep.* **44:** 1735-1742.

19. Williams, S.G. *et al.* 1992. Typus and typhuslike rickettsiae associated with opossums and their fleas in Los Angeles County, California. *J. Clin. Microbiol.* **30:** 1758–1762.

20. Parola, P., C.D. Paddock & D. Raoult. 2005. Tick-borne rickettsioses around the world: emerging diseases challenging old concepts. **18:** 719–756.

21. Philip, R.N. & E.A. Casper. 1981. Serotypes of spotted fever group rickettsiae isolated from *Dermacentor andersoni* (Stiles) in western Montana. *Am. J. Trop. Med. Hyg.* **30:** 230–238.

22. Gage, K.L. *et al.* 1994. DNA typing of rickettsiae in naturally infected ticks using a polymerase chain reaction/restriction fragment length polymorphism system. *Am. J. Trop. Med. Hyg.* **50:** 247–260.

23. Price, W. H. 1954. The epidemiology of Rocky Mountain spotted fever. II. Studies on the biological survival mechanism of *Rickettsia rickettsii*. *Am. J. Hyg.* **60:** 292–319.

24. Ammerman, N.C. *et al.* 2004. Spotted fever group *Rickettsia* in *Dermacentor variablis*, Maryland. *Emerg. Infect. Dis.* **10:** 1478–1481.

25. Gordon, J.C., S.W. Gordon, E. Peterson & R.N. Philip. 1984. Epidemiology of Rocky Mountain spotted fever in Ohio, 1981: serologic evaluation of canines and rickettsial isolation from ticks associated with human case exposure sites. *Am. J. Trop. Med. Hyg.* **33:** 1026–1031.

26. Burgdorfer, W. 1988. Ecological and epidemiological considerations of Rocky Mountain spotted fever and scrub typhus. *The Biology of Rickettsial Diseases*, Vol. I. D.H. Walker, Ed. 33–50. CRC Press. Boca Raton, FL.

27. Lane, R.S., R.N. Philip & E.A. Casper. 1981. Ecology of tick-borne agents in California. II. Further observations on rickettsiae. *Rickettsiae and Rickettsial Diseases*. W. Burgdorfer & R.L. Anacker, Eds.: 575–584. Academic Press. New York, NY.

28. Wikswo, M.E. *et al.* 2008. Detection and identification of spotted fever group rickettsiae in *Dermacentor* species from southern California. *J. Med. Entomol.* **45:** 509–516.

29. Sangioni, L.A. *et al.* 2005. Rickettsial infection in animals and Brazilian spotted fever endemicity. *Emerg. Infect. Dis.* **11:** 265–270.

30. Pinter, A. & M.B. Labruna. 2006. Isolation of *Rickettsia rickettsii* and *Rickettsia bellii* in cell culture from the tick *Amblyomma aureolatum* in Brazil. *Ann. N.Y. Acad. Sci.* **1078:** 523–530.

31. Philip, C.B. 1959. Some epidemiological considerations in Rocky Mountain spotted fever. *Public Health Rep.* **74:** 595–600.

32. Shepard, C.C. & R.A. Goldwasser. 1960. Fluorescent antibody staining as a means of detecting Rocky Mountain spotted fever infection in individual ticks. *Am. J. Hyg.* **72:** 120–129.

33. Linneman, C.C. *et al.* 1980. Rocky Mountain spotted fever in Clermont County, Ohio. II. Distribution of population and infected ticks in an endemic area. *Am. J. Epidemiol.* **111:** 31–36.

34. Sumner, J.W. *et al.* 2007. Gulf Coast ticks (*Amblyomma maculatum*) and *Rickettsia parkeri*, United States. *Emerg. Infect. Dis.* **13:** 751–753.

35. Nava, S. *et al.* 2008. *Rickettsia parkeri* in Argentina. *Emerg. Infect. Dis.* **14:** 1894–1897.

36. Mixson, T.R. *et al.* 2006. Prevalence of *Ehrlichia*, *Borrelia*, and rickettsial agents in *Amblyomma americanum* (Acari: Ixodidae) collected from nine states. *J. Med. Entomol.* **43:** 1261–1268.

37. Centers for Disease Control and Prevention. 2008. Notice to readers: final 2007 reports of nationally notifiable infectious diseases. *M.M.W.R.* **57:** 903–913.

38. Paddock, C.D. *et al.* 2008. *Rickettsia parkeri* rickettsiosis and its clinical distinction from Rocky Mountain spotted fever. *Clin. Infect. Dis.* **47:** 1188–1196.

39. Graf, P.C.F. *et al.* 2008. Prevalence of seropositivity to spotted fever group rickettsiae and *Anaplasma phagocytophilum* in a large, demographically diverse U.S. sample. *Clin. Infect. Dis.* **46:** 70–77.

40. Marshall, G.S. *et al.* 2003. Antibodies reactive to *Rickettsia rickettsii* among children living in the southeast and south central regions of the United States. *Arch. Pediatr. Adolesc. Med.* **157:** 443–448.

41. Apperson, C.S. *et al.* 2008. Tick-borne diseases in North Carolina: is "*Rickettsia amblyommii*" a possible cause of rickettsiosis reported as Rocky Mountain spotted fever? *Vector-Borne Zoonotic Dis.* **8:** 1–10.

42. Chapman, A.S. *et al.* 2006. Rocky Mountain spotted fever in the United States, 1997–2002. *Vector-Borne and Zoonotic Dis.* **6:** 170–178.

43. Paddock, C.D. *et al.* 2008. Rocky Mountain spotted fever in Argentina. *Am. J. Trop. Med. Hyg.* **78:** 687–692.

44. deSousa, R.A. *et al.* 2008. Host- and microbe-related risk factors for and pathophysiology of fatal *Rickettsia conorii* infection in Portuguese patients. *J. Infect. Dis.* **198:** 576–585.

45. Fernández-Soto, P., R. Pérez-Sánchez, R. Álamo-Sanz & A. Encinas-Grandes. 2006. Spotted fever group rickettsiae in ticks feeding on humans in northwestern Spain: Is *Rickettsia conorii* vanishing? *Ann. N.Y. Acad. Sci.* **1078:** 331–333.

46. Márquez, F.J. *et al.* 2008. Spotted fever group *Rickettsia* in brown dog ticks *Rhipicephalus sanguineus* in southwestern Spain. *Parasitol. Res.* **103:** 119–122.

47. Burgdorfer, W., S.F. Hayes & A.J. Mavros. 1981. Nonpathogenic rickettsiae in *Dermacentor andersoni*: a limiting factor for the distribution of *Rickettsia rickettsii*. *Rickettsiae and Rickettsial Diseases*. W. Burgdorfer & R. L. Anacker, Eds.: 585–594. Academic Press. New York, NY.

48. Macaluso, K.R., D.E. Sonenshine, S.M. Ceraul & A.F. Azad. 2002. Rickettsial infection in *Dermacentor variabilis* (Acari: Ixodidae) inhibits transovarial transmission of a second *Rickettsia*. *J. Med. Entomol.* **39:** 809–813.

49. Maver, M.B. 1911. Transmission of spotted fever by means other than Montana and Idaho ticks. *J. Infect. Dis.* **8:** 322–326.

50. Parker, R.R., C.B. Philip & W.L. Jellison. 1933. Rocky Mountain spotted fever. Potentialities of tick transmission in relation to the geographical occurrence in the United States. *Am. J. Trop. Med.* **13:** 341–379.

51. Burgdorfer, W., J.C. Cooney & L.A. Thomas. 1974. Zoonotic potential (Rocky Mountain spotted fever and tularemia) in the Tennessee Valley region. II. Prevalence of *Rickettsia rickettsi* and *Francisella tularensis*. *Am. J. Trop. Med. Hyg.* **23:** 109–117.

52. Stromdahl, E.Y. *et al.* 2008. *Rickettsia amblyommii* infecting *Amlyomma americanum* larvae. *Vector-Borne Zoonotic Dis.* **8:** 1–10.

53. Parker, R.R., G.M. Kohls, G.W. Cox & G.E. Davis. 1939. Observations on an infectious agent from *Amblyomma maculatum*. *Public Health Rep.* **54:** 1482–1484.

54. Burgdorfer, W. *et al.* 1975. *Rhipicephalus sanguineus*: vector of a new spotted fever group rickettsia in the United States. *Infect. Immun.* **12:** 205–210.

55. Feng, W.C., & J.L. Waner. 1980. Serological cross-reaction and cross-protection in guinea pigs infected with *Rickettsia rickettsii* and *Rickettsia montana*. *Infect. Immun.* **28:** 627–629.

56. Todd, W.J., W. Burgdorfer & A.J. Mavros. 1982. Establishment of cell cultures persistently infected with spotted fever group rickettsiae. *Can. J. Microbiol.* **28:** 1412–1416.

57. Ogata, H. *et al.* 2006. Genome sequence of *Rickettsia bellii* illuminates the role of amoebae in gene exchanges between intracellular pathogens. *PLoS Genet.* **2:** e76.

58. McKiel, J.A., E.J. Bell & D.B. Lackman. 1967. *Rickettsia canada*: a new member of the typhus group rickettsiae isolated from *Haemaphysalis leporispalustris* ticks in Canada. *Can. J. Microbiol.* **13:** 503–510.

59. Philip, R.N., R.S. Lane & E.A. Casper. 1981. Serotypes of tick-borne spotted fever group rickettsiae from western California. *Am. J. Trop. Med. Hyg.* **30:** 722–727.

60. Philip, C.B., & L.E. Hughes. 1953. Disease agents found in the rabbit tick, *Dermacentor parumapertus*, in the southwestern United States. *Sixth Int. Cong. Microbiol, Rome* **5:** 541–548.

61. Hughes, L.E. *et al.* 1976. Isolation of a spotted fever group *Rickettsia* from the Pacific Coast tick, *Ixodes pacificus*, in Oregon. *Am. J. Trop. Med. Hyg.* **25:** 513–516.

62. Pusterla, N. *et al.* 2000. Helminthic transmission and isolation of *Ehrlichia risticii*, the causative agent of Potomac horse fever, by using trematode stages from freshwater snails. *J. Clin. Microiol.* **38:** 1293–1297.

63. Gibson, K.E., Y. Rikihisa, C. Zhang & C. Martin. 2005. *Neorickettsia risticii* is vertically transmitted in the trematode *Acanthatrium oregonense* and horizontially transmitted to bats. *Environ. Microbiol.* **7:** 203–212.

64. Perlman, S.J., M.S. Hunter & E. Zchori-Fein. 2006. The emerging diversity of *Rickettsia*. *Proc. R. Soc. B.* **273:** 2097–2106.

65. Policastro, P.F., U.G. Munderloh, E.R. Fischer & T. Hackstadt. 1997. *Rickettsia rickettsii* growth and temperature-inducible protein expression in embryonic tick cell lines. *J. Med. Microbiol.* **46:** 839–845.

66. Oaks, S.C. & J.V. Osterman. 1969. The influence of temperature and pH on the growth of *Rickettsia conorii* in irradiated mammalian cells. *Acta Virol.* **23:** 67–72.

67. Schaechter, M., F.M. Bozeman & J.E. Smadel. 1957. Study on the growth of rickettsiae. II. Morphologic observations of living rickettsiae in tissue culture cells. *Virol.* **3:** 160–172.

68. Labruna, M.B. *et al.* 2004. *Rickettsia* species infecting *Amblyomma cooperi* ticks from an area in the state of São Paulo, Brazil, where Brazilian spotted fever is endemic. *J. Clin. Microbiol.* **42:** 90–98.

69. Beati, L., P.F. Humair, A. Aeschlimann & D. Raoult. 1994. Identification of spotted fever group rickettsiae

isolated from *Dermacentor marginatus* and *Ixodes ricinus* ticks collected in Switzerland. *Am. J. Trop. Med. Hyg.* **51:** 138–148.

70. Kurtti, T.J. *et al*. 2005. Factors influencing the infectivity and growth of *Rickettsia peacockii* (Rickettsiales: Rickettsiaceae), an endosymbiont of the Rocky Mountain wood tick, *Dermacentor andersoni* (Acari, Ixodidae). *J. Invert. Pathol.* 90: 177–186.

71. Raoult, D. *et al*. 2001. A flea-associated *Rickettsia* pathogenic for humans. *Emerg. Infect. Dis.* **7:** 73–81.

72. Horta, M.C., M.B. Labruna, E.L. Durigon & T.T.S. Schumaker. 2006. Isolation of *Rickettsia felis* in the mosquito cell line C6/36. *Appl. Environ. Microbiol.* **72:** 1705–1707.

73. Pornwiroon, W., S.S. Pourciau, L.D. Foil & K.R. Macaluso. 2006. *Rickettsia felis* from cat fleas: isolation and culture in a tick-derived cell line. *Appl. Environ. Microbiol.* **72:** 5589–5595.

74. Karpathy, S., G.A. Dasch & M.E. Eremeeva. 2007. Molecular typing of isolates of *Rickettsia rickettsii* by use of DNA sequencing of variable intergenic regions. *J. Clin. Microbiol.* **45:** 2545–2553.

75. Furman, D.P. & E.C. Loomis. 1984. The ticks of California (Acari: Ixodida). *Bull. California Insect Surv.* **25:** 37–40.

76. Paddock, C.D. 2006. *Rickettsia parkeri* as a paradigm for multiple causes of tick-borne rickettsioses in the Western Hemisphere. *Ann. N.Y. Acad. Sci.* **1063:** 315–326.

77. Simser, J.A., A.T. Palmer, U.G. Munderloh & T.J. Kurtti. 2001. Isolation of a spotted fever group *Rickettsia*, *Rickettsia peacockii*, in a Rocky Mountain wood tick, *Dermacentor andersoni*, cell line. *Appl. Environ. Microbiol.* **67:** 546–552.

78. Baldridge, G.D. *et al*. 2004. Sequence and expression analysis of the *ompA* gene of *Rickettsia peacockii*, an endosymbiont of the Rocky Mountain wood tick, *Dermacentor andersoni*. *Appl. Environ. Microbiol.* **70:** 6628–6636.

79. Simser, J.A., M.S. Rahman, S.M. Dreher-Lesnick & A. F. Azad. 2005. A novel and naturally occurring transposon, ISRpe1, in the *Rickettsia peacockii* genome disrupting the *rickA* gene involved in actin-based motility. *Molec. Microbiol.* **58:** 71–79.

80. Robertson, R.G. & C.L. Wisseman. 1973. Tick-borne rickettsiae of the spotted fever group in west

Pakistan. II. Serological evidence of isolates from west Pakistan and Thailand: evidence for two new species. *Am. J. Epidemiol.* **97:** 55–64.

81. Baird, R.W. *et al*. 1992. Characterization and comparison of Australian human spotted fever group rickettsiae. *J. Clin. Microbiol.* **30:** 2896–2902.

82. Graves, S.R., B.W. Dwyer, D. McColl & J.E. McDade. 1991. Flinders Island spotted fever: a newly recognized endemic focus of tick typhus in Bass Strait. *Med. J. Aust.* **154:** 99–103.

83. Rezina, R., J. Řeháček, P. Áč & M. Majerská. 1968. Two stains of rickettsiae of Rocky Mountain spotted fever group recovered from *Dermacentor marginatus* ticks in Czechoslovakia. Results of preliminary serological identification. *Acta Virol.* **13:** 142–145.

84. Adams, J.R., E.T. Schmidtmann & A.F. Azad. 1990. Infection of colonized cat fleas, *Ctenocephalides felis* (Bouche) with a *Rickettsia*-like microorganism. *Am. J. Trop. Med. Hyg.* **43:** 400–409.

85. Beati, L., J.P. Finidori, B. Gillot & D. Raoult. 1992. Comparison of serologic typing, sodium dodecyl sulfate-polyacrylamide gel electrophoresis protein analysis, and genetic restriction fragment length polymorphism analysis for identification of rickettsiae: characterization of two new rickettsial strains. *J. Clin. Microbiol.* **30:** 1922–1930.

86. Bacellar, F., R.L. Regnery, M.S. Núncio & A.R. Filipe. 1995. Genotypic evaluation of rickettsial isolates recovered from various species of ticks in Portugal. *Epidemiol. Infect.* **114:** 169–178.

87. Rydkina, E. *et al*. 1999. New rickettsiae in ticks collected in territories of the former Soviet Union. *Emerg. Infect. Dis.* **5:** 811–814.

88. Ibarra, V. *et al*. 2006. *Rickettsia slovaca* infection: DEBONEL/TIBOLA. *Ann. N.Y. Acad. Sci.* **1078:** 206–214.

89. Simser, J.A. *et al*. 2002. *Rickettsia monacensis* sp. nov., a spotted fever group rickettsia, from ticks (*Ixodes ricinus*) collected in a European city park. *Appl. Environ. Microbiol.* **68:** 4559–4566.

90. Philip, R.N. *et al*. 1978. Serologic typing of rickettsiae of the spotted fever group by microimmunofluorescence. *J. Immunol.* **121:** 1961–1968.

91. Raoult, D. 2004. A new tick-borne rickettsiosis in the U.S.A. *Clin. Infect. Dis.* **38:** 812–813.

Status of the "East Side Hypothesis" (Transovarial Interference) 25 Years Later

Sam R. Telford, III

Division of Infectious Diseases, Cummings School of Veterinary Medicine, Tufts University, 200 Westboro Road, North Grafton, Massachusetts 01536, USA

Rocky Mountain spotted fever (RMSF) cases in the notorious Bitterroot Valley outbreak of the early 20th century were peculiarly distributed, with virtually all reported from the west side of the valley. Such a distribution remained unexplained until Burgdorfer and colleagues (1981) reported that endosymbiotic rickettsiae were prevalent in wood ticks on the east side of the Bitterroot River valley but not on the west side. The "East Side agent" was said to prevent the transovarial transmission of *Rickettsia rickettsii*, thereby severely limiting the prevalence of the latter. This hypothesis has been considered one of the most innovative explanations for an epidemiological conundrum and, indeed, has generally been accepted as a fact in the medical entomology literature. I review the evidence for the interference hypothesis, and suggest that the distribution of the Bitterroot Valley RMSF outbreak might actually have its basis in habitat or microclimate-related factors, as opposed to reflecting interspecific competition by closely related rickettsiae.

Key words: Rocky Mountain spotted fever; *Rickettsia*; *Rickettsia rickettsii*; ticks; *Dermacentor*; *Rickettsia peacockii*; interference; transovarial transmission; Bitterroot Valley

Introduction

Between 1873 and 1910, 295 cases of what is now known as Rocky Mountain spotted fever occurred in the northern Bitterroot Valley of Montana, of which 64% proved fatal.[1] Although this disease was not as great a public health burden in Montana at the time as typhoid, diphtheria, or smallpox, its dramatic clinical presentation, great case-fatality rate, and unknown etiology stimulated intensive investigation of the cause.[2] The first epidemiological analyses formally established that virtually all such cases occurred in individuals who lived or worked in the western side of the valley.[3] Subsequent compilations of case reports even into the 1950s confirm such an unusual distribution, although there were some clearly identified exposures on the east side leading to typical RMSF.[4] No reasonable explanation of the peculiar distribution of RMSF in the Bitterroot Valley had been advanced, until the hypothesis of transovarial interference by nonpathogenic rickettsiae was presented.[5] A typical representation of this hypothesis is: Wood ticks (*Dermacentor andersoni*), the vector of RMSF, contain only nonpathogenic rickettsiae on the eastern side of the Bitterroot Valley, and these interfere with transovarial passage of *R. rickettsii*, a critical mode of perpetuation for this agent. Prevalence of *R. rickettsii* infection in host-seeking ticks is thereby greatly reduced.

Ecological or evolutionary theory has precedences for the idea that two closely related organisms might have interactions that prevent the stable coexistence of one or the other. At the level of geological time, "incumbent replacement" applies, that is, a preexisting species will tend to exclude others regardless of adaptation;[6] a species becomes common only when the preexisting species becomes ecologically moribund or extinct. The political extension of this (e.g., American presidential elections)

Address for correspondence: Sam R. Telford III, Division of Infectious Diseases, Cummings School of Veterinary Medicine, Tufts University, 200 Westboro Road, North Grafton, MA 01536. Voice: +508-887-4236; fax: +508-839-7911. sam.telford@tufts.edu

Rickettsiology and Rickettsial Diseases-Fifth International Conference: Ann. N.Y. Acad. Sci. 1166: 144–150 (2009).
doi: 10.1111/j.1749-6632.2009.04522.x © 2009 New York Academy of Sciences.

is well-known. In general ecological theory, Gause's Law of competitive exclusion states that two species competing for the same resource cannot stably coexist. A bacteriological example may be found in the observation that preexisting eperythrozoa exclude *Bartonella* spp. infection[7] within rodent hosts; such interactions are now well recognized and explained by diverse immunological mechanisms including antigenic cross-reactivity and cytokine balance. Accordingly, the rickettsial interference hypothesis has been well received because it is consistent with general biological laws.

The evidence that serves as the basis for rickettsial transovarial interference, however, has not been critically examined. Biological laws tend to be generalizable; thus, if rickettsial interference operates for *R. rickettsii*, such effects should be detected for other transovarially-maintained tick-borne rickettsiae or even nonrickettsial tick-borne infections. Indeed, our observations that interference does not characterize *Francisella* spp.[8] led me to reread the original report of the East Side hypothesis and search for reports that corroborated or refuted it.

Reanalysis

What exactly did Burgdorfer and colleagues (1981) say? The original suggestion was within the proceedings of the 1980 Conference on Rickettsiae and Rickettsial Diseases held at the Rocky Mountain Laboratories, published by Academic Press. This text is not commonly represented in libraries, and the reprint of the famous paper is not available online. Thus, relatively few investigators are likely to have read the original paper. The data comprise the report that 80% of ticks from the east side of the Bitterroot River contained a transovarially maintained spotted fever group *Rickettsia* that was nonpathogenic for guinea pigs; 8–16% of ticks from the west side contained this agent. It was concluded that "Inability of virulent *R. rickettsii* to invade ovarial tissues harboring the East Side agent is a typical example of 'interference' known to occur among many animal, plant, and bacterial viruses ... it appears that development of *R. rickettsii* does not take place in epithelial and germinative ovarial cells that are infected by the East Side agent." (Ref. 5, p. 592).

The experiments that served as the evidence for interference were simple and elegant. Two groups of larvae derived from female ticks that transmitted the East Side agent (now known as *Rickettsia peacockii*[9]) were used: 'line 2,' of which 98% of progeny were infected by R. peacocki; and 'line 21'; of which 94% of progeny were infected by R. peacocki. These larvae were fed on guinea pigs that were rickettsemic, and the resulting nymphs were 100% infected by *R. rickettsii* (as determined by allowing 50–100 nymphs to feed on guinea pigs that subsequently died). The fed nymphs were allowed to molt to adults and then dissected to determine the infection status of various tissues. Using fluorescent antibody (FA), 9/10 of line 2 and 8/10 of line 31 were found to have heavy *R. rickettsii* infections of all tissues except ovaries. The effect was not absolute: 1/10 of line 2 and 2/10 of line 31 had *R. rickettsii* in ovaries; "2 of these females were negative and 1 only mildly positive for the East Side agent.[5]" In the critical experiment analyzing the efficiency of transovarial rickettsial passage, 10 females of line 2 and 8 females of line 31 (all hemolymph test positive for *R. rickettsii*) were allowed to feed and oviposit. Ten eggs from each egg batch were tested by FA as were carcasses of the ovipositing females. The result was that 7/10 of line 2 and 4/8 of line 31 did not transmit *R. rickettsii* through the egg but "their ovarial tissues and eggs were heavily infected with the East Side agent." However, 3/10 of line 2 and 4/8 of line 31 laid eggs "either all of which or at least some were infected by *R. rickettsii*." It was concluded that "Those females that transmitted *R. rickettsii* to all eggs examined were negative for the East Side agent; the others were rather mildly infected for both the East Side agent and *R. rickettsii*." (Ref. 5, p. 590).

Transovarial interference, then, is not absolute but relative. The presence of *R. peacockii* within a tick matrilineage tends to greatly reduce the probability that *R. rickettsii* will subsequently pass by transovarial transmission (TOT) when it is acquired by feeding on a rickettsemic animal. The presence of *R. peacockii* does not at all preclude the infection of a tick by *R. rickettsii*, but the ovaries usually fail to support both species of rickettsiae. But, the fact that some oocytes are indeed dually infected would seem to erect difficult scenarios for molecular mechanisms to explain transovarial interference, such as the alteration of a critical entry receptor.[10] Such a change would be oocyte specific because other tick tissues (as the gut epithelium) may be invaded by either *Rickettsia* spp., but not all oocytes would undergo such change because they are receptive to the second *Rickettsia*, as documented by the "mild" ovarial dual infections reported in Burgdorfer *et al.* (1981). It is conceptually difficult to erect the hypothesis that there is a receptor on or a change that occurs within most, but not all oocytes.

Other experiments are alluded to within the same paper, in which *R. rhipicephali* or *R. montanensis* excluded *R. rickettsii*, but the data were not presented (nor have they subsequently been published, to my knowledge). Recent experiments using capillary feeding established the phenomenon with *R. montanensis* and *R. rhipicephali*, wherein *R. montanensis*-infected *D. variabilis* ticks failed to transovarially pass the latter species and vice versa.[10] In contrast, a report of a triply infected field-collected tick suggests that coinfection by 2 *Rickettsia* spp., at least 1 of which was likely to have been acquired by TOT, occurs but demonstrating such associations requires careful analysis of amplicons from PCR screening assays.[11] The generality of TOT interference among tick-perpetuated *Rickettsia* spp. might be supported through field studies of the more common nonpathogenic (or rather, pathogenicity undescribed[12]) *Rickettsia* spp. as well as known human pathogens such as *R. conorii*, *R. sibirica*, *R. japonica*, or *R. australis*.

Our understanding of the diversity of tick endobionts has been facilitated by molecular detection methods and phylogenetic analysis. In characterizing *R. peacockii*, a *Francisella* sp. was found to be ubiquitous within *D. andersoni* populations.[9] The presence or absence of this bacterium did not affect the transovarial passage of *R. peacockii*, thereby suggesting that the transovarial interference phenomenon is not simply due to an inability of oocytes to thrive when more than one endobiont is present. Our observations of another distinct *Francisella* sp. endobiont of *D. variabilis* indicate that two closely related *Francisella* spp., presumably facultatively intracellular bacteria, may be simultaneously passed within the same egg batch,[8] thereby arguing against the generality of transovarial interference for another clade of tick-perpetuated agents. On the other hand, one strain of *Anaplasma marginale* excluded another[13] from transovarial passage. Whether spirochetes of the *Borrelia burgdorferi* sensu lato complex may be passed transovarially by ticks coinfected by relapsing fever-like species such as *B. miyamotoi* (which are apparently maintained by TOT) is not known. Nor have such associations been established for arboviral perpetuation, for example, tick-borne encephalitis virus with Kemerovo group viruses in *Ixodes ricinus*.

Measuring Transovarial Transmission

The literature is conflicting with respect to how efficient and how stable TOT is for *R. rickettsii*. Price[14] and colleagues[15] indicated that 35% of infected female ticks gave rise to infected progeny, whereas Burgdorfer[16] and Burgdorfer and Brinton[17] found virtually 100% of infected females gave rise to infected progeny. The efficiency of TOT may relate to the degree of infection within the tick, with "massively infected" ticks universally giving rise to infected progeny and "mild" infections giving rise to variable TOT rates.[1] It may also be that TOT measurements are greatly affected by the specifics for each experimental situation, such as the genetics of the tick colony, the strain and passage history of *R. rickettsii*,[15] the mode of infection (even guinea pig strain and health status), other known factors that affect vector competence for other pathogens (e.g., extrinsic incubation temperature), as well as assays (fluorescent antibody versus chick embryo inoculation vs. PCR).

Varying reports of TOT efficiency notwithstanding, the existing literature appears to be poorly precise with respect to the concept of inheritance and the perpetuation of a pathogen. In a very detailed paper, Price[14] reported 30–40% of infected female ticks gave rise to infected egg batches; but "in about 50% of the instances 1 egg in every 5–10 was infected; 15% showed at least 1 egg infected out of every 2–4; and 35% . . . passed the rickettsiae to about 1 egg out of 20–40." This demonstrates that even the measurement of "TOT" needs to be critically examined. Indeed, arbovirologists have more precisely defined TOT[18] by requiring 2 separate measurements: Vertical transmission rate (VTR) = Filial infection rate (FIR) × Transovarial transmission rate (TOTR). The filial infection rate is the proportion of eggs that are positive if the egg batch is positive. The TOTR is the proportion of females giving rise to infected batches of eggs regardless of what proportion of the eggs in each batch is infected. This precision is important for quantitative analysis of perpetuation, particularly for estimating the basic reproduction number. The actual number of "secondary cases" produced by 1 infected tick is not quantifiable if the nebulous "35% of females" are TOT positive but "35% of females give rise to an average of 300 infected larvae each" is a precise number.

Note also that power calculations suggest that more attention needs to be paid to the number of eggs sampled for estimating FIR. At Price's lower estimate of "1 egg out of 20 to 40" (say 5%), the 95% confidence interval for the true proportion of infected eggs obtained by testing 50 eggs (typical for the above-cited reports) is 1.2–16.6%, but by testing 200, the 95% CI is a more precise 2.4–9.0%. Accordingly, TOT interference needs to be reassessed using VTR, and giving attention to statistical significance.

How Important Is TOT?

The epidemiological relevance of transovarial interference depends on how important TOT is to the perpetuation of *R. rickettsii*, a question debated since Ricketts' seminal work. Although the ecology of RMSF remains to be fully understood, it is apparent that there are important contributions for both horizontal and vertical components of transmission.[4,19,20] Whether *R. rickettsii* can be perpetuated in a natural focus solely by transmission to and from rodents by subadult ticks (by either systemic infection or co-feeding) is not known. Epidemic typhus rickettsiae are apparently perpetuated in the absence of TOT,[21] although unlike wood ticks, the louse vector has great vectorial capacity given that it focuses all bites on humans and there is a mechanism for long-term persistence through recrudescent typhus (Brill Zinsser disease).

On the other hand, it seems unlikely that *R. rickettsii* can be maintained solely by TOT for more than a few years, because infection of ticks reduces their fitness; particularly with respect to reproductive success.[15,17] However, as with reports of the efficiency of TOT, there are conflicting data on how commonly infection may prevent reproduction. Price[14] and Burgdorfer[16] failed to comment on excessive mortality in their TOT experiments, whereas Burgdorfer and Brinton[17] and Niebylski and colleagues[15] report clear effects on survival to oviposition as well as fecundity of those that did oviposit. (The latter report also provides evidence for negative effects of transstadial rickettsial passage as well and made the interesting suggestion that *R. peacockii* may confer a selective advantage on *D. andersoni* by protecting it from *R. rickettsii*-mediated reproductive

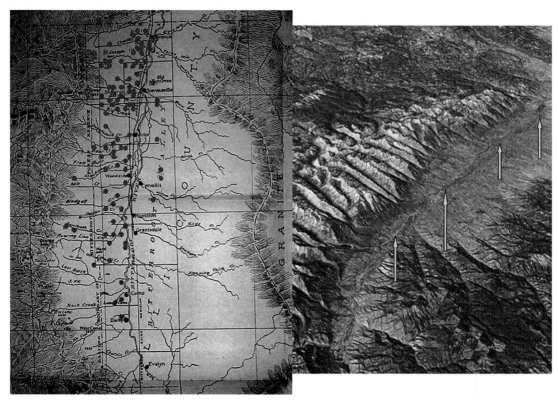

Figure 1. *Left side*, epidemiological map of Wilson and Chowning (1904); *Right side*, topographic detail (from http://130.166.124.2/montana_panorama_atlas/page27/files/page27-1003-full.html) of the Bitterroot Valley; arrows show track of the Bitterroot River. The west side of the valley clearly comprises foothills and other rocky terrain; the east side of the valley, particularly at the northern and central portions of the valley, is flat agricultural terrain.

inhibition. Selective sweeps, therefore, might explain the great prevalence of "non-pathogenic" rickettsiae within ticks from across the world.) As suggested in the discussion on the estimation of TOT rates, the details in the individual experiments may largely explain such discrepancies. The apparent variability in the controlled laboratory environment would suggest that the enzootic cycle may be even more variable, that is, in some sites during some years, infection may be detrimental to the tick population but in other sites, there is no net effect on tick population dynamics.

Where does this analysis leave the TOT interference hypothesis? Its epidemiological relevance remains unclear given the difficulty with which ecologic correlates of risk can be de-

termined, a situation that is not unique to RMSF. Ecologically, more work seems needed, although field studies are hindered by low prevalence of *R. rickettsii* in host-seeking ticks. Use of molecular tools, and particularly the cloning and sequencing of rickettsial amplicons during field surveys, may provide more information on the extent of coinfection in ticks. Mathematical modeling to determine the basic reproduction number of *R. rickettsii* might help resolve the controversy of the relative contributions of horizontal versus vertical transmission. Thus, the TOT interference hypothesis is left as an intriguing idea that deserves to be true but for which the data remains inconclusive, particularly with respect to its influence on the perpetuation of *R. rickettsii*.

So How Do We Explain the Bitterroot Valley?

If TOT interference does not necessarily explain the distribution of RMSF cases in the Bitterroot Valley, what does? Visits to Hamilton, Montana, and to the Rocky Mountain Laboratories provide a visual clue to a likely explanation, as does juxtaposition of the epidemiological map produced by Wilson and Chowning[3] with an aerial view of the topography (Fig. 1). The west side of the Bitterroot Valley comprises foothills of the Bitterroot Range, with rocky canyons and rugged terrain. The east side of the Bitterroot Valley is largely flat agricultural land or, now, successional growth from long-cleared forest. The two sides would have different microclimates as well as mammal faunas. Whereas the dozens of rocky canyons in the foothills would provide multiple microfoci, the lack of geographical barriers to dispersal would reduce the stability of microfoci of transmission in the eastern part of the valley. Monitoring of relative humidity and temperature in sites on either side would be instructive; those on the east side might experience great ranges of temperatures or humidity, whereas those on the west side would be stabilized by the rocky physiography. Extrinsic incubation temperatures, in particular, might greatly differ between the two sites; it is noteworthy that infected ticks held at lower temperatures (4°C) were less likely to be negatively affected by infection than those held at room temperature (21°C).[15] Although tick densities and exposures may be similar overall between the two sides of the Bitterroot Valley, it is likely that the ticks themselves feed on different potential reservoir animals or experience different environmental factors, and thus the prevalence of *R. rickettsii* may differ. This suggestion is as testable as the TOT interference hypothesis.

Acknowledgments

My laboratory has been generously supported by the National Institute of Health (NIH) (RO1 AI 064218).

Conflicts of Interest

The author declares no conflicts of interest.

References

1. Burgdorfer, W. 1977. Tick borne diseases in the United States: Rocky Mountain spotted fever and Colorado tick fever. A review. *Acta. Tropica* **34**: 103–126.
2. Harden, V.A. 1990. *Rocky Mountain Spotted Fever. A History of a Twentieth Century Disease*. Johns Hopkins Press. Baltimore. p. 375.
3. Wilson, L.B. & W.M. Chowning. 1904. Studies in pyroplasmosis hominis (Spotted fever or tick fever of the Rocky Mountains). *J. Infect Dis.* **I**: 31–33.
4. Philip, C.B. 1959. Some epidemiological considerations in Rocky Mountain spotted fever. *Publ. Health Repts* **74**: 595–600.
5. Burgdorfer, W., S.F. Hayes & A.J. Mavros. 1981. Nonpathogenic rickettsiae in Dermacentor andersoni: a limiting factor for the distribution of Rickettsia rickettsii. *Rickettsiae and Rickettsial Diseases*. W. Burgdorfer & R.L. Anacker, Eds.: 585–594, 650. Academic Press. New York, NY.
6. Rosenzweig, M.L. & R.D. McCord. 1991. Incumbent replacement: evidence for longterm evolutionary progress. *Paleobiology* **17**: 202–213.
7. Tyzzer, E.E. 1941. Interference in mixed infections of *Bartonella* and eperythrozoon in mice. *Am. J. Pathol.* **17**: 141–153.
8. Goethert, H.K. & S.R. Telford. 2005. A new *Francisella* (*Beggiatales: Francisellaceae*) inquiline within *Dermacentor variabilis* Say (*Acari: Ixodidae*). *J. Med. Entomol.* **42**: 502–505.
9. Niebylski, M.L. *et al.* 1997. *Rickettsia peacockii* sp nov, a new species infecting wood ticks, *Dermacentor andersoni*, in western Montana. *Int. J. Syst. Bacteriol.* **47**: 446–452.
10. Macaluso, K.R., D.E. Sonenshine, S.M. Ceraul & A.F. Azad. 2002. Rickettsial infection in *Dermacentor variabilis* (*Acari: Ixodidae*) inhibits transovarial transmission of a second *Rickettsia*. *J. Med. Entomol.* **39**: 809–813.
11. Carmichael, J.R. & P.A. Fuerst. 2006. A rickettsial mixed infection in a *Dermacentor variabilis* tick from Ohio. *Ann. N. Y. Acad. Sci.* **1078**: 334–337.
12. Parola, P., C.D. Paddock & D. Raoult. 2005. Tick borne rickettsioses around the world: emerging diseases challenging old concepts. *Clin. Microbiol. Rev.* **18**: 719–756.
13. De la Fuente, J., E. Blouin & K.M. Kocan. 2003. Infection exclusion of the rickettsial pathogen *Anaplasma marginale* in the tick vector *Dermacentor variabilis*. *Clin. Diag. Lab. Immunol.* **10**: 182–184.

14. Price, W.H. 1954. The epidemiology of Rocky Mountain spotted fever. II. Studies on the biological survival mechanism of *Rickettsia rickettsii*. *Am. J. Hyg.* **60:** 292–319.

15. Niebylski, M.L., M.G. Peacock & T.G. Schwan. 1999. Lethal effect of *Rickettsia rickettsii* on its tick vector (Dermacentor andersoni). *Appl. Environ. Microbiol* **65:** 773–778.

16. Burgdorfer, W. 1963. Investigation of transovarial transmission of *Rickettsia rickettsii* in the wood tick, Dermacentor andersoni. *Exp. Parasitol.* **14:** 152–159.

17. Burgdorfer, W. & L.P. Brinton. 1975. Mechanisms of transovarial infection of spotted fever rickettsiae in ticks. *Ann. N. Y. Acad. Sci.* **266:** 61–72.

18. Turell, M.J. Horizontal and vertical transmission of viruses by insect and tick vectors. *The Arboviruses: Epidemiology and Ecology*, Vol. 1. T.P. Monath, Ed.: 127–152. CRC Press Inc. Boca Raton, FL.

19. McDade, J.E. & V.F. Newhouse. 1986. Natural history of *Rickettsia rickettsii*. *Ann. Rev. Microbiol.* **40:** 287–309.

20. Burgdorfer, W. 1988. Ecological and epidemiological considerations of Rocky Mountain spotted fever and scrub typhus. *Biology of Rickettsial Diseases*, Vol. 1. D.H. Walker, Ed.: 33–50, 146. CRC Press. Boca Raton, FL.

21. Houhamdi, L. *et al.* 2002. An experimental model of human body louse infection with *Rickettsia prowazekii*. *J. Infect. Dis.* **186:** 1639–1646.

Rickettsioses in Australia

Stephen Graves[a,c] and John Stenos[b]

[a]*Director and* [b]*Supervising Scientist. Australian Rickettsial Reference Laboratory, Geelong, Victoria, Australia*

[c]*Director of Microbiology, Hunter Area Pathology Service, Newcastle, NSW, Australia*

The rickettsial diseases of Australia are described in their chronological order of discovery. The include epidemic typhus (*R. prowazekii*); murine typhus (*R. typhi*) found Australia-wide; scrub typhus (*O. tsutsugamushi*) only in tropical, northen Australia; Q. fever (*C. burnetti*) found Australia-wide; Queensland tick typhus (*R. australis*) along the east coast of Australia; Flinders Island spotted fever (*R. honei*) in southeast Australia; Variant Flinders Island spotted fever (*R. honei*, strain "marmionii") in eastern Australia; *Rickettsia felis*, Western Australia; eight new RFG rickettsiae from ticks (of unknown pathogenicity); and two nonhuman pathogens in *A. platys* (dogs) and *A. marginale* (cattle).

Key words: rickettsioses; Australia

The first rickettsial disease recognized in Australia was epidemic typhus (*Rickettsia prowazekii*), which was regularly introduced into Australia via the body lice of convicts and early European migrants. This era lasted from 1788 to 1869 (last known typhus case). There was rarely secondary spread on shore as the warm, sunny climate of Australia allowed residents to wash themselves and their clothes regularly. However, there was a small outbreak on the Victorian goldfields in 1853.[1] Outbreaks of Brill's disease (recrudescent epidemic typhus) have been described in Australia,[2] and further cases should be anticipated as Australia currently receives immigrants from countries that are endemic for *R. prowazekii*.

The second rickettsial disease recognized in Australia was murine typhus (R. *typhi*), although it was initially called "endemic" typhus, to distinguish it from "epidemic" typhus. Hone,[3] a public health doctor in Adelaide, South Australia, recognized cases of a typhus-like illness among men loading wheat onto ships, and residents of poor quality housing. In both environments, rodents were present, and this association was noted. This was in fact the first published report of murine typhus in the world (1922). Patients were not lice-infested, and mortality was much lower than in epidemic typhus. As the years progressed, the same disease was observed in Queensland, during a mouse plague,[4] and in Western Australia, associated with handling wheat.[5] The main differential diagnosis was recrudescent epidemic typhus; especially when the patient was an Australian soldier having returned from Europe post World War I. The disease is still being diagnosed in Western Australia,[6] and, recently, the first case in Victoria was reported.[7]

The third rickettsial disease recognized in Australia was scrub typhus (*Orientia tsutsugamushi*). As new settlers in Australia pushed north into tropical Queensland, they encountered many endemic febrile illnesses. Often these were referred to by their regional name (e.g., "Mossman" Fever). In fact, they were a mixture of diseases (malaria, leptospirosis, dengue, etc.), 1 of which was scrub typhus. As 1 of the key tasks of settlement was clearing the native vegetation (scrub), the disease was ultimately called

Address for correspondence: Dr Stephen Graves, Division of Microbiology, Hunter Area Pathology Service, Newcastle, Locked Bag #1 HRMC, NSW, 2310 Australia. Stephen.graves @hnehealth.nsw.gov.au

Rickettsiology and Rickettsial Diseases-Fifth International Conference: Ann. N.Y. Acad. Sci. 1166: 151–155 (2009).
doi: 10.1111/j.1749-6632.2009.04530.x © 2009 New York Academy of Sciences.

"scrub typhus." In 1935, 2 papers were published that identified a typhus-like disease, by positive OXK Weil-Felix serology, among patients in Cairns and Tully (both towns in north Queensland).[8,9] It was not epidemic typhus, so the authors initially called it "endemic typhus" (despite this name having already been used by Hone, to describe the typhus disease he had recognized, and which was later called murine typhus). Later, it was called "*tsutsugamushi* fever" when it was considered to be the same disease as that in Japan.[10] Ultimately, it was named scrub typhus. Today, the disease is still seen regularly in all regions of tropical Australia, including the Kimberley region of Western Australia,[11,12] the "top-end" of the Northern Territory,[13] north Queensland, and the Torres Strait Islands.[14]

The fourth rickettsial disease recognized in Australia was Q Fever (*Coxiella burnetii*). Q (query) Fever was an undiagnosed fever occurring among abattoir workers in Brisbane, Australia; it was first described by Derrick,[15] who inoculated the agent into guinea pigs, which then became febrile. The involvement of Burnet[16] resulted in its recognition as a rickettsial disease. Independently, workers in Montana, USA, who were studying a human pathogen obtained from a tick (*Dermacentor andersoni*), named their isolate the "Nine Mile" strain.[17] These 2 isolates were later shown to be the same microbe,[18] causing the same disease (Q Fever). Reflecting the contributions of both US workers (Cox *et al.*) and Australian workers (Burnet *et al.*), it was named *Coxiella burnetii*. It is found in many species of Australian ticks, especially those from bandicoots[19] and kangaroos.[20] Human infection, mostly in New South Wales and Queensland, is usually associated with aerosol spread from dried excreta of goats, cattle, and sheep. Recent Q Fever research in Australia has centered around Marmion's group in Adelaide. They have developed and tested a Q Fever vaccine, which is now produced and given routinely to selected persons in Australia such as abattoir workers. The vaccine is very effective.[21] Australia is the only country to have a human Q Fever vaccine available for general use. It has resulted in a significant reduction in occupational Q Fever.[22] Recent work has described the post-Q Fever fatigue syndrome[23] and its relationship to persistent *C.burnetii* antigen in patients.[24]

The fifth rickettsial disease recognized in Australia was Queensland Tick Typhus (*R. australis*), but it was the first spotted fever group (SFG) rickettsiosis detected. Soldiers training in the bush in Queensland during World War II who were infected by tick bite developed an eschar, fever and vesicular rash (the differential diagnosis being chicken pox).[25] The *Rickettsia* was isolated and later shown to be a genetic outlier in the SFG. It has been isolated from *Ixodes holcyclus* and *I. tasmani* ticks. Cases have occurred only down the east coast of Australia, from the tip of the continent and Torres Strait Island to the southeastern corner (Wilson's promontory, in Victoria). While the disease is generally considered to be mild, serious illness and death has occurred.[26]

The sixth (and final, at the time of writing) rickettsial disease is Flinders Island Spotted Fever (FISF), (*R. honei*), which is also a member of the SFG, albeit a mainstream member from a genetic viewpoint. The disease was recognized by Stewart,[27] the only doctor on Flinders Island, which is located in Bass Strait, between mainland Australia and the island state of Tasmania, at the southeast corner of the continent. It is a relatively mild disease, and no deaths have yet been recorded. The microbe was isolated from a patient during acute illness,[28] eventually described as a new species,[29] and to much surprise, was recognized as being widespread in the reptile tick *Aponoma* (now *Bothriocroton*) *hydrosauri*.[30] *R. honei* was named to honor Frank Hone, Australia's first rickettsiologist, who described murine typhus in 1922. The reptile ticks on lizards and snakes were heavily colonized, with 63% positive for the rickettsia. Attempts at infecting laboratory-bred and immunologically naïve blue-tongued lizards with ticks carrying *R.honei* were not successful (unpublished data). The disease FISF is now known to be more

TABLE 1. Spotted Fever Group Rickettsiae Detected in Australian Ticks

Rickettsia (proposed name)	Tick Species	Vertebrate Host	In Pure Culture?	Location in Australia
"*R.antechini*"	*Ixodes antechini*	*Antechinus* (marsupial mouse)	No	SW
"*R.argus*" (sp. nov)[a]	*Argus dewae* (soft-tick)	Gould's Wattled Bat	Yes	SE
"*R. derrickii*"	*Bothriocroton hydrosaurii*[b] (reptile tick)	Snakes/Lizards; Humans	No	SE
"*R. gravesii*" (sp.nov)[39][a]	*Amblyomma triguttatum*[b] *A. limbatum*	Kangaroo; Humans; Euro, Wallaroo; Bandicoot; Bettong; Possum	Yes	NW & SW
"*R.guntherii*"	*Haemaphysalis humerosa*	Northern Brown Bandicoot	No	NE
"*R. sauri*"	*Bothriocroton hydrosaurii*[b] (reptile tick)	Snakes/Lizards; Humans	No	SE
"*R. tasmanensis*"	*Ixodes tasmanii*[b]	Tasmanian Devil (marsupial); Humans	No	SE
"*Koala Rickettsia*"[40]	*Ixodes tasmanii*[b]	Koalas	No	Eastern

This table represents work by Nathan Unsworth, Helen Owen, Inger-Marie Vilcins, and Leonard Izzard.
[a]in culture.
[b]Tick species that bite humans.

widely spread in Australia (Tasmania, South Australia, Queensland, Torres Strait Islands)[31] and may be worldwide (Thailand, Sri Lanka, Italy).

Recently, a genetic variant of *R. honei*, the "marmionii" strain (named in honor of the Australian rickettsiologist Marmion), was discovered causing acute disease in several patients in eastern Australia.[32] Only one patient had a history of tick bite, and the tick (*Haemaphysalis novaeguineae*) was shown to contain the "marmionii" strain.[33] This strain has never been detected in the reptile tick, so its epidemiology is clearly different from that of the parent strain of *R.honei*. This latter *Rickettsia* has also been detected in the blood of 3% of chronically unwell patients (many with chronic fatigue) in Melbourne, Australia,[34] suggesting that this microbe may establish a chronic infection with possible relapse in some patients. It is not yet known if the presence of rickettsial DNA and/or positive rickettsial serology in these patients is causally related to their symptoms of chronic illness, or simply a reactivation phenomenon, which is sometimes seen in herpes virus reactivation during other illnesses.

There is 1 small island in Torres Strait (Darnley Island) that has 3 endemic rickettsiae: *R.australis*, *O.tsutsugumushi*, and *R.honei* (marmionii strain). [35]

Rickettsiales Associated with Australian Animals

Rickettsia felis has been detected in 4 species of fleas from dogs and cats in Western Australia,[36] but there have been no human cases yet described.

Anaplasma platys, transmitted by the dog tick *Rhipicephalus sanguineus* and dog louse *Heterodoxus spiniger*, is present in some Australian dogs,[37] especially in aboriginal communities.

Anaplasma marginale in cattle is transmitted by the ticks *Boophilus microplus* and *R. sanguineus*.[38]

No *Ehrlichia* sp. has yet been detected in Australia.

Several new spotted fever group *Rickettsia* have been detected in Australian ticks (Table 1). Two of these are growing in pure culture (*R. gravesii*, sp.nov), obtained from the kangaroo tick in Western Australia and *R. argus* sp. nov isolated from the soft tick *Argus dewae*. None is yet known to be a human pathogen.

In conclusion, our understanding of the epidemiology of rickettsiae and rickettsial diseases in Australia is still evolving and far from complete.

Conflicts of Interest

The authors declare no conflicts of interest.

References

1. Cumston, J.H.L & F. McCallum. 1927. The history of the intestinal infections and typhus fever in Australia 1788–1923. Melbourne Government Pinter, Service Publication #36, Australian Department of Health.

2. Tonge, J.I. 1959. Brill's Disease (recrudescent epidemic typhus) in Australia. *Med. J. Aust.* **19:** 919–921.

3. Hone, F.S. 1922. A series of cases closely resembling typhus fever. *Med. J. Aust.* 1–13.

4. Wheatland, F.T. 1926. A fever resembling a mild from of typhus fever. *Med. J. Aust.* 201–266.

5. Saint, E.G., A.F. Drummond & I.O. Thorburn. 1954. Murine typhus in Western Australia. *Med. J. Aust.* 731–737.

6. Beaman, M.H. & N. Marinovitch. 1999. Murine typhus in metropolitan Perth. *Med. J. Aust.* **170:** 93–94.

7. Jones, S.L. *et al.* 2004. Murine typhus: the first reported case from Victoria. *Med. J. Aust.* **180:** 482.

8. Langan, A.M. & R.Y. Matthew. 1935. The establishment of "Mossman", "Coastal" and other previously unclassified fevers of north Queensland as endemic typhus. *Med. J. Aust.* 145–148.

9. Unwin, M.L. 1935. "Coastal Fever" and endemic tropical typhus in north Queensland: recent investigations, clinical and laboratory findings. *Med. J. Aust.* 303–308.

10. Heaslip, W.G. 1941. Tsutsugamushi fever in north Queensland, Australia. *Med. J. Aust.* 380–392.

11. Quinlan, M.L & T. Chappell. 1993. Scrub typhus in Western Australia. *Communicable Diseases Intelligence (Australian Government)* **17:** 570–571.

12. Graves, S.R., L. Wang, Z. Nack & S. Jones. 1999. Rickettsia serosurvey in Kimberley, Western Australia. *Am. J. Trop. Med. Hyg.* **60:** 786–789.

13. Ralph, A., M. Raines, P. Whelan & B.J. Currie. 2004. Scrub typhus in the Northern Territory: exceeding the boundaries of Litchfield National park. *Communicable Diseases Intelligence (Australian Government)* **28:** 267–269.

14. Faa, A.G. *et al.* 2003. Scrub typhus in the Torres Strait Islands of North Queensland, Australia. *Emerg. Infect. Dis.* **9:** 480–482.

15. Derrick, E.H. 1937. "Q" Fever, a new fever entity: clinical features, diagnosis and laboratory investigations. *Med. J. Aust.* 281–299.

16. Burnet, F.M. & M. Freeman. 1937. Experimental studies on the virus of "Q" fever. *Med. J. Aust.* 299–305.

17. Davis, G.E. & H.R. Cox. 1938. A filter-passing infectious agent isolated from ticks. Isolation from *Dermacentor andersoni*, reactions in animals and filtration experiments. *Public Health Reports* **53:** 2259–2267.

18. Burnet, F.M. & M. Freeman. 1939. A comparative study of rickettsial strains from an infection of ticks in Montana (USA) and from Q Fever. *Med. J. Aust.* 887–891.

19. Derrick, E.H. & D.J.W. Smith. 1940. Studies in epidemiology of Q Fever. 2. The isolation of three strains of *Rickettsia burnetii* from the bandicoot *Isoodon torosus*. *Aust. J. Exp. Biol. Med. Sci.* **18:** 99–102.

20. Pope, J.H., W. Scott & R. Dwyer. 1960. *Coxiella burnetii* in kangaroos and kangaroo ticks in Western Queensland. *Aust. J. Exp. Biol.* **38:** 17–28.

21. Marmion, B.P. *et al.* 1990. Vaccine prophylaxis of abattoir – associated Q Fever: eight years' experience in Australian abattoirs. *Epidemiol. Infect.* **104:** 275–287.

22. Marmion, B.P. 2007. Q Fever: the long journey to control by vaccination. *Med. J. Aust.* **186:** 164–165.

23. Marmion, B.P. *et al.* 1996. Protracted debility and fatigue after Q Fever. *Lancet* **347:** 977–978.

24. Marmion, B.P. *et al.* 2005. Long-term persistence of *Coxiella burnetii* after acute primary Q Fever. *Q.J. Med.* **98:** 7–20.

25. Andrews, R., J.M. Bonnin & S. Williams. 1946. Tick typhus in north Queensland. *Med. J. Aust.* 253–258.

26. McBride, W.J.H., J.P. Hanson, R. Miller & D. Wenck. 2007. Severe spotted fever group rickettsiosis, Australia. *Emerg. Infect. Dis.* **13:** 1742–1744.

27. Stewart, R.S. 1991. Flinders Island Spotted Fever: a newly recognised endemic focus of tick typhus in Bass Strait. Part 1. Clinical & Epidemiology Features. *Med. J. Aust.* **154:** 94–99.

28. Graves, S.R. *et al.* 1993. Spotted Fever Group rickettsial infection in south-eastern Australia: isolation of rickettsiae. *Comp. Immun. Microbiol. Infect. Dis.* **16:** 223–233.

29. Stenos, R., V. Roux, D. Walker & D. Raoult. 1998. *Rickettsia honei* sp.nov. the aetiological agent of Flinders Island spotted fever in Australia. *Int. J. Systematic Bacteriology.* **48:** 1399–1404.

30. Stenos, J., S.R. Graves, V.L. Popov & D.H. Walker. 2003. *Aponomma hydrosauri*, the reptile-associated tick reservoir of *Rickettsia honei* on Flinders Island, Australia. *Am. J. Trop. Med. Hyg.* **69:** 314–317.

31. Unsworth, N.B. *et al.* 2005. Not only 'Flinders Island' spotted fever. *Pathology* **37:** 242–245.

32. Unsworth, N.B. *et al.* 2007. Flinders Island Spotted Fever rickettsioses caused by "marmionii" strain of *Rickettsia honei*, east Australia. *Emger. Infect. Dis.* **13:** 566–573.

33. Lane, A.M., M.D. Shaw, E.A. McGraw & S.L. O'Neill. 2005. Evidence of a spotted fever-like *Rickettsia* and a potential new vector from north eastern Australia. *J. Med. Entomol.* **42:** 918–921.

34. Unsworth, N.B. *et al*. 2008. Markers of exposure to spotted fever rickettsiae in patients with chronic illness, including fatigue, in two Australian populations. *Q.J. Med.* **101:** 269–274.

35. Unsworth, N.B., J. Stenos, A.G. Faa & S.R. Graves. 2007. Three rickettsioses, Darnley Island, Australia. *Emerg. Infect. Dis.* **13:** 1105–1107.

36. Schloderer, D. *et al*. 2006. *Rickettsia felis* in fleas, Western Australia. *Emerg. Infect. Dis.* **12:** 841–843.

37. Brown, G.K. *et al*. 2006. Detection of *Anaplasma platys* and *Babesia canis vogeli* and their impact on platelet numbers in free-roaming dogs associated with remote aboriginal communities in Australia. *Aust. Vet. J.* **84:** 321–325.

38. Callow, L.L. 1984. *Animal Health in Australia. Vol.5. Protozoal and Rickettsial Diseases*. Australian Government Publishing Service. Canberra, 177–200.

39. Owen, H. *et al*. 2006. Detection and identification of a novel spotted fever group rickettsiae in Western Australia. *Ann. N.Y. Acad. Sci.* **1078:** 197–199.

40. Vilcins, I-M.E., J.M. Old & E.M. Deane. 2008. Detection of a spotted fever group Rickettsia in the tick *Ixodes tasmani* collected from koalas in Port Macquarie, Australia. *J. Med. Entomol.* **45:** 745–750.

Ecology of Rickettsia in South America

Marcelo B. Labruna

Department of Preventive Veterinary Medicine and Animal Health, Faculty of Veterinary Medicine, University of São Paulo, São Paulo, Brazil

Until the year 2000, only three *Rickettsia* species were known in South America: (i) *Rickettsia rickettsii*, transmitted by the ticks *Amblyomma cajennense,* and *Amblyomma aureolatum*, reported in Colombia, Argentina, and Brazil, where it is the etiological agent of Rocky Mountain spotted fever; (ii) *Rickettsia prowazekii*, transmitted by body lice and causing epidemic typhus in highland areas, mainly in Peru; (iii) *Rickettsia typhi*, transmitted by fleas and causing endemic typhus in many countries. During this new century, at least seven other rickettsiae were reported in South America: *Rickettsia felis* infecting fleas and the tick-associated agents *Rickettsia parkeri, Rickettsia massiliae, Candidatus* "Rickettsia amblyommii," *Rickettsia bellii, Rickettsia rhipicephali*, and *Candidatus* "Rickettsia andeanae." Among these other rickettsiae, only *R. felis*, *R. parkeri*, and *R. massiliae* are currently recognized as human pathogens. *R. rickettsii* is a rare agent in nature, infecting ≤1% individuals in a few tick populations. Contrastingly, *R. parkeri, Candidatus* "*R. amblyommii," R. rhipicephali*, and *R. bellii* are usually found infecting 10 to 100% individuals in different tick populations. Despite rickettsiae being transmitted transovarially through tick generations, low infection rates for *R. rickettsii* are possibly related to pathogenic effect of *R. rickettsii* for ticks, as shown for *A. aureolatum* under laboratory conditions. This scenario implies that *R. rickettsii* needs amplifier vertebrate hosts for its perpetuation in nature, in order to create new lines of infected ticks (horizontal transmission). In Brazil, capybaras and opossums are the most probable amplifier hosts for *R. rickettsii*, among *A. cajennense* ticks, and small rodents for *A. aureolatum*.

Key words: *Rickettsia*; ecology; tick; lice; flea; South America

Introduction

Until the year 2000, only three *Rickettsia* species were known to occur in South America, being two typhus group (TG) species (*Rickettsia prowazekii* and *Rickettsia typhi*) and only one spotted fever group (SFG) species (*Rickettsia rickettsii*). These three species are pathogenic for humans to whom *R. prowazekii* is transmitted by lice, *R. typhi* by fleas, and *R. rickettsii* by ticks. During this new century, at least 7 other *Rickettsia* species were reported in South America: *Rickettsia felis* infecting fleas in Argentina, Brazil, Chile, Peru, and Uruguay, *Rickettsia parkeri* in-fecting ticks in Uruguay and Brazil, *Rickettsia massiliae* infecting ticks in Argentina, *Candidatus* "Rickettsia amblyommii" infecting ticks in Argentina, Brazil, and French Guyana, *Rickettsia bellii* infecting ticks in Argentina and Brazil, *Rickettsia rhipicephali* infecting ticks in Brazil, and *Candidatus* "Rickettsia andeanae" infecting ticks in Peru. Among these, all species are classified into the SFG except for *R. bellii*, which in neither a TG nor a SFG species.

Rickettsia rickettsii

Rickettsia rickettsii is the most pathogenic *Rickettsia* species of the world.[1] It has been reported in Canada, United States, Mexico, Costa Rica, Panama, Colombia, Brazil, and Argentina.[2,3] The disease caused by *R. rickettsii* is generally

Address for correspondence: Marcelo B. Labruna, Faculdade de Medicina Veterinária e Zootecnia, Universidade de São Paulo. Av. Prof. Dr. Orlando Marques de Paiva, 87, São Paulo, Brazil 05508-270. Voice: +55-11-3091-1394; fax: +55-011-3091-7928. labruna@usp.br

Rickettsiology and Rickettsial Diseases-Fifth International Conference: Ann. N.Y. Acad. Sci. 1166: 156–166 (2009).
doi: 10.1111/j.1749-6632.2009.04516.x © 2009 New York Academy of Sciences.

called Rocky Mountain spotted fever (RMSF), because it was first reported in the Rocky Mountain region of the United States, but it is also called as Brazilian spotted fever (BSF) in Brazil. Different tick species have been implicated as vectors of *R. rickettsii* accordingly to different geographic areas. Whereas the ticks *Dermacentor andersoni* and *Dermacentor variablilis* are the main vectors in the United States,[2] *Amblyomma cajennense* has been implicated to be the most important vector in South America. *Amblyomma aureolatum* is also a recognized vector within the metropolitan area of São Paulo city,[4] where *Rhipicephalus sanguineus* is a suspected vector.[5]

RMSF has been reported in Brazil since the 1920s. After various reports during the 1930s and 1940s, much fewer reports were released from the 1950s to early 1980s. From the end of the 1980s to the beginning of the present century, there has been a clear re-emergence of the disease in Brazil. For example, from 1988 to 1997, there were 25 laboratory-confirmed cases distributed among 6 municipalities in the state of São Paulo. During the subsequent decade, from 1998 to 2007, there were 255 confirmed cases distributed among 54 municipalities of the state. Indeed, this increase is partially attributed to a much more efficient surveillance, especially after the disease became nationally notifiable in 2001. However, ecological factors seem to have played a major role, as discussed below. In the southeastern region of Brazil, composed by four states (São Paulo, Minas Gerais, Rio de Janeiro, and Espírito Santo), there were 334 laboratory-confirmed cases of RMSF from 1995 to 2004, with a 31% fatality-ratio. Only in the state of São Paulo, 128 additional cases (case fatality: 29%) were confirmed from 2005 to 2007 (official data from the São Paulo State Health Secretary).

A. cajennense is one of the most common tick species in southeastern Brazil, where it is far the most frequent human-biting tick. Comparing to *A. cajennense,* other tick species are seldom found biting humans in southeastern Brazil.[6] The most abundant primary hosts for *A. cajen-* *nense* in southeastern Brazil are horses and capybaras (*Hydrochoerus hydrochaeris*), which are infested by all tick's parasitic stages. Humans are also attacked by all parasitic stages, usually by hundreds of larvae, dozens of nymphs, or/and a few adult specimens. Fortunately, serologic-based studies on horses and capybaras (sentinels for RMSF within the distribution area of *A. cajennense* in Brazil) have indicated that very few populations of *A. cajennense* are infected by SFG rickettsiae.[7,8] This finding is corroborated by the low number of RMSF cases in the southeastern region of Brazil, in contrast to the large human population that is exposed to infestations by *A. cajennense* in almost the entire rural area of this region. Even in RMSF-endemic areas in Brazil, infection rates by *R. rickettsii* among *A. cajennense* populations are usually very low, around 1%,[9] or low enough for some studies to have failed to find a *R. rickettsii*-infected tick specimen.[7]

A. aureolatum has been implicated as the vector of *R. rickettsii* in the São Paulo metropolitan area since the 1930s.[10] The adult stage of this tick uses Carnivore species (mostly the domestic dog) as primary host while immature stages seem to use Passeriformes birds and a few rodent species as primary hosts.[11] Humans are attacked only by the adult stage, usually by a single adult tick, because population density of this tick species is usually low.[12] One recent study found 0.9% (6/669) *A. aureolatum* ticks to be infected by *R. rickettsii*.[4] In most of the sites of transmission of *R. rickettsii* by *A. aureolatum, A. cajennense* is scarce or absent, whereas *R. sanguineus* is sometimes abundant.[5,12]

In vertebrate hosts, *R. rickettsii* causes acute infection lasting for only a few days or weeks, with no persistent maintenance of the agent.[13] Thus, vertebrate hosts cannot be considered reservoirs of *R. rickettsii* in nature. Studies in the United States demonstrated that *R. rickettsii* is transmitted transovarially and transstadially in several tick species occurring in North America, including its main tick vectors *D. andersoni, D. variabilis,* and *R. sanguineus*.[2,13,14] These laboratory studies indicated that ticks are the main reservoir of *R. rickettsii* in nature.[15] However, other factors must account for the usually low *R. rickettsii*-infection rates in ticks, ranging from 0.05 to 1.3% in the United States and Brazil.[4,7,9,13]

Burgdorfer and Brinton[16] and Nielbisky[17] showed that *R. rickettsii* displays some degree of pathogenicity to both *D. anndersoni* and *D. variabilis* ticks, thus uninfected ticks would have advantage over infected ticks in a tick population during consecutive generations. This rickettsial pathogenicity is possibly the major cause of very low infection rates of *R. rickettsii*-infected ticks in nature. Thus, even that ticks are the main reservoir of *R. rickettsii* in nature, the *R. rickettsii* pathogenicity for ticks precludes its enzootic maintenance solely by transovarial and transstadial transmissions in ticks.[17] In this case, the participation of amplifier hosts (vertebrate animals that develop a rickettsemia for some days) is crucial when new uninfected ticks become infected and start new lineages of infected ticks within the tick population.[2] In the United States, several small rodent species have been implicated to act as amplifier hosts of *R. rickettsii*, as for example, *Microtus pennsylvanicus* for *D. variabilis* in the eastern part of the country.[13,15,18]

In general, a vertebrate host species has to fulfill the following five requirements in order to be considered an efficient amplifier host for *R. rickettsii* in a given RMSF-endemic area:

1. It has to be abundant in the *R. rickettsii*-endemic area.
2. It has to be a major host for the tick vector.
3. It has to be susceptible to the *R. rickettsii* infection.
4. Once infected by *R. rickettsii*, the host has to develop a rickettsemia of sufficient length and degree to infect ticks that feed on this host.
5. It has to be a prolific species, in order to have a continuous introduction of nonimmune animals in the host population.

M. pennsylvanicus is an efficient amplifier host species for *R. rickettsii* in the United States because it is abundant in many *R. rickettsii*-endemic areas in the eastern part of the country, where it is also a primary host for the immature stages of *D. variablilis*.[15] In addition, *M. pennsylvanicus* has been shown to be highly susceptible to *R. rickettsii*, as it developed rickettsemia for 6 to 8 days in concentrations sufficient to infect nearly 100% of uninfected *Dermacentor* larvae that fed on them.[18] Finally, as any other small rodent, *M. pennsylvanicus* is highly prolific, as average females have between one and five litters in a year, producing about five pups in each litter.[19] This last requirement is very important if one considers that once living in an endemic area, each individual host will develop only one rickettsemia (lasting for a few days or weeks) during its lifetime, since after the rickettsemia, the animal develops strong immunity against the agent, precluding a second rickettsemia.[20,21]

In Brazil, at least two animals are incriminated to act as efficient amplifier hosts for *A. cajennense*: capybaras and opossums (*Didelphis* spp.). Capybaras are abundant and act as primary hosts for *A. cajennense* in all RMSF-endemic areas of the state of São Paulo, where *A. cajennense* is the vector, in contrast to many other non-endemic areas for RMSF with abundant populations of *A. cajennense* sustained by horses in the absence of capybaras. Earlier studies in the 1940s showed that capybaras are susceptible to the *R. rickettsii* infection, with rickettsemia lasting for several weeks.[22] Capybaras are prolific, generating a mean of six pups per female per year.[23] Finally, a recent study in our laboratory has shown that after being experimentally infected with *R. rickettsii*, rickettsemic capybaras infected 20–25% of the *A. cajennense* nymphs that fed on them, as shown by PCR performed on the adult ticks that molted from the nymphs.[24]

Coupled to these evidences, the major environmental modification implicated to have contributed to the re-emergence of RMSF in the state of São Paulo is the explosive increase of capybara populations during the last few decades. There are no official numbers about the temporal distribution of capybaras in São Paulo, however it is well known that this large rodent was considered threatened with extinction during the 1950s; during subsequent decades capybaras increased in populations in many areas, and nowadays it is considered a major cause of crop damage in the state,[25] besides various complaints of high environmental burdens by *A. cajennense* due to increased capybara populations. An increase in capybara populations is considered to be a result of extensive reforestation of areas near water courses (capybaras have a strong affinity to water, which they use for mating and avoiding predators) and strict laws prohibiting wildlife hunting in Brazil. Since these reforestation areas lack natural predators of capybaras (e.g., jaguars, anacondas, and alligators), and the nearby crops (e.g., corn, sugarcane) provide an abundant food supply, capybaras encountered an anthropogenic habitat where they can reach population densities much higher than those usually seen in its natural habitats in Pantanal and Amazon.[25]

Opossums (*Didelphis* spp.) are abundant in all RMSF-endemic areas of Brazil, where they can be infested by a large number of *A. cajennense* immature ticks, sometimes with close to 1,000 immature *Amblyomma* ticks (mostly *A. cajennense*) per opossum.[26] The susceptibility of opossums to the *R. rickettsii* infection has been demonstrated since the 1930s, when the first isolations of *R. rickettsii* from naturally infected wildlife were performed, being one from *Didelphis aurita* (reported as *Didelphis marsupialis*)[27] from the state of Minas Gerais and another from *D. aurita* from the state of São Paulo.[28] Interestingly, in the United States the opossum *Didelphis virginiana* was experimentally shown to develop a rickettsemia lasting for 3 to 4 weeks after being experimentally inoculated with *R. rickettsii*.[29] This has been the longest rickettsemic period ever reported for *R. rickettsii* infection; other animals develop rickettsemia usually lasting for 1 to 2 weeks.[18,20] Opossums are also prolific, the female births 5 to 9 young between 1 and 3 times per year. Finally, a recent study in our laboratory has shown that *R. rickettsii*-experimentally-infected opossums (*Didelphis aurita*) developed rickettsemia lasting for 3 to 4 weeks, when ~5–20% of the *A. cajennnense* immature ticks that fed on them became infected by *R. rickettsii*, as shown by PCR performed on the ticks after molting.[30]

For *A. aureolatum*, there is little available ecological information, although the rodent *Euryzygomatomys spinosus* is largely suspected to be an amplifier host for *R. rickettsii*. This rodent is abundant in RMSF-endemic areas in the São Paulo metropolitan area, where it is suspected to be a primary host for the immature stages of *A. aureolatum*.[31] *E. spinosus* is also a prolific species, but there is no available information regarding its susceptibility to *R. rickettsii*. However, *E. spinosus* is phylogenetically closely related to guinea pigs (*Cavea aperea porcellus*), as they both belong to the same Rodent infraorder, the Caviomorpha. Since guinea pigs are highly susceptible to *R. rickettsii* and also develop rickettsemia in a sufficient magnitude to infect feeding ticks,[18] it is possible that *E. spinosus* would give similar results and act as amplifier hosts for *R. rickettsii* in RMSF-endemic areas of the São Paulo metropolitan area, as suggested recently.[31]

In a recent study in our laboratory, each of six guinea pigs, experimentally infected with *R. rickettsii*, were simultaneously infested by larvae of *A. cajennense* and *A. aureolatum* (tick species were infested separately, into two feeding chambers glued to the back of each guinea pig). After feeding during the guinea pig febrile period, engorged larvae of the two species were collected and allowed to molt to nymphs in an incubator. The resultant nymphs were tested by PCR (10–20 nymphs per species per guinea pig) giving the following results: 80 to 100% of the *A. aureolatum* nymphs from six guinea pigs were PCR positive, whereas only 10 to 60% of the *A. cajennense* nymphs were PCR positive.[32] These results clearly indicate that *A. cajennense* are much less susceptible to the *R. rickettsii* infection, even after they fed on animals developing rickettsemia with sufficient magnitude to infect 100% of the *A. aureolatum* ticks. As an important note, part of the *A. cajennense* ticks used in this study were derived from uninfected females collected in a RMSF-endemic area in the state of São Paulo, thus they represented a tick population that has been incriminated in transmitting *R. rickettsii* to humans. An ongoing study in our laboratory has also shown that *R. rickettsii* is moderately pathogenic for *A. aureolatum* ticks, especially engorged females (M. B. Labruna, unpublished data).

Considering that not all *A. cajennense* ticks become infected by *R. rickettsii* after feeding on a highly competent experimental amplifier host (i.e., guinea pig), the fact that only a minority of the *A. cajennense* ticks sustained the rickettsial infection after feeding on *R. rickettsii*-infected opossums or capybaras means that these wild animals are also competent amplifier hosts for *R. rickettsii*. This partial susceptibility of *A. cajennense* for *R. rickettsii* infection might explain why so few populations of this tick species are found naturally infected by *R. rickettsii*, despite its widespread distribution in central and southeastern Brazil. Also, it might explain the scarcity of human cases in RMSF-endemic areas where humans are often attacked by *A. cajennense*; usually in mass attack by hundreds or thousands of ticks. Interestingly, Parker and colleagues[14] showed under experimental conditions that *A. cajennense* was an efficient vector of *R. rickettsii*, with successful transstadial transmission of the agent. However, a subsequent study revealed that the *A. cajenennse* tick colony used in the study of Parker and colleagues[14] was, in fact, another tick species, described later as *Amblyomma imitator*.[33] Even though, Monteiro and Fonseca[34] demonstrated transovarial transmission, and Brumpt[35] demonstrated transstadial transmission of *R. rickettsii* in *A. cajennense*, but always without quantification analysis.

In contrast to *A. cajennense*, *A. aureolatum* seems to be a very efficient reservoir of *R. rickettsii* because usually 100% of the ticks became infected after feeding on a competent amplifier host (i.e., guinea pigs). In addition, Pinter and Labruna[36] reported 100% transstadial transmission (larvae to nymphs) of *R. rickettsii* in *A.*

aureolatum. However, population densities of *A. aureolatum* are generally low, and humans are seldom infested by this tick. In a two-year study in a RMSF-endemic area of the São Paulo metropolitan area, dogs were found to be continuously infested by adults of *A. aureolatum*, with mean infestations around 2 ticks per dog; during this same period, human infestation was documented only once by a single tick specimen.[12] This might explain why RMSF cases are also sporadically reported even in this area, besides the high vectoral competence of *A. aureolatum*.

RMSF continues to be a threatening disease because high lethality rates are still occurring. The disease has shown to have a complex ecology with participation of different vertebrate animals and tick species from the United States to Argentina. Besides capybaras and opossums, other potential animal species have been implicated to act as amplifier hosts in Brazil, as is the case of rabbits (*Sylvilagus brasiliensis*) and the domestic dog.[37] More studies are needed to determine the role of the dog tick, *R. sanguineus*, in the ecology of RMSF in South America. This tick is widespread in all South American countries, and a recent study found *R. rickettsii*-infected *R. sanguineus* ticks in Brazil.[5] Further ecological studies in each of the RMSF-endemic areas are needed in order to understand the dynamics of the occurrence of the disease, and consequently, to generate subsidies for adoption of more rational preventive and control methods.

Rickettsia prowazekii and Rickettsia typhi

R. prowazekii is the etiologic agent of epidemic typhus, the second most severe rickettsiosis of the world. The only known vector of *R. prowazekii* in South America is the human body lice, *Pediculus humanus corporis*. During the last decades, the occurrence of epidemic typhus in South America has been confirmed only in Peru, especially in the Calca-Cuzco zones.[38] *R. prowazekii* is highly lethal for lice, in which the bacterium is transstadially but not transovarially transmitted.[39] Unlike other rickettsiosis, humans surviving from *R. prowazekii*-acute infection usually develop asymptomatic latent infection for many years, with the possibility of a later recrudescence that could start new epidemics by infecting new lice. A recent study reported the isolation of *R. prowazekii* from *Amblyomma* ticks in Mexico, suggesting a participation of ticks in the ecology of epidemic typhus.[40]

The occurrence of *R. typhi* in South America has been reported since the first decades of the last century.[41] *R. typhi* is the etiologic agent of murine typhus, a rarely lethal, however, very incapacitating rickettsiosis. *R. typhi* is classically vectored by the flea species *Xenopsylla cheops*, but the occurrence of transovarial transmission of *R. typhi* in fleas seem to be a rare event.[42] *R. typhi* is widely distributed in the world, however, it has been largely neglected in South America during the last decades. Except for a few recent studies reporting endemic typhus in Brazil and Colombia,[43,44] there has been no clinical or ecological study of *R. typhi* in South America. This situation will possibly remain stable because there has been no interest of South American laboratories to implement proper techniques for diagnosis of TG rickettsia. For example, the Brazilian reference laboratories for the diagnosis of RMSF employ serological methods with SFG antigens, but most of the time no TG antigen is available. Since there is little or no cross-reactivity between TG and SFG rickettsiae, possibly several cases of TG rickettsiosis have been undiagnosed in Brazil.

Rickettsia parkeri

R. parkeri was first shown to cause spotted fever in humans in the United States in 2004, 65 years after this rickettsia was first isolated from the tick *Amblyomma maculatum* in that country.[45] Currently, *R. parkeri* is a recognized human pathogen with several confirmed cases in the United States, where it is transmitted by *A.*

maculatum.[46,47] One retrospective study in the United States provided serological evidence, for a number of RMSF cases (presumably caused by *R. rickettsii*) were caused by *R. parkeri*, suggesting that rickettsiosis due to *R. parkeri* has been misidentified with RMSF in that country.[48] There has been convincing evidence that *R. parkeri* is the agent responsible for previously reported cases of SFG rickettsiosis in southern Uruguay, with transmission by the tick *Amblyomma triste*.[46,49]

Recent studies have shown that nearly 10% of both *A. maculatum* and *A. triste* ticks are infected by *R. parkeri* in the United States and Uruguay, respectively.[49,50] In the study of the United States, all tick populations tested were shown to be infected by *R. parkeri*, indicating that this agent is widely distributed among the *A. maculatum* distribution area in that country. One study in Brazil also reported ~10% infection rate by *R. parkeri* in an *A. triste* population, besides human infection by this agent in Brazil remains to be reported.[51] Overall, all populations of both *A. maculatum* and *A. triste* tested so far have been found infected by *R. parkeri*. Since *A. maculatum* is distributed from southern United States to the northwestern part of South America, whereas *A. triste* is likely to be established in most countries of South America,[52] it is possible that *R. parkeri* is also widely distributed in the Americas. Interestingly, these two tick species are morphologically, genetically, and ecologically very closely related, indicating that further studies are needed to test if they represent different strains of a single species or if they have just gone through speciation. Thus, human cases by *R. parkeri* in South America have been possibly undiagnosed or misdiagnosed with *R. rickettsii*, since this rickettsia seems to cause a milder disease culminating in no lethality to date, what turns even more difficult a definitive diagnosis.

The intimate relation of *R. parkeri* with its primary vectors, added by high infection rates among tick populations (if compared to *R. rickettsii*), are indicative that ticks are very efficient reservoirs of this rickettsia, although further studies are needed to evaluate the role of amplifier hosts in the ecology of this rickettsia.

Rickettsia felis

Since the end of the last century, cases of flea-borne spotted fever have been reported throughout the world, implicating *R. felis* as the etiological agent.[53] Like its main host (fleas of the genus *Ctenocephalides*), *R. felis* seems to be cosmopolitan. In South America, *R. felis* has been reported infecting *Ctenocephalides* spp. fleas in Argentina, Brazil, Chile, Peru, and Uruguay, but human infection by *R. felis* has been reported only in Brazil so far.[54,55]

Laboratory studies showed that *R. felis* is successfully maintained in flea populations by transstadial and transovarial transmission.[56] Field studies with different *Ctenocephalides* spp. populations in the above-mentioned South American countries have shown that 13.5 to 90% of the individual fleas are infected by *R. felis*.[54,55] Indeed, such high infection rates indicate that *R. felis* is not pathogenic for fleas under natural conditions of South America.

Ctenocephalides fleas are the most prevalent and abundant fleas of dogs and cats in South America and possibly in the world. Since the vast majority of the *Ctenocephalides* populations are infected by *R. felis*, usually at high infection rates, one would expect that flea-borne spotted fever would occur more frequently than currently recognized. However, one study showed no serologic evidence of *R. felis* infection in dogs, cats, and opossums that were parasitized by *R. felis*-infected fleas in different areas of the state of São Paulo.[57] In another study, cats artificially infested by *R. felis*-infected fleas took a minimum of 2 to 4 months to seroconvert while other cats did not seroconvert, despite various previous contact with infected fleas.[58] A study in Chile showed serologic evidence of *R. felis* infection in 16/22 (72.7%) cats that sustained a *R. felis*-infected flea population.[54] These studies show that despite of the widespread distribution of *R. felis*, cases of human or animal infection by

this agent are rare or irregular. Possibly, *Ctenocephalides* fleas are not a very efficient vector of *R. felis*. Previous analyses of infected fleas showed that *R. felis* colonizes the midgut, muscles, fat body, tracheal matrix, and reproduction organs, but not the salivary glands.[59] The presence of *R. felis* DNA in feces of infected fleas has also been reported.[56] A more recent study demonstrated the presence of *R. felis* in flea salivary glands for the first time, but it is not known if the agent is also present in flea saliva.[60] If *R. felis* is not transmitted via flea saliva, possible transmission mechanisms could be through the ingestion of infected fleas or contact of damaged skin or mucosa with fresh flea feces containing viable *R. felis*. In addition, it is possible that due to unknown reasons, only a minority of humans and animals are susceptible to the *R. felis* infection.

Other Rickettsia Species

Several other *Rickettsia* species have been reported infecting South American ticks recently (Table 1). All these rickettsia but *R. bellii* are considered to be SFG rickettsiae. No human infection by these rickettsiae has been reported in South America. The finding of *R. massiliae* in Argentina[61] deserves attention because until this report, *R. massiliae* was known to occur only in the Old World, where it was first described in 1993 infecting *Rhipicephalus* spp. ticks in Europe and Africa.[62] More than 10 years later, this rickettsia was first shown to be pathogenic for humans in Europe.[63] Due to the widespread distribution of *R. sanguineus* in South America, it is possible that undiagnosed or misdiagnosed cases of *R. massiliae* are occurring in this continent. Regarding the other rickettsiae described in Table 1, at least among animals, there has been serological evidence of canine infection by *Candidatus* "R. amblyommii" and *R. rhipicephali*,[64] and capybara infection by *R. bellii*.[8]

Since these other rickettsiae usually infect ticks at high infection rates (10 to 100%), they are possibly non-pathogenic for ticks. In

TABLE 1. Other *Rickettsia* spp. Reported Infecting Ticks in South America

Rickettsia	Tick species[Reference]	Country
R. rhipicephali	*Haemaphysalis juxtakochi*[67]	Brazil
R. bellii	*Amblyomma dubitatum* (reported as *A. cooperi*),[68] *A. aureolatum*,[4] *A. ovale*,[69] *A. oblongoguttatum*,[69] *A. rotundatum*,[69] *A. humerale*,[69] *A. scalpturatum*,[69] *A. neumanni*,[70] *H. juxtakochi*,[67] *Ixodes loricatus*[65]	Argentina, Brazil
R. massiliae	*Rhipicephalus sanguineus*[61]	Argentina
Candidatus "R. amblyommii"	*A. cajennense*,[69] *A. coelebs*,[69,71] *A. neumanni*[70]	Argentina, Brazil, French Guyana
Candidatus "R. andeanae"	*I. boliviensis*,[72] *A. maculatum*[72]	Peru
Rickettsia sp. strain Argentina	*A. parvum*[73]	Argentina
Rickettsia sp. strain COOPERI*	*A. dubitatum* (reported as *A. cooperi*)[68]	Brazil
Rickettsia sp. strain AL#	*A. longirostre*[74]	Brazil
Rickettsia sp. strain ARANHA#	*A. longirostre*[75]	Brazil

*This rickettsia is possibly a different strain of *R. parkeri*
#These rickettsiae are possibly different strains of Candidatus "R. amblyommii"

addition, transovarial transmission seems to be a rule for them, as it has been shown for *R. bellii* in *I. loricatus*.[65] These other rickettsiae might also have a role in the *R. rickettsii* ecology, since once prevailing at higher infection rates in some tick populations, these rickettsiae could prevent the establishment of *R. rickettsii* infection in these tick populations by the interference mechanism, as previously reported for some tick populations in the United States.[13,66]

Acknowledgments

Financial support by Fundação de Amparo a Pesquisa do Estado de São Paulo (FAPESP) and Conselho Nacional de Desenvolvimento Científico e Tecnologógico (CNPq).

Conflicts of Interest

The author declares no conflicts of interest.

References

1. Parola, P., C.D. Paddock & D. Raoult. 2005. Tick-borne rickettsioses around the world: emerging diseases challenging old concepts. *Clin. Microbiol. Rev.* **18:** 719–756.
2. Dumler, J.S. & D.H. Walker. 2005. Rocky Mountain spotted fever-changing ecology and persisting virulence. *N. Engl. J. Med.* **353:** 551–553.
3. Paddock, C.D. *et al.* 2008. Rocky mountain spotted fever in Argentina. *Am. J. Trop. Med. Hyg.* **78:** 687–692.
4. Pinter, A. & M.B. Labruna. 2006. Isolation of *Rickettsia rickettsii* and *Rickettsia bellii* in cell culture from the tick *Amblyomma aureolatum* in Brazil. *Ann. N.Y. Acad. Sci.* **1078:** 523–529.
5. Moraes-Filho, J. *et al.* 2009. New epidemiological data on Brazilian spotted fever in an endemic area of the state of São Paulo, Brazil. *Vector Borne Zoonotic Dis.* **9:** 73–78.
6. Guglielmone, A.A. *et al.* 2006. Ticks (Ixodidae) on humans in South America. *Exp. Appl. Acarol.* **40:** 83–100.
7. Sangioni, L.A. *et al.* 2005. Rickettsial infection in animals and Brazilian Spotted Fever endemicity. *Emerg. Infect. Dis.* **11:** 265–270.
8. Pacheco, R.C. *et al.* 2007. Rickettsial infection in capybaras (*Hydrochoerus hydrochaeris*) from São Paulo, Brazil: serological evidence for infection by *Rickettsia bellii* and *Rickettsia parkeri*. *Biomedica* **27:** 364–371.
9. Guedes, E. *et al.* 2005. Detection of *Rickettsia rickettsii* in the tick *Amblyomma cajennense* in a new Brazilian spotted fever-endemic area in the state of Minas Gerais. *Mem. Inst. Oswaldo Cruz* **100:** 841–845.
10. Gomes, L.S. 1933. Typho exanthematico de São Paulo. *Brasil-Medico* **17:** 919–921.
11. Guglielmone, A.A. *et al.* 2003. *Amblyomma aureolatum* (Pallas, 1772) and *Amblyomma ovale* Koch, 1844 (Acari: Ixodidae): hosts, distribution and 16S rDNA sequences. *Vet. Parasitol.* **113:** 273–288.

12. Pinter, A. *et al*. 2004. Study of the seasonal dynamics, life cycle, and host specificity of *Amblyomma aureolatum* (Acari: Ixodidae). *J. Med. Entomol.* **41:** 324–332.

13. Burgdorfer, W. 1988. Ecological and epidemiological considerations of Rocky Mountain spotted fever and scrub typhus. *Biology of Rickettsial Diseases.* D.H. Walker, Ed.: 33–50. CRC Inc. Boca Raton, FL.

14. Parker, R., C.B. Philip & W.L. Jellinson. 1933. Rocky Mountain spotted fever. Potentialities oof tick transmission in relation to geographic occurrence in the United States. *Am. J. Trop. Med.* **13:** 241–378.

15. McDade, J.E. & V.F. Newhouse. 1986. Natural history of *Rickettsia rickettsii*. *Annu. Rev. Microbiol.* **40:** 287–309.

16. Burgdorfer, W. & L.P. Brinton. 1975. Mechanisms of transovarial infection of spotted fever rickettsiae in ticks. *Ann. N. Y. Acad. Sci.* **266:** 61–72.

17. Niebylski, M.L., M.G. Peacock & T.G. Schwan. 1999. Lethal effect of *Rickettsia rickettsii* on its tick vector (*Dermacentor andersoni*). *Appl. Environ. Microbiol.* **65:** 773–778.

18. Burgdorfer, W., K.T. Friedhoff & J.L. Lancaster. 1966. Natural history of tick-borne spotted fever in the USA. Susceptibility of small mammals to virulent *Rickettsia rickettsii*. *Bull. Wld. Hlth. Org.* **35:** 149–153.

19. Meikle, D.B., M.D. Spritzer, & N.G. Solomon. 2006. Social dominance among male meadow voles is inversely related to reproductive success. *Ethology* **112:** 1027–1037.

20. Lundgreen, D.L. & B.D. Thorpe. 1966. Infectious diseases in wild animals in Utah. VII. Experimental infection of rodents with *Rickettsia rickettsii*. *Am. J. Trop. Med. Hyg.* **15:** 799–806.

21. Philip, C.B. 1959. Some epidemiological considerations in Rocky Mountain spotted fever. *Pub. Health Rep.* **74:** 595–600.

22. Travassos, J. & A. Vallejo. 1942. Comportamento de alguns cavídeos (*Cavia aperea* e *Hydrochoerus capybara*) às inoculações experimentais do vírus da febre maculosa. Possibilidade desses cavídeos representarem o papel de depositários transitórios do vírus na natureza. *Mem. Inst. Butantan* **15:** 73–86.

23. Ojasti, J. 1973. *Estudio Biologico del Chigüire o Capibara.* FONAIAP, Caracas, Venezuela.

24. Souza, C. *et al*. 2008. Experimental infection of capybaras *Hydrochaeris hydrochoerus* by *Rickettsia rickettsii* and evaluation of the transmission of the infection to *Amblyomma cajennense* [Abstract]. Presented at the *6th International Conference on Ticks and Tick-borne Pathogens.* Buenos Aires, Argentina, September 23.

25. Verdade, L.M. & K.M.P.M.B. Ferraz. 2006. Capybaras in an anthropogenic habitat in southeastern Brazil. *Braz. J. Biol.* **66:** 371–378.

26. Perez, C. 2007. Bioecologia e manejo do carrapato-estrela, *Amblyomma cajennense* (Fabricius) (Acari: Ixodi-

dae), vetor da febre maculosa brasileira. Ph.D. thesis, University of São Paulo, Piracicaba, São Paulo, Brazil.

27. Moreira, J.A. & O. Magalhães. 1935. Thypho exanthematico em Minas Gerais. *Brasil-Médico* **44:** 465–470.

28. Travassos, J. 1937. Identification d'un virus semblable a celui du "Typhus exanthématique de Sao Paulo", isolé de la sarigue marsupiale (*Didelphis paraguayensis*). *Compt. Rend. Soc. Biol.* **126:** 1054–1056.

29. Bozeman, F.M. *et al*. 1967. Ecology of Rocky Mountain spotted fever. II. Natural infection of wild mammals and birds in Virginia and Maryland. *Am. J. Trop. Med. Hyg.* **16:** 48–59.

30. Horta, M.C. *et al*. 2009. Experimental infection of opossums *Didelphis aurita* by *Rickettsia rickettsii* and evaluation of the transmission of the infection to ticks *Amblyomma cajennense*. *Vector Borne Zoonotic Dis.* **9:** 109–117.

31. Pinter, A. 2007. Aspectos ecológicos da febre maculosa brasileira em um foco endêmico no Estado de São Paulo. Ph.D thesis, University of São Paulo, São Paulo, Brazil.

32. Labruna, M.B. *et al*. 2008. Comparative susceptibility of larval stages of *Amblyomma aureolatum*, *Amblyomma cajennense*, and *Rhipicephalus sanguineus* to infection by *Rickettsia rickettsii*. *J. Med. Entomol.* **45:** 1156–1159.

33. Kohls, G.M. 1958. *Amblyomma imitator*, a new species of ticks from Texas and Mexico, and remarks on the synonymy of *A. cajennense* (Fabricius) (Acarina – Ixodidae). *J. Parasitol.* **44:** 430–433.

34. Monteiro, J.L. & F. Fonseca. 1932. Typho exantemático de S. Paulo. XI. Novas experiências sobre a transmissão experimental por carrapatos (*Boophilus microplus* e *Amblyomma cajennense*). *Mem. Inst. Butantan* **7:** 35–40.

35. Brumpt, E. 1933. Transmission de la fiévre pourprée des Montagnes rocheuses par la tique américaine *Amblyomma cajennense*. *Compt. Rend. Senac. Soc. Biol.* **114:** 416–419.

36. Pinter, A. & M.B. Labruna. 2006. Competência vetorial de *Amblyomma aureolatum* na transmissão da bacteria *Rickettsia rickettsii* [Abstract]. Presented at the *14 Congresso Brasileiro de Parasitologia Veterinária & 2 Simposio Latino-Americano de Rickettsioses, Ribeirão preto, Brazil.* Abstract Book, p. 368.

37. Dias, E. & A.V. Martins. 1939. Spotted fever in Brazil. *Am. J. Trop. Med.* **19:** 103–108.

38. Anaya, E. 2004. Prevenção e controle das rickettsioses no Peru. In *Consulta de especialistas OPAS/OMS sobre rickettsioses nas Américas.* Relatório final: 40–43. Organização Pan-Americana da Saúde. Rio de Janeiro, Brazil.

39. Murray E.S. & S.B. Torrey. 1975. Virulence of *Rickettsia prowazekii* for head lice. *Ann. N.Y. Acad. Sci.* **266:** 25–34.

40. Medina-Sanchez, A. *et al.* 2005. Detection of a typhus group *Rickettsia* in *Amblyomma* ticks in the state of Nuevo Leon, Mexico. *Ann. N. Y. Acad. Sci.* **1063:** 327–332.

41. Travassos, J., P.M. Rodrigues & L.N. Carrijo. 1949. Tifo murino em São Paulo. Identificação da *Rickettsia mooseri* isolada de um caso humano. *Mem. Inst. Butantan* **21:** 77–106.

42. Azad, A.F. 1990. Epidemiology of murine typhus. *Annu. Rev. Entomol.* **35:** 553–570.

43. Silva, L.J. & P.M.O. Papaiordanou. 2004. Tifo murino (endêmico) no Brasil: relato de caso e revisão. *Rev. Inst. Med. Trop. S. Paulo* **46:** 283–285.

44. Hidalgo, M. *et al.* 2008. Murine typhus in Caldas, Colombia. *Am. J. Trop. Med. Hyg.* **78:** 321–322.

45. Paddock, C.D. *et al.* 2004. *Rickettsia parkeri:* A newly recognized cause of spotted fever rickettsiosis in the United States. *Clin. Infect. Dis.* **38:** 805–811.

46. Paddock, C.D. 2005. *Rickettsia parkeri* as a paradigm for multiple causes of tick-borne spotted fever in the western hemisphere. *Ann. N. Y. Acad. Sci.* **1063:** 315–326.

47. Whitman, T.J. *et al.* 2007. *Rickettsia parkeri* infection after tick bite, Virginia. *Emerg. Infect. Dis.* **13:** 334–336.

48. Raoult, D. & C.D. Paddock. 2005. *Rickettsia parkeri* infection and other spotted fevers in the United States. *N. Engl. J. Med.* **353:** 626–627.

49. Venzal, J.M. *et al.* 2004. *Rickettsia parkeri* in *Amblyomma triste* from Uruguay. *Emerg. Infec. Dis.* **10:** 1493–1495.

50. Sumner, J.W. *et al.* 2007. Gulf Coast ticks (*Amblyomma maculatum*) and *Rickettsia parkeri*, United States. *Emerg. Infect. Dis.* **13:** 751–753.

51. Silveira, I. *et al.* 2007. First report of *Rickettsia parkeri* in Brazil. *Emerg. Infect. Dis.* **13:** 1111–1113.

52. Guglielmone *et al.* 2003. Ticks (Acari: Ixodida) of the Neotropical Zoogeographic Region. *International Consortium on Ticks and Tick-borne Diseases.* Atalanta, Houten, The Netherlands.

53. Parola, P., B. Davoust & D. Raoult. 2005. Tick- and flea-borne rickettsial emerging zoonoses. *Vet. Res.* **36:** 469–492.

54. Labruna, M.B. *et al.* 2007. *Rickettsia felis* in Chile. *Emerg. Infect. Dis.* **13:** 1794–1795.

55. Nava, S. *et al.* 2008. *Rickettsia felis* in *Ctenocephalides felis* from Argentina. *Vector Borne Zoonotic Dis.* **8:** 465–466.

56. Wedincamp, J. & L.D. Foil. 2002. Vertical transmission of *Rickettsia felis* in the cat flea (*Ctenocephalides felis* Bouché). *J. Vector Ecol.* **27:** 96–101.

57. Horta, M.C. *et al.* 2007. *Rickettsia* infection in five areas of the State of São Paulo, Brazil. *Mem. Inst. Oswaldo Cruz* **102:** 793–801.

58. Wedincamp, J. & L.D. Foil. 2000. Infection and seroconversion of cats exposed to cat fleas (*Ctenocephalides felis* Bouche) infected with *Rickettsia felis*. *J. Vector Ecol.* **25:** 123–126.

59. Adams, J.R., E.T. Schmidtmann & A.F. Azad. 1990. Infection of colonized cat fleas, *Ctenocephalides felis* (Bouché), with a rickettsia-like microorganism. *Am. J. Trop. Med. Hyg.* **43:** 400–409.

60. Macaluso, K.R. *et al.* 2008. Identification of *Rickettsia felis* in the salivary glands of cat fleas. *Vector Borne Zoonotic Dis.* **8:** 391–396.

61. Cicuttin, G.L. *et al.* 2004. Primera detección de *Rickettsia massiliae* en la Ciudad de Buenos Aires, Resultados preliminares. *Rev. Argentina Zoonosis* **1:** 8–10.

62. Beati, L. & D. Raoult. 1993. *Rickettsia massiliae* sp. nov., a new spotted fever group Rickettsia. *Int. J. Syst. Bacteriol.* **43:** 839–840.

63. Vitale, G. *et al.* 2006. *Rickettsia massiliae*: first isolation from the blood of a patient. *Emerg. Infect. Dis.* **12:** 174–175.

64. Labruna, M.B. *et al.* 2007. Prevalence of *Rickettsia* infection in dogs from the urban and rural areas of Monte Negro Municipality, western Amazon, Brazil. *Vector Borne Zoonotic Dis.* **7:** 249–255.

65. Horta, M.C. *et al.* 2006. Natural infection, transovarial transmission, and transstadial survival of *Rickettsia bellii* in the tick *Ixodes loricatus* (Acari: Ixodidae) from Brazil. *Ann. N. Y. Acad. Sci.* **1078:** 285–290.

66. Macaluso, K.R. *et al.* 2002. Rickettsial infection in *Dermacentor variabilis* (Acari:Ixodidae) inhibits transovarial transmission of a second rickettsia. *J. Med. Entomol.* **39:** 808–813.

67. Labruna, M.B. *et al.* 2007. Isolation of *Rickettsia rhipicephali* and *Rickettsia bellii* from ticks *Haemaphysalis juxtakochi* in the state of Sao Paulo, Brazil. *Appl. Environ. Microbiol.* **73:** 869–873.

68. Labruna, M.B. *et al.* 2004. *Rickettsia* species infecting *Amblyomma cooperi* ticks from an area in the State of São Paulo, Brazil, where Brazilian spotted fever is endemic. *J. Clin. Microbiol.* **42:** 90–98.

69. Labruna, M.B. *et al.* 2004. *Rickettsia bellii* and *Rickettsia amblyommii* in *Amblyomma* ticks from the state of Rondônia, Western Amazon, Brazil. *J. Med. Entomol.* **41:** 1073–1081.

70. Labruna, M.B. *et al.* 2007. Infection by *Rickettsia bellii* and *Candidatus* "Rickettsia amblyommii" in *Amblyomma neumanni* ticks from Argentina. *Microb. Ecol.* **54:** 126–133.

71. Parola, P. *et al.* 2007. A tick-borne rickettsia of the spotted-fever group, similar to *Rickettsia amblyommii*, in French Guyana. *Ann. Trop. Med. Parasitol.* **101:** 185–188.

72. Blair, P.J. *et al*. 2004. Characterization of spotted fever group rickettsiae in flea and tick specimens from northern Peru. *J. Clin. Microbiol.* **42:** 4961–4967.

73. Pacheco, R.C. *et al*. 2007. Detection of a novel spotted fever group rickettsia in *Amblyomma parvum* ticks (Acari: Ixodidae) from Argentina. *Exp. Appl. Acarol.* **43:** 63–71.

74. Ogrzewalska, M. *et al*. 2008. Ticks (Acari: Ixodidae) infesting wild birds in an Atlantic Forest area in the state of São Paulo, Brazil, with isolation of *Rickettsia* from the tick *Amblyomma longirostre*. *J. Med. Entomol.* **45:** 770–774.

75. Labruna, M.B. *et al*. 2004. Molecular evidence for a spotted fever group Rickettsia species in the tick *Amblyomma longirostre* in Brazil. *J. Med. Entomol.* **41:** 533–537.

Characterization of Rickettsial Diseases in a Hospital-Based Population in Central Tunisia

Naoufel Kaabia and Amel Letaief

Infectious Diseases Unit, Farhat Hached, University Hospital Sousse – Tunisia

In Tunisia, 2 rickettsial groups, spotted fever group and typhus group, have been described since the beginning of the 20th century. Mediterranean spotted fever (MSF), also known as Boutonneuse fever, caused by *Rickettsia conorii* and transmitted by the dog tick *Rhipicephalus sanguineus,* is the most frequent rickettsial infection observed. Its seroprevalence in our region is 9% among blood donors and 23% in hospitalized febrile patients. Typhus group rickettsioses, caused by *R. typhi* and *R. prowazekii,* are less frequently reported than in the 1970s. Only sporadic cases of typhus were reported in the last decade. However, *R. typhi* antibodies were present in 3.6% among healthy people and 40% in patients with acute fever of undetermined origin. In the unit of Infectious Diseases at Farhat Hached University Hospital in Sousse, during 2007, 5% of hospitalized patients had eruptive fever, and half of the cases met clinical criteria of MSF and/or were confirmed by rickettsial serology. The majority of cases (90%) were noted in hot seasons, and contact with domestic animals was found in 76%. The most common symptoms were fever (present in all cases), skin rash (in 85% to 98% of cases), and headache (in 69.5% of cases). The clinical triad (fever + rash + "tache noire") was noted in 32 to 61%. Normal blood cells or leukopenia, cytolysis, and thrombopenia were the most frequent biological abnormalities. Complications and malignant forms of rickettsial infections were reported in 3.5 to 6% among hospitalized adult patients. When specific serology was performed, MSF was confirmed in 15%, and we noted an emergence of murine typhus (MT) mistaken for *R. conorii* or viral infection. *Rickettsia felis* was identified in 1 patient, whereas 17% of cases remained undetermined. *Rickettsia conorii Malish* was identified by PCR in skin biopsies. Doxycycline was the antibiotic of choice for rickettsial infections; it was prescribed in the majority of patients, associated with fever defervescence, in a mean of 72 hours. The mean length of stay among hospitalized patients with rickettsial infections was 5.9 days. In conclusion, in our region, MSF and murine typhus are endemic. Doxycycline should be prescribed in patients with acute fever and skin rash, especially in hot seasons. These rickettsioses were characterized by benign prognosis. More skin biopsies are needed to identify other SFG rickettsies.

Keys words: Rickettsia conorii; Rrickettsia typhi; Rickettsia prowazekii; Rickettsia felis; epidemiology; Tunisia

Introduction

Tunisia is a North African country with ten million inhabitants and 165,000 km^2 of superficies. In Tunisia, however, rickettsioses have been described since the beginning of the 20th century,[1,2] and few and fragmentary reports have been published. The most human tick borne rickettsioses known to occur in our region are Mediterranean spotted fever (MSF) and murine typhus.[3,4] Indeed, seroprevalence of antibodies against *Rickettsia conorii* and *Rickettsia typhi* among blood donors were 9 and 3.6%, respectively.[5] This article will provide a descriptive overview of rickettsial infections in hospitalized patients in central Tunisia. The

Address for correspondence: Dr. Amel Letaief, Infectious Diseases Unit, Farhat Hached Hospital, 4000, Sousse, Tunisia. amel.letaief@famso.rnu.tn

Rickettsiology and Rickettsial Diseases-Fifth International Conference: Ann. N.Y. Acad. Sci. 1166: 167–171 (2009).
doi: 10.1111/j.1749-6632.2009.04521.x © 2009 New York Academy of Sciences.

diagnosis of rickettsiosis was confirmed by either clinical criteria or positive serology.[6]

Prevalence of Rickettsioses in Hospitalized Patients

Rickettsioses are endemic in our region and constitute a frequent cause of hospitalization in hot season. In a prospective study conducted in the year 1995, among 300 patients hospitalized with fever, infectious diseases were confirmed or suspected in 220 cases—in this group, when serology of rickettsial infections were performed systematically, 6% of patients had acute rickettsioses, and seroprevalence of *R. conorii* and *R. typhi* were 22.6% and 15.6%, respectively.[7] In 2007, from 605 hospitalized patients of our unit of Infectious Diseases at Farhat Hached University Hospital in Sousse, half of the cases met clinical criteria of MSF and/or were confirmed by rickettsial serology.[8] In the same unit during the summer of 2004, when serology of rickettsial infections and *Coxiella burnetii* was systematically performed in 47 patients—hospitalized for acute fever with undetermined origin—rickettsioses were confirmed in 58%, and acute Q fever in 8%.[9]

Epidemiological, Clinical, and Laboratory Features

Spotted Fever Group (SFG)

The majority of cases with SFG rickettsioses were seen during the hot season; indeed, 90% of cases were hospitalized between May and October. On the other hand, the few cases observed in winter were neither clinically typical cases of MSF, nor were they confirmed by specific serology. Patients were adults with a mean age of 39 years, mostly from rural areas, with a predominance of males associated with professional exposure, and contact with domestic animals was noted in 76%. However, tick bites are reported by less than 5% of patients. Before admission, most patients (86%) had seen a doctor, and 57% received antibiotics; frequently, this form of treatment was ineffective against rickettsioses. In admission, fever was present in all cases—its mean duration was 5 ± 1.3 days—and its onset was abrupt in all cases. The most frequent symptoms were headache, chills, and myalgia (Table 1). The presence of eschar facilitated the diagnosis of MSF; however, its presence was noted in 61% of cases, but if all rickettsial infections were considered, eschar was noted in only 32% of cases. There was 1 unique eschar in the majority of cases, usually located in hidden areas. In 3% of cases, 2 eschars were noted, even in confirmed MSF. In 85% to 98% of patients, 4 to 5 days following the onset of fever, there appears to be a generalized maculopapular and, sometimes, purpuric rash that involves the palms and soles but spares the face, and it disappears within 6 days. The clinical triad of fever, skin rash, and eschar was noted in 32% to 61% of patients. Recently, in a prospective study conducted at the ophthalmology unit at Monastir, 30 patients with confirmed MSF underwent a complete ophthalmic examination. Eighty-three percent of them had unilateral or bilateral posterior segment involvement, and white retinal lesions were frequent, but only 30% of the patients had ocular complaints. The majority of these abnormalities resolved after 3 to 10 weeks, and final visual acuity was restored in 93% of affected eyes[10] Leukopenia and/or normal blood cells, thrombopenia, and moderate elevation of transaminases were the most frequent laboratory findings noted in 79, 67.5, and 83.5%, respectively (Table 1). In addition, 5% had an elevated creatine level.[4,8,11]

Typhus Group

Typhus group infection was thought to have disappeared in the 1970s. When *R. typhi* and *R prowazekii* antigens were added in serologic tests, more cases of murine typhus were confirmed.

TABLE 1. Clinical and Laboratory Features in Hospitalized Patients with Rickettsioses

	2000–2007 patients with rickettsiosis[8] N (%)	1987–2006 patients with MSF[11] N (%)
Clinical data		
Fever	119 (100)	200 (100)
Headache	82 (69,5)	153 (76)
Asthenia	63 (52,9)	–
Arthralgia/Myalgia	48 (40,3)	116 (58)
Cough	27 (22,7)	35 (17.5)
Gastrointestinal symptoms	25 (21)	33 (16.5)
Rash	102 (86,4)	197 (98.5)
Eschar	38 (31,9)	126 (63)
Conjunctivitis	22 (18.4)	12 (6)
Laboratory findings		
Leukopenia and/or normal blood cells	79/117 (67.5)	158 (79)
Thrombocytopenia	50/114 (44)	135 (67.5)
Elevation of transaminases	69/109 (63)	148/177 (83.5)
Hyponatremia	68 (57)	113/167 (58)
Elevated ESR	53/92 (57.5)	150/162 (92.5)

MSF = Mediterranean spotted fever; ESR = elevated erythrocyte sedimentation rate.

R. typhi antibodies were found in 23% of hospitalized patients with fever of undetermined origin.[9] MT was often mistaken for *R. conorii* or viral infection.[9,12] Most cases of MT were noted during summer and in patients of rural areas, and the main clinical features were sudden onset of fever, absence of eschar (in all cases), maculopapular rash, prostration, meningismus, and pneumonia. The frequent laboratory findings were moderate thrombopenia and elevated transaminases.[12,13]

Epidemic typhus (ET) had been epidemic in Tunisia until the 1970s. Using non-specific serology tests, no confirmed cases of ET were reported. The last reported cases of ET were in the 1980s, with 7 serologically-confirmed cases occurred in elderly patients in the cold season.[14] Although ET cases have not been reported in recent years, an epidemiological survey is necessary.

Severe Forms and Complications

Although MSF is considered a benign disease, complications and severe forms of the infections were reported among 5 to 6% of a hospitalized-based population, involving the central nervous, gastrointestinal, cardiovascular and renal systems.[15] In our region, rickettsioses have been described as a typically moderate illness. Indeed, severe forms were noted in 3.5% of patients, with favorable outcome—no sequela and no patient death.[4,8] In contrast, in Algerian series of MSF, severe forms of disease and death rates occurred, reaching 40% and 6%, respectively.[16] The principal risk factor for severe forms of disease occurrence was advanced age.[11] The most frequent, severe form involved the cerebral nervous system. Meningismus was noted in 4.5 to 11% of patients, and meningitis was noted in 3.5% of patients. When lumbar puncture was performed, it showed lymphocytic meningitis and normal glucose concentration. In rare cases, we noted meningoencephalitis. After antibiotic treatment, neurological manifestations improved in all cases.[4,8] Other rare complications were reported: as acute renal failure,[17] myocarditis in <1%[11], and sensorineural hearing and vision loss.[8,10] Recently, cases of angina pectoris[18] and pulmonary thrombosis were reported as complications of MSF.[19]

Diagnosis Tools

In practice, serology is the best tool to confirm diagnosis. In our hospital, immunofluorescent assay (IFA) is performed to detect only *R. conorii* antibodies. Often patients had only 1 early serology, which confirmed MSF in only 30 to 37% of patients, and late serology was performed in one half of the cases. Therefore, diagnostic score helps physicians diagnose MSF. It was recently presented as a helpful tool even when using clinical and epidemiological criteria only.[20]

When specific serology, Western blot (WB) and a cross-absorption test, were performed in Unité des Rickettsies in Marseille, diagnosis of murine typhus and MSF were confirmed in patients, 24% and 15%, respectively, whereas 17% of cases remained undetermined.[9] In this same study, we reported for the first time serological evidence of *Rickettsia felis* infection in humans in Tunisia. None of the sera tested showed antibodies against *Bartonella henselae*, *Bartonella quintana, and human granulocytic anaplasma*. To identify species of rickettsies, 14 skin biopsies were performed in patients with clinical criteria of MSF (PCR showed 4 cases to be positive for *R. conorii Malish*), and, in our country, this is the first isolation of rickettsia in humans.[9]

Treatment

In our region, tetracycline and doxycycline remained the treatment of choice prescribed in 50 to 85% of patients.[8,11] The mean duration of treatment was 5 to 7 days, and apyrexia was noted 3 days after the beginning of antibiotic treatment. No side effects were noted.

Conclusion

Rickettsioses, especially MSF and murine typhus, are the most common causes of hospitalized patients with acute fever in Tunisia in hot season. Therefore, empirical antibiotic treatment with cyclines should be prescribed early, before diagnostic confirmation. In contrast to Algeria, rickettsial infections in our region were benign, with a low rate of severe forms and mortality. Finally, more skin biopsies are needed to identify other SFG rickettsies.

Conflicts of Interest

The authors declare no conflicts of interest.

References

1. Conor, A. & A. Bruch. 1910. Une fièvre boutonneuse observée en Tunisie. *Bulletin de la Société de Pathologie Exotiques et Filiales* **8:** 492–496.
2. Conseil, E. 1907. Le typhus exanthématique en Tunisie. *Archives de l'institut Pasteur de Tunis* **2:** 145–154.
3. Kennou, M.F. & E. Edlinger. 1984. Current data on rickettsial diseases in Tunisia. *Arch. Inst. Pasteur Tunis* **61:** 427–433.
4. Jemni, L., H. Hmouda, M. Chakroun & M. Ernez. 1994. Mediterranean spotted fever in central Tunisia. *J. Travel Med.* **1:** 106–108.
5. Letaïef, A.O. *et al.* 1995. Seroepidemiological survey of rickettsial infections among blood donors in central Tunisia. *Trans. R Soc. Trop. Med. Hyg.* **89:** 266–268.
6. Brouqui, P. *et al.* 2004. Guidelines for the diagnosis of tick-borne bacterial diseases in Europe. *Clin. Microbiol. Infect.* **10:** 1108–1132.
7. Letaief, O.A. *et al.* 1997. Etude séroépidémiologique chez 300 malades fébriles hospitalisés dans un service de médecine et maladies infectieuses. *Méd. Mal. Infect RICAI* **27:** 663–666.
8. Kaabia, N. *et al.* 2008. Rickettsial infection in hospitalized patients in central Tunisia: Report of 119 cases. *Clin. Microbiol. Infect.* in press.
9. Kaabia, N. *et al.* 2006. Serologic study of rickettsioses among acute febrile patients in central Tunisia. *Ann. N. Y. Acad. Sci.* **1078:** 176–179.
10. Khairallah, M. *et al.* 2004. Posterior segment manifestations of *Rickettsia conorii* infection. *Ophtalmology* **3:** 529–534.
11. Ben Romdhane, F. *et al.* 2008. Mediterranean spotted fever: a report of 200 cases in Tunisia. *P028 5th International Meeting on Rickettsiae and Rickettsial Diseases*, May 18–20, Marseille, France.
12. Letaïf, O.A. *et al.* 2005. Clinical and murine typhus in central Tunisia: a report of seven cases. *Int. J. Infect. Dis.* **145:** 1–4.
13. Toumi, A. *et al.* 2007. Meningitis revealing *Rickettsia typhi* infection. *Rev. Med. Interne.* **28:** 131–133.

14. Ernez, M., M. Chakroun, A. Letaief & L. Jemni. 1995. Clinical and biological features of exanthematous typhus. *Presse Med.* **24:** 1358

15. Raoult, D. & V. Roux. 1997. Rickettsioses as paradigms of new emerging infectious diseases. *Clin. Microbiol. Rev.* **10:** 694–719.

16. Mouffok, N. *et al.* 2006. Reemergence of rickettsiosis in Oran, Algeria. *Ann. N. Y. Acad. Sci.* **1078:** 180–184.

17. Skhiri, H. *et al.* 2004. Acute kidney failure in association with boutonneuse fever: Discription of three cases. *Med. Tropical.* **64:** 58–60.

18. Maaloul, I., F. Kanoun, M. Ben Jemaa & S. Ben Hamed. 1995. Angina pectoris and Mediterranean spotted fever. *Med. Mal. Infect.* **25:** 949–950.

19. Ben Brahim, H. *et al.* 2006. Pulmonary thrombosis as a complication of a Mediterranean spotted fever. *Rev. Med. Interne.* **27:** 973–975.

20. Letaïef, A. *et al.* 2003. Evaluation of clinical diagnosis scores for boutonneuse fever. *Ann. N. Y. Acad. Sci.* **990:** 327–330.

Epidemiology and Clinical Aspects of Rickettsioses in Thailand

Y. Suputtamongkol,[a] C. Suttinont,[b] K. Niwatayakul,[c]
S. Hoontrakul,[d] R. Limpaiboon,[e] W. Chierakul,[f]
K. Losuwanaluk,[g] and W. Saisongkork[h]

[a]*Department of Medicine, Faculty of Medicine Siriraj Hospital, Mahidol University,
Bangkok,* [b]*Maharat Nakhon Ratchasima Hospital, Nakhon Ratchasima Province,* [c]*Loei
Hospital, Loei Province,* [d]*Chumphon Hospital, Chumphon Province,* [e]*Udonthani
Hospital, Udonthani Province,* [f]*Department of Clinical Tropical Medicine, Faculty of
Tropical Medicine, Mahidol University, Bangkok,* [g]*Banmai Chaiyapod Hospital,
Bureerum Province, and* [h]*National Institue of Health, Ministry of Public Health of
Thailand, Nondhaburi Province, Thailand*

Scrub typhus and murine typhus are widespread in Thailand. Clinical manifestations of both diseases are nonspecific and vary widely. Acute undifferentiated fever (AUF), with or without organ dysfunction, is a major clinical presentation of these two diseases. The epidemiology and clinical manifestations including severe complications of scrub typhus and murine typhus in Thailand are summarized. Sixteen hundred and sixty-three patients with AUF were studied in six hospitals in Thailand between 2000 and 2003. Scrub typhus and murine typhus were diagnosed in 16.1% and 1.7% of them, respectively. Clinical spectrum of murine typhus was similar to scrub typhus. Hepatic dysfunction and pulmonary involvement were common complications. Multi-organ dysfunction mimicking sepsis syndrome occurred in 11.9% of patients with scrub typhus. The mortality of severe scrub typhus varied from 2.6% to 16.7%. Awareness that scrub typhus and murine typhus are prominent causes of AUF in adults in Thailand improves the probability of an accurate clinical diagnosis. Early recognition and appropriate treatment reduces morbidity and mortality. Results from recent clinical studies from Thailand indicated that rational antimicrobial therapy would be doxycycline in mild cases and a combination of either cefotaxime or ceftriaxone and doxycycline in severe cases. Azithromycin could be considered as an alternative treatment when doxycycline allergy is suspected. This would be either curative, or have no ill effect, in the majority of instances. Failure to improve or defervesce within 48 hours would indicate the need to perform a thorough re-evaluation of clinical findings and initial laboratory investigation results, as well as a need to change antibiotic.

Key words: scrub typhus; murine typhus; Thailand

Introduction

Human rickettsioses, known to occur in Thailand, include mainly scrub typhus and murine typhus.[1,2] Serological documented cases of spotted fever group (SFG) rickettsioses have been reported since 1994.[3–5] Although specific etiologic agents of these SFG rickettsioses have not been isolated from humans, several SFG rickettsiae have been identified from ticks in Thailand.[5,6] Scrub typhus is caused by *Orientia tsutsugamushi*, an obligate intracellular gram-negative bacterium that has a different cell wall structure and genetic makeup from those of rickettsiae.[7] It is transmitted to humans by the bite of the larval stage of trombiculid mites (chiggers). The endemic areas

Address for correspondence: Yupin Suputtamongkol, Department of Medicine, Faculty of Medicine at Siriraj Hospital, Mahidol University, Bangkok 10700, Thailand. Voice: +66-2-419-7203; fax: +66-2-412-5994. siysp@mahidol.ac.th

Rickettsiology and Rickettsial Diseases-Fifth International Conference: Ann. N.Y. Acad. Sci. 1166: 172–179 (2009).
doi: 10.1111/j.1749-6632.2009.04514.x © 2009 New York Academy of Sciences.

of scrub typhus include rural areas of Southeast Asia throughout the Asia Pacific rim and Northern Australia. More than a billion people are at risk of infection, and about one million cases occur annually.[2] Murine typhus is another rickettsial disease resulting from an infection with *Rickettsia typhi*. The main vector is the rat flea *Xenopsylla cheopis*, and rodents, mainly *Rattus norvegicus* and *R. rattus*, act as reservoirs.[2] Murine typhus has a worldwide distribution. Most people become infected when flea feces containing *R. typhi* contaminate disrupted skin, although infections may also result from flea bites. The report incidence of both scrub typhus and murine typhus has increased during the previous decade.[2,8] Clinical manifestations of both diseases vary widely from a mild and self-limited febrile illness to a more severe course that may be fatal.[2,8] Scrub typhus and murine typhus were recently recognized as common causes of acute undifferentiated fever both in indigenous population and ill travelers returning from the tropics.[2,4,8]

Despite the availability of a low cost and effective antibiotic treatment, both scrub typhus and murine typhus continue to cause significant morbidity and mortality in otherwise healthy adults and children. The greatest challenge to a clinician is diagnosing these infections early in their courses, when antibiotic therapy is most effective. The purpose of this presentation is to summarize the epidemiologic situations and clinical manifestations including severe complications of scrub typhus and murine typhus in Thailand.

Epidemiology of Scrub Typhus and Murine Typhus in Thailand

Scrub typhus was first reported in humans from the central region of Thailand in 1952,[9] and *O. tsutsugamushi* was first isolated from rodents trapped from the same area in 1955.[10] *Leptotrombidium deliensis* is the primary vector of *O. tsutsugamushi*. However, several other species have been implicated as vectors such as *L. Chiangraiensis*, *L. imphalum*, and *Blankaartia acuscutel-*

laris.[11] The rodents, including *Bandicota indica*, *R. losea*, and *R. rattus*, served as main maintenance hosts for the vector mites.[1,9,12] *R. typhi* was first isolated from patients with acute fever of unknown origin in Thailand in 1964.[1] *R. rattus, R. exulans,* and *X. cheopsis* are the main reservoirs of *R. typhi* in Thailand.[1]

Nationwide sero-epidemiological studies indicate that both *O. tsutsugamushi* and *R. typhi* infection are widespread in Thailand.[1] The seropositivity rates of *O. tsutsugamushi* among soldiers and patients with acute febrile illness varied from 5.4% to 21%.[1,4] These surveys have found high point prevalence, varied from 13% to 31% of inhabitants in suburban Bangkok,[13] to 59–77% of inhabitants of three villages in the northern and northeastern region, respectively.[14] According to the unpublished records of the Public Health Ministry of Thailand, fewer than 100 cases of scrub typhus were reported annually before 1983, 750–900 cases/year were reported between 1988 and 1991, and 3000–5000 cases/year have been reported since 2001.

The data regarding murine typhus is scarcer. However, *R. typhi* has been isolated from rats and their ectoparasites from the same study areas as scrub typhus.[1] *R. typhi* antibody was detected in 7.6% to 21% of sera from asymptomatic population in the northeastern and northern parts of this country.[1,15] The seropositivity rates of *R. typhi* varied from 1.8 to 6.6% among patients with acute febrile illness.[4,15,16]

We conducted an epidemiological and clinical study of 1663 patients with acute febrile illness without an obvious focus of infection (acute undifferentiated fever), between October 2000 and March 2003 in six hospitals in rural Thailand; four hospitals in the northeastern region, one hospital in the central region, and one hospital in the southern region. There were 268 (16.1%) and 28 (1.7%) patients with laboratory-confirmed scrub typhus and murine typhus, respectively. The diagnosis of scrub typhus was made by PCR (101 out of 141 patients tested) or by indirect immunofluorescent antibody (IFA) against combined Karp, Kato, and

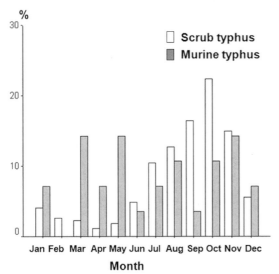

Figure 1. Monthly distribution of scrub typhus compared to murine typhus.

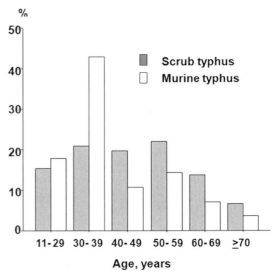

Figure 2. Age distribution of scrub typhus compared to murine typhus.

Gilliam strain of *O. tsutsugamushi* (74 patients by a fourfold rising in titer to ≥ 1:400, 76 patients by a single titer to ≥ 1:400, 17 patients by a fourfold rising in titer, or stable titers of at least 1:200). Murine typhus was diagnosed by a fourfold rising in specific *R. typhi* IFA titer to ≥ 1:400 in 18 patients, by a single titer to ≥ 1:400 in three patients, and by a stable titer of at least 1:200 in 7 patients. Blood culture for aerobic bacteria, serological tests for leptospirosis, and dengue infection were negative in all of these patients. Scrub typhus, murine typhus, and SFG rickettsioses were diagnosed in 7.8%, 2.4%, and 5%, respectively, in a subgroup of patients who were enrolled in a clinical trial of suspected severe leptospirosis.[17]

Results of this study confirmed the seasonal variation of scrub typhus. Most patients were diagnosed during the end of the rainy season and the beginning of winter, whereas murine typhus was evenly diagnosed in all seasons (Fig. 1). Patients with scrub typhus ranged in age from 11 to 92 years compared to 16 to 70 years in patients with murine typhus. The age distribution when compared between these two diseases is shown in Figure 2. The male-to-female ratio was 2:1 in both diseases. Although most patients had occupational exposure to rodent and arthropod bites (such as rice farmers or military personnel), only 41 (15.3%) patients with scrub typhus and 4 (14.3%) patients with murine typhus recalled a history of insect bites during the two weeks before the illness. The demographic and epidemiological data compared between scrub typhus and murine typhus is shown in Table 1.

Clinical Features

The median duration of fever was seven and five days in patients with scrub typhus and murine typhus, respectively. Headache, generalized myalgia, and calf pain were very common in both groups. History of abdominal pain and vomiting were more common in patients with scrub typhus than in patients with murine typhus. The classic manifestation of scrub typhus, including generalized lymphadenopathy, maculopapular rash, and splenomegaly, were not common in this case series. Eschar was found in 56 (20.9%) patients. Lists of clinical manifestations and laboratory results, including chest radiography on admission of patients with scrub typhus compared to murine typhus, are shown in Tables 2 and 3, respectively.

TABLE 1. Epidemiological Data Compared Between Scrub Typhus and Murine Typhus

	Scrub typhus No (%)	Murine typhus No (%)	*P*-value
Total	268 (16.1)	28 (1.7)	
Season			0.007
Summer (Jan–Apr)	27 (10.2)	8 (28.6)	
Rainy (May–Aug)	80 (30.1)	10 (35.7)	
Winter (Sept–Dec)	159 (59.8)	10 (35.7)	
Male	176 (65.7)	18 (64.3)	0.88
Mean (SD) Age, yrs	46 (16)	39 (15)	0.04
Age group			0.12
11–29	41 (15.5)	5 (18.5)	
30–39	56 (21.2)	12 (44.4)	
40–49	53 (20.1)	3 (11.1)	
50–59	59 (22.3)	4 (14.8)	
60–69	37 (14)	2 (7.4)	
≥70	18 (6.8)	1 (3.7)	
Occupational exposure to rodents/other animals[a]			0.03
- High exposure	188 (70.1)	26 (92.9)	
- Low/no exposure	13 (4.9)	1 (3.6)	
- Unknown exposure	67 (25)	1 (3.6)	

[a]High exposure = rice farmers, gardeners and their families, labors; low/no exposure = office workers; unknown = housewife, monk

TABLE 2. Symptoms and Signs of Patients with Scrub Typhus and Murine Typhus

	Scrub typhus, *n* (%)	Murine typhus, *n* (%)	*P*-value
Median (range) days of fever	7 (1–20)	5 (2–14)	0.20
Headache	228 (84.4)	24 (85.7)	0.86
Myalgia	206 (76.3)	20 (71.4)	0.57
Calf pain	111 (41.1)	13 (46.4)	0.59
Sore throat	113 (41.9)	10 (35.7)	0.53
Cough	123 (45.6)	9 (32.1)	0.17
Chest pain	47 (17.4)	4 (14.3)	0.67
Nausea	138 (51.1)	11 (39.3)	0.23
Vomiting	130 (48.1)	7 (25)	0.02
Abdominal pain	72 (26.7)	2 (7.1)	0.02
Diarrhea	62 (23)	5 (17.9)	0.54
Constipation	30 (11.1)	1 (3.6)	0.21
Alteration of consciousness	25 (9.3)	2 (7.1)	0.71
Rash	24 (8.9)	2 (7.1)	0.76
Injected pharynx	23 (8.5)	3 (0.7)	0.009
Calf muscle tenderness	27 (10)	9 (32.1)	0.001
Lymphadenopathy			
- Generalized	4 (7.8)	0	0.68
- Cervical LN enlargement	42 (15.6)	8 (28.6)	0.08
Lung's crepitation	19 (17)	1 (3.6)	0.29
Abdominal tenderness	47 (17.5)	5 (17.9)	0.96
Hepato/splenomegaly	39/1 (14.4/0.4)	0/0	0.03

TABLE 3. Laboratory Investigations on Admission of Patients with Scrub Typhus and Murine Typhus

Mean (SD)	Scrub typhus	Murine typhus	*P*-value
Hct, %	37.4 (6.7)	39.6 (6.9)	0.10
Total WBC count, $\times 10^3$	11.1 (5.2)	7.9 (2.9)	0.002
Platelet, $\times 10^3 \times 10^9$	173.65 (93.82)	216.81 (93.36)	0.03
Urine protein >1+, n (%)	27 (17)	2 (8.3)	0.28
Total bilirubin, mg/dl	2.5 (4.7)	2.0 (5.5)	0.71
AST, IU/L	147.3 (202.6)	81.8 (61.8)	0.12
ALT, IU/L	117.6 (251.8)	74.5 (68.3)	0.41
Alkaline phosphatase, IU/L	307.6 (302.1)	228.5 (174.9)	0.22
Urea, mg/dl	24.9 (23.2)	13.2 (6.1)	<0.001
Creatinine, mg/dl	1.9 (2.8)	1.1 (0.3)	<0.001
Chest radiography, *n* (%)			
Total study	119	15	0.75
- Normal	37 (31.6)	4 (26.7)	
- Bilateral reticular infiltration	60 (51.3)	9 (60)	
- Cardiomegaly	36 (30.8)	5 (33.3)	
- Congestive heart failure	23 (19.7)	1 (6.7)	
- Pleural effusion	15 (12.8)	0	
- Hilar node enlargement	2 (1.7)	1 (6.7)	
- Atelectatsis	1 (0.9)	0	

Complications such as hepatic dysfunction (defined as jaundice or total bilirubin ≥2.5 mg/dl, or high serum aspartate aminotransferase [AST] and/or alanine aminotransferase [ALT] level to more than 120 U/L, or high alkaline phosphatase level to more than 350 U/L, or mixed abnormalities), renal dysfunction (defined as oliguria or abnormal serum urea and/or creatinine level), hypotension (defined as systolic BP <90 mmHg on admission), congestive heart failure, or pulmonary involvement (defined as abnormal chest radiography) were common in both scrub and murine typhus. Only 32% of patients with scrub typhus and 39% of patients with murine typhus did not have any complication on admission.

In patients with scrub typhus, hepatic dysfunction was the most common complication. Pulmonary involvement was found in approximately half of study group. The chest radiographic abnormalities were similar to those previously reported, except that hilar lymphadenopathy was not as common as previously reported.[18] Cardiac involvement such as cardiomegaly defined by cardiac-to-thoracic ratio > 0.5 on postero-anterior (PA),

chest radiography or >0.6 on antero-posteria (AP), chest radiography (36/119, 30.3%), or congestive heart failure (23/119, 19.3%) were common abnormal radiographic findings. However, this finding was not associated with hypotension on admission. Approximately 12% of the patients presented with multi-organ dysfunction (MOD) mimic community-acquired septicemia in this case series.

Hepatic dysfunction and pulmonary involvement were also common complications found in this small case series of murine typhus. However, there was no patient who presented with multi-organ dysfunction. The complications on admission compared between scrub typhus and murine typhus are shown in Table 4.

Overall, 7 (2.6%) patients with scrub typhus died. The causes of death in all except 1 patient were multi-organ failure including respiratory failure. ARDS was not a prominent cause of death. The cause of death (bleeding hepatoma) was unrelated to scrub typhus in 1 patient. The description of fatal cases is shown in Table 5. Scrub typhus was not included in the differential diagnosis, and no effective treatment was given in 4 out of 6 patients who died. There

TABLE 4. Clinical Syndromes of Patients with Scrub Typhus and Murine Typhus

	Scrub typhus, n (%)	Murine typhus, n (%)	P-value
Acute febrile illness	88 (32.8)	11 (39.3)	0.49
Hepatic dysfunction			0.25
- None	106 (43.1)	16 (66.7)	
- Jaundice	8 (3.3)	0	
- High AST/ALT	58 (23.6)	2 (8.3)	
- High alkaline phosphatase	30 (12.2)	4 (16.7)	
- Mixed dysfunction	44 (17.8)	2 (8.3)	
Pulmonary involvement	63 (52.5)	9 (60)	0.69
Congestive heart failure	24 (20)	1 (6.7)	0.46
Hypotension	32 (13.9)	4 (14.3)	0.93
Renal dysfunction	54 (20.5)	0	0.008
Thrombocytopenia	49 (20.9)	1 (3.7)	0.03
Sepsis syndrome (MOD)	32 (11.9)	0	0.06

TABLE 5. Characteristics of Seven Fatal Cases of Scrub Typhus

No.	Age (yrs)/sex	Days of fever/ admission	IFA titer IgM/IgG	Complications	Antibiotic treatment
1.	67, F	7/3	1:1600/1:200	Jaundice, high AST/ALT Acute renal failure Hypotension, congestive heart failure	Penicillin G sodium, Gentamicin
2.	66, M	7/3	1:6400/1:6400	Jaundice, mixed liver dysfunction Acute renal failure	Ampicillin, Gentamicin, Cefotaxime
3.	78, M	10/15	1:6400/1:800	Jaundice, high AST, ALT Hypotension, thrombocytopenia Mechanical ventilation	Ceftazidime, Amikacin, Doxycycline
4.	35, M	6/1	1:6400/1:6400	Jaundice, high alkaline phosphatase Acute renal failure	Cefotaxime
5.	62, F	7/6	1:6400/1:1600	Acute renal failure Hypotension Thrombocytopenia	Co-trimoxazole Cefotaxime
6.	65, F	21/2	1:6400/1:1600	Jaundice, mixed liver dysfunction Cardiomegaly	Penicillin G sodium Oral doxycycline
7.	54, M	3/9	1:200/1:1600	Hepatoma bleeding Cause of dead unrelated to scrub typhus	Oral Doxycycline

was no death among patients with murine typhus.

Discussion

The epidemiology of scrub typhus and murine typhus are different. Scrub typhus occurs mainly in rural areas and is endemic in specific geographical areas. Murine typhus is an urban disease with worldwide distribution. However, in endemic areas such as Thailand, these two diseases coexist. Although they were both underreported in Thailand because of the general lack of physician awareness and the general lack of a widely available specific serological test, the number of scrub typhus and murine typhus are now increasingly documented in this country.[4] In accordance with studies elsewhere in Thailand, we observed seasonal variations in the distribution of scrub typhus[1] but not in the distribution of murine typhus.[1,19] The role of rodents and their ectoparasites as the most probable vectors of scrub typhus and murine typhus was well documented in this country. Cats and cat fleas (*Ctenocephalides felis*) have been found to be involved in the transmission of murine typhus in Texas.[8] No epidemiological study has been conducted to determine the role of cats and cat fleas in the transmission of murine typhus in Thailand.

Acute undifferentiated fever was the most common clinical presentation of both scrub typhus and murine typhus. It is difficult to distinguish these two typhuses on the epidemiologic and clinical grounds. Eschar is the only clinical sign that differentiates scrub typhus from other infectious disease, including murine typhus. Typical manifestations of scrub typhus (i.e., generalized lymphadenopathy, rash, and splenomegaly) were less common in Thai patients compared to those reported from Far East Asia such as China or Korea.[18] In addition, severe scrub typhus can manifest as multiorgan dysfunction, which mimics septicemia from other bacteria and leptospirosis. Ignorance of the diagnosis of severe scrub typhus in these patients could lead to delayed diagnosis and high mortality, as shown in this case series. Scrub typhus was diagnosed in 18 out of 51 (35.3%) of patients who were presented with septic shock in one of our study hospitals between November 2001 and January 2002.[20] The mortality was 16.7% in this subgroup of scrub typhus patients with septic shock.

Acute fever, headache, and myalgia, especially calf muscle pain, were the predominant symptoms, with rash occurring in 7% of this case series of adult murine typhus from Thailand. Complications such as hepatic dysfunction or pulmonary involvement of murine typhus were similar to scrub typhus, except congestive heart failure and thrombocytopenia were less common in murine typhus than in scrub typhus. Although we did not find a patient with murine typhus who presented with multi-organ dysfunction in this study, the number of cases was too small to rule out the possibility of this occurring. Fatal murine typhus was reported elsewhere.[21]

Awareness that scrub typhus and murine typhus are prominent causes of acute febrile illness without foci of infection in adults improves the probability of an accurate clinical diagnosis. Early recognition and appropriate treatment reduce morbidity and mortality. Results from recent clinical studies from Thailand indicate that rational antimicrobial therapy would be doxycycline in mild cases[22] and a combination of either cefotaxime or ceftriaxone and doxycycline in severe cases.[17] Azithromycin could be considered as an alternative treatment whenever doxycycline allergy is suspected.[22] This would be either curative, or have no ill effect, in the majority of instances. Failure to improve or defervesce within the next 48 hours would indicate the need to perform a thorough reevaluation of the clinical findings and the initial laboratory investigation results, as well as a need to change antibiotic.

Acknowledgments

The authors thank the doctors, nurses, and medical technologists of Udonthani Hospital, Maharat Nakhon Ratchasima Hospital, Loei Hospital, Ratchaburi Hospital, Banmai Chaiyapod Hospital, and Chumphon Hospital for their cooperation and help during the study period. Thailand Research Fund and the Ministry of Public Health, Thailand and the Wellcome Trust of Great Britain funded this study.

Conflicts of Interest

The authors declare no conflicts of interest.

References

1. Puranavei, S. *et al*. 1968. SEATO medical research study on rickettsial diseases in Thailand. Annual Research Progress Report, US Army Medical Research

Unit, Royal Thai Army Medical Service, Bangkok, Thailand. p. 444–448.

2. Watt, G. & P. Parola. 2003. Scrub typhus and tropical rickettsioses. *Curr. Opin. Infect. Dis.* **16:** 429–436.

3. Sirisanthana, T. *et al.* 1994. First case of spotted fever group rickettsioses in Thailand. *Am. J. Trop. Med. Hyg.* **50:** 682–686.

4. Suttinont, C. *et al.* 2006. Causes of acute, undifferentiated, febrile illness in rural Thailand: results of a prospective observational study. *Ann. Trop. Med. Parasitol.* **100:** 363–370.

5. Parola, P. *et al.* 2003. Emerging rickettsioses of the Thai-Myanmar border. *Emerg. Infect. Dis.* **9:** 657–663.

6. Robertson, R.G. & C.L. Weisseman. 1973. Tick-borne rickettsiae of the spotted fever group in west Pakistan. II. Serological classification of isolates from west Pakistan and Thailand: evidence of two new species. *Am. J. Epidemiol.* **97:** 55–64.

7. Tamura, A., N. Ohashi, H. Urakami & S. Miyamura. 1995. Classification of *Rickettsia tsutsugamushi* in a new genus, *Orientia* gen. nov., as *Orientia tsutsugamushi* comb. Nov. *Int. J Syst. Bacteriol.* **45:** 589–591.

8. Civen, R. & N. Van. 2008. Murine typhus: an unrecognized suburban vector borne disease. *Clin. Infect. Dis.* **46:** 913–918.

9. Trishnananda, M., C. Vasuvat & C. Harinasuta. 1964. Investigation of scrub typhus in Thailand. *J. Trop. Med. Hyg.* **67:** 215–219.

10. Traub, R., P. Johnson, M. Mirsse & R. Elbel. 1954. Isolation of *Rickettsia tsutsugamushi* from rodents from Thailand. *Am. J. Trop. Med. Hyg.* **3:** 356–359.

11. Lerdthusnee, K. *et al.* 2003. Vector competence of *Leptotrombidium Chiangraiensis* chiggers and transmission efficacy and isolation of *Orientia tsutsugamushi*. *Ann. N. Y. Acad. Sci.* **990:** 25–35.

12. Coleman, R.E. *et al.* 2003. Occurrence of Orientia tsutsugamushi in small mammals from Thailand. *Am. J. Trop. Med. Hyg.* **69:** 519–524.

13. Strickman, D., P. Tanskul, C. Eamsila & D.J. Kelly. 1994. Prevalence of antibodies to rickettsiae in the human population of suburban Bangkok. *Am. J. Trop. Med. Hyg.* **5:** 149–153.

14. Johnson, D.E., J.W. Crum, S. Hanchalay & C. Dasengruchi. 1982. Sero-epidemiological survey of *Rickettsia tsutsugamushi* infection in a rural Thai village. *Trans. R. Soc. Trop. Med. Hyg.* **76:** 1–3.

15. Sangkasuvan, V. *et al.* 1969. Murine typhus in Thailand. *Trans. R Soc. Trop. Med. Hyg.* **63:** 639–643.

16. Silpapojakul, S. *et al.* 1987. Murine typhus in southern Thailand. *J. Med. Asso. Thai.* **70:** 55–62.

17. Suputtamongkol, Y. *et al.* 2004. An open, randomized, controlled trial of penicillin, doxycycline, and cefotaxime for patients with severe leptospirosis. *Clin. Infect. Dis.* **39:** 1417–1424.

18. Jeong, Y.J. *et al.* 2007. Scrub typhus: clinical, pathologic, and imaging findings. *Radiographics* **27:** 161–172.

19. Silpapojakul, S., P. Chayakul, S. Krisanapan & K. Silpapojakul. 1993. Murine typhus in Thailand: clinical features, diagnosis and treatment. *Q. J. Med.* **86:** 43–47.

20. Thap, L.C. *et al.* 2002. Septic shock secondary to scrub typhus: characteristics and complications. *Southeast Asian Trop. Med. Public Health* **33:** 780–786.

21. Pether, J.V. *et al.* 1994. Fatal murine typhus from Spain. *Lancet* **344:** 897–898.

22. Phimda, K. *et al.* 2007. Doxycycline versus Azithromycin for treatment of leptospirosis and scrub typhus. *Antimicrob Agents Chemother.* **51:** 3259–3263.

Erratum for Ann. N. Y. Acad. Sci. 1063: 425–428

Rickettsioses: From Genome to Proteome, Pathobiology, and Rickettsiae as an International Threat

Karim E. Hechemy, José A. Oteo, Didier A. Raoult, David J. Silverman, and José R. Blanco, Eds.

In the article in Reference 1 on page 427, the first line of the second paragraph should read *A. phagocytophilum* (Webster strain) instead of *A. phagocytophilum* (MRK strain).

We apologize for this error.

Reference

1. SCORPIO, D.G., F.D. VON LOEWENICH, C. BOGDAN & J.S. DUMLER. 2006. Innate immune tissue injury and murine HGA: tissue injury in the murine model of granulocytic anaplasmosis relates to host innate immune response and not pathogen load. *Ann. N.Y. Acad. Sci.* **1063:** 425–428.

Rickettsiology and Rickettsial Diseases-Fifth International Conference: Ann. N.Y. Acad. Sci. 1166: 180 (2009).
doi: 10.1111/j.1749-6632.2009.04923.x © 2009 New York Academy of Sciences.